Alterations of Consciousness in the Emergency Department

Guest Editor
CHAD KESSLER, MD, FACEP, FAAEM

EMERGENCY MEDICINE CLINICS OF NORTH AMERICA

www.emed.theclinics.com

Consulting Editor
AMAL MATTU, MD

August 2010 • Volume 28 • Number 3

SAUNDERS an imprint of ELSEVIER, Inc.

W.B. SAUNDERS COMPANY

A Division of Elsevier Inc.

1600 John F. Kennedy Boulevard • Suite 1800 • Philadelphia, Pennsylvania 19103-2899

http://www.theclinics.com

EMERGENCY MEDICINE CLINICS OF NORTH AMERICA Volume 28, Number 3
August 2010 ISSN 0733-8627, ISBN-13: 978-1-4377-2444-8

Editor: Patrick Manley
Developmental Editor: Donald Mumford

Emergency Medicine Clinics of North America (ISSN 0733-8627) is published quarterly by Elsevier Inc., 360 Park Avenue South, New York, NY, 10010-1710. Months of issue are February, May, August, and November. Business and Editorial Offices: 1600 John F. Kennedy Boulevard, Suite 1800, Philadelphia, PA 19103-2899. Customer Service Office: 6277 Sea Harbor Drive, Orlando, FL 32887-4800. Periodicals postage paid at New York, NY, and additional mailing offices. Subscription prices are $127.00 per year (US students), $247.00 per year (US individuals), $414.00 per year (US institutions), $180.00 per year (international students), $354.00 per year (international individuals), $499.00 per year (international institutions), $180.00 per year (Canadian students), $305.00 per year (Canadian individuals), and $499.00 per year (Canadian institutions). International air speed delivery is included in all *Clinics'* subscription prices. All prices are subject to change without notice. **POSTMASTER:** Send address changes to *Emergency Medicine Clinics of North America*, Elsevier Periodicals Customer Service, 11830 Westline Industrial Drive, St. Louis, MO 63146. Customer Service (orders, claims, online, change of address): Elsevier Periodicals Customer Service, 11830 Westline Industrial Drive, St. Louis, MO 63146. Tel: 1-800-654-2452 (U.S. and Canada); 314-453-7041 (outside U.S. and Canada). Fax: 314-453-5170. E-mail: journalscustomerservice-usa@elsevier.com (for print support); journalsonline support-usa@elsevier.com (for online support).

Reprints. For copies of 100 or more of articles in this publication, please contact the Commercial Reprints Department, Elsevier Inc., 360 Park Avenue South, New York, NY 10010-1710. Tel.: 212-633-3812; Fax: 212-462-1935; E-mail: reprints@elsevier.com.

Emergency Medicine Clinics of North America is covered in *MEDLINE/PubMed (Index Medicus), Current Contents/Clinical Medicine, EMBASE/Excerpta Medica, BIOSIS, SciSearch, CINAHL, ISI/BIOMED,* and *Research Alert.*

Printed and bound by CPI Group (UK) Ltd, Croydon, CR0 4YY
Transferred to Digital Print 2011

Contributors

CONSULTING EDITOR

AMAL MATTU, MD, FAAEM, FACEP
Program Director, Emergency Medicine Residency; Professor, Department of Emergency Medicine, University of Maryland School of Medicine, Baltimore, Maryland

GUEST EDITOR

CHAD KESSLER, MD, FACEP, FAAEM
Section Chief, Emergency Medicine, Jesse Brown Veterans Affairs Hospital; Assistant Professor, Departments of Internal Medicine and Emergency Medicine; Associate Program Director, Combined Internal Medicine/Emergency Medicine Residency, The University of Illinois School of Medicine at Chicago, Chicago, Illinois

AUTHORS

STEVEN E. AKS, DO, FACMT, FACEP
Director, Toxikon Consortium; Division of Toxicology, Department of Emergency Medicine, Cook County Hospital (Stroger); Associate Professor of Emergency Medicine, Rush University, Chicago, Illinois

JEFFREY J. BAZARIAN, MD, MPH
Associate Professor, Department of Emergency Medicine, Center for Neural Development and Disease, University of Rochester School of Medicine and Dentistry, Rochester, New York

BRIAN J. BLYTH, MD
Assistant Professor, Department of Emergency Medicine, Center for Neural Development and Disease, University of Rochester School of Medicine and Dentistry, Rochester, New York

SEAN M. BRYANT, MD
Associate Professor, Department of Emergency Medicine, Cook County Hospital (Stroger); Assistant Fellowship Director, Toxikon Consortium; Associate Medical Director, Illinois Poison Center, Chicago, Illinois

JENNIFER J. CASALETTO, MD, FACEP
Associate Professor, Department of Emergency Medicine; Residency Program Director, Virginia Tech-Carilion School of Medicine, Roanoke, Virginia

CHRISTINE S. CHO, MD, MPH, FAAP
HS Assistant Clinical Professor, Department of Pediatrics, University of California, San Francisco; Division of Emergency Medicine, Children's Hospital & Research Center Oakland, Oakland, California

COL ROBERT DE LORENZO, MD, MSM, FACEP, MC, USA
Professor of Military and Emergency Medicine, Uniformed Services University of the Health Sciences, Bethesda, Maryland; Chief, Department of Clinical Investigation, MCHE-CI, Brooke Army Medical Center, Fort Sam Houston, Texas

E. WESLEY ELY, MD, MPH
Division of Allergy, Pulmonary, and Critical Care, Department of Internal Medicine, Center for Health Services Research, Vanderbilt University Medical Center, Nashville, Tennessee

JASON W.J. FISCHER, MD, MSc
Emergency Medicine Ultrasound Fellow, Department of Emergency Medicine, Alameda County Medical Center; Pediatric Emergency Medicine Fellow, Division of Emergency Medicine, Children's Hospital & Research Center Oakland, Oakland, California

JIN H. HAN, MD, MSc
Department of Emergency Medicine, Vanderbilt University Medical Center, Nashville, Tennessee

BLAINE HANNAFIN, MD
Attending Physician, Department of Emergency Medicine, Chandler Regional Hospital, Chandler, Arizona

ANDY JAGODA, MD, FACEP
Professor and Chair of Emergency Medicine, Mount Sinai School of Medicine, New York, New York

CHAD KESSLER, MD, FACEP, FAAEM
Section Chief, Emergency Medicine, Jesse Brown Veterans Affairs Hospital; Assistant Professor, Departments of Internal Medicine and Emergency Medicine; Associate Program Director, Combined Internal Medicine/Emergency Medicine Residency, The University of Illinois School of Medicine at Chicago, Chicago, Illinois

JASMINE KOITA, MD
Department of Emergency Medicine, Mount Sinai School of Medicine, New York, New York

CHRISTINE KULSTAD, MD
Assistant Program Director; Clinical Assistant Professor, Department of Emergency Medicine, Advocate Christ Medical Center, Oak Lawn, Illinois

SHARON E. MACE, MD
Professor, Department of Emergency Medicine, Cleveland Clinic Lerner College of Medicine of Case Western Reserve University; Faculty, Emergency Medicine Residency Program, MetroHealth Medical Center; Director, Pediatric Education/Quality Improvement; Director, Observation Unit; Research Director, Rapid Response Team, Cleveland Clinic, Cleveland, Ohio

TIMOTHY J. MEEHAN, MD, MPH
Fellow in Medical Toxicology, Toxikon Consortium; Clinical Instructor, Department of Emergency Medicine, University of Illinois - Chicago, Chicago, Illinois

HELEN OUYANG, MD, MPH
Department of Emergency Medicine, Brigham and Women's Hospital; Massachusetts General Hospital, Department of Emergency Medicine, Boston, Massachusetts

HENRY Z. PITZELE, MD
Associate Director, Section of Emergency Medicine, Jesse Brown Veterans Affairs Medical Center; Clinical Assistant Professor, Department of Emergency Medicine, University of Illinois at Chicago, Chicago, Illinois

CHARLES V. POLLACK Jr, MA, MD, FACEP, FAAEM, FAHA
Professor and Chairman, Department of Emergency Medicine, Pennsylvania Hospital, University of Pennsylvania, Philadelphia, Pennsylvania

JAMES QUINN, MD, MS
Associate Professor of Surgery/Emergency Medicine, Division of Emergency Medicine, Stanford University, Palo Alto, California

SYLVANA RIGGIO, MD
Professor of Psychiatry and Neurology, Mount Sinai School of Medicine, New York, New York

DOUGLAS RUND, MD
Professor; Chair of the Department of Emergency Medicine, Ohio State University Medical Center, Columbus, Ohio

DAVID E. SLATTERY, MD, FACEP, FAAEM
Assistant Professor, Department of Emergency Medicine, University of Nevada School of Medicine, Las Vegas, Nevada

VAISHAL M. TOLIA, MD, MPH
Assistant Professor, Department of Emergency Medicine, University of California San Diego, San Diego, California

JENNY M. TRISTANO, MD
Internal Medicine/Emergency Medicine Residency Program, University of Illinois at Chicago, Chicago, Illinois

AMANDA WILSON, MD
Departments of Psychiatry and Emergency Medicine, Vanderbilt University Medical Center, Nashville, Tennessee

JAMES L. YOUNG, MD
Clinical Assistant Professor; Associate Chair for Clinical Services, Department of Psychiatry; Director of Psychiatric Emergency Services, OSU Harding Hospital, Ohio State University Medical Center, Columbus, Ohio

Contents

The Emergency Department Approach to Syncope: Evidence-based Guidelines and Prediction Rules 487

Chad Kessler, Jenny M. Tristano, and Robert De Lorenzo

Syncope is a sudden, transient loss of consciousness associated with inability to maintain postural tone followed by spontaneous recovery and return to baseline neurologic status. Global cerebral hypoperfusion is the final pathway common to all presentations of syncope, but this symptom presentation has a broad differential diagnosis. It is important to identify patients whose syncope is a symptom of a potentially life-threatening condition. This article reviews the current status of syncope from the emergency department perspective, focusing on the current evidence behind the various clinical decision rules derived during the past decade.

Pediatric Syncope: Cases from the Emergency Department 501

Jason W.J. Fischer and Christine S. Cho

Pediatric syncope is a common presentation in the emergency department. Most causes are benign, but an evaluation must exclude rare life-threatening disorders. The lack of objective findings can pose a challenge. This case-based review emphasizes the importance of a detailed history and physical examination with electrocardiogram in determining high-risk patients.

Seizures as a Cause of Altered Mental Status 517

David E. Slattery and Charles V. Pollack Jr

The differential diagnosis and empiric management of altered mental status and seizures often overlap. Altered mental status may accompany seizures or simply be the manifestation of a postictal state. This article provides an overview of the numerous causes of altered mental status and seizures: metabolic, toxic, malignant, infectious, and endocrine causes. The article focuses on those agents that should prompt the emergency physician to initiate unique therapy to abate the seizure and correct the underlying cause.

Central Nervous System Infections as a Cause of an Altered Mental Status? What is the Pathogen Growing in Your Central Nervous System? 535

Sharon E. Mace

There are several central nervous system (CNS) infections (meningitis, encephalitis, and brain abscess), any of which may present with an altered level of consciousness. Because CNS infections can have a devastating outcome, it is important to recognize the presence of a CNS infection and begin treatment as soon as possible because early appropriate therapy may, in some cases, limit morbidity and mortality.

Traumatic Alterations in Consciousness: Traumatic Brain Injury 571

Brian J. Blyth and Jeffrey J. Bazarian

Mild traumatic brain injury (mTBI) refers to the clinical condition of transient alteration of consciousness as a result of traumatic injury to the brain. The

priority of emergency care is to identify and facilitate the treatment of rare but potentially life-threatening intracranial injuries associated with mTBI through the judicious application of appropriate imaging studies and neurosurgical consultation. Although post-mTBI symptoms quickly and completely resolve in the vast majority of cases, a significant number of patients will complain of lasting problems that may cause significant disability. Simple and early interventions such as patient education and appropriate referral can reduce the likelihood of chronic symptoms. Although definitive evidence is lacking, mTBI is likely to be related to significant long-term sequelae such as Alzheimer disease and other neurodegenerative processes.

Psychiatric Considerations in Patients with Decreased Levels of Consciousness 595

James L. Young and Douglas Rund

When patients present to the emergency department with changes in behavior and levels of consciousness, psychiatric causes often move to the top of the list of diagnostic considerations. It is important to thoroughly assess such patients for medical causes. Although it is not common for primary psychiatric conditions to present with altered levels of consciousness, severe cases may present in this fashion. Altered mental states may also be caused by adverse reactions to psychiatric medications. In this article, the authors review some of the psychiatric causes of decreased levels of consciousness, as well as certain adverse drug reactions to psychotropic medications.

Delirium in the Older Emergency Department Patient: A Quiet Epidemic 611

Jin H. Han, Amanda Wilson, and E. Wesley Ely

Delirium is defined as an acute change in cognition that cannot be better accounted for by a preexisting or evolving dementia. This form of organ dysfunction commonly occurs in older patients in the emergency department (ED) and is associated with a multitude of adverse patient outcomes. Consequently, delirium should be routinely screened for in older ED patients. Once delirium is diagnosed, the ED evaluation should focus on searching for the underlying cause. Infection is one of the most common precipitants of delirium, but multiple causes may exist concurrently.

Is Salt, Vitamin, or Endocrinopathy Causing this Encephalopathy? A Review of Endocrine and Metabolic Causes of Altered Level of Consciousness 633

Jennifer J. Casaletto

Altered level of consciousness describes the reason for 3% of critical emergency department (ED) visits. Approximately 85% will be found to have a metabolic or systemic cause. Early laboratory studies such as a bedside glucose test, serum electrolytes, or a urine dipstick test often direct the ED provider toward endocrine or metabolic causes. This article examines common endocrine and metabolic causes of altered mentation in

the ED via sections dedicated to endocrine-, electrolyte-, metabolic acidosis-, and metabolism-related causes.

Drugs of Abuse: The Highs and Lows of Altered Mental States in the Emergency Department **663**

Timothy J. Meehan, Sean M. Bryant, and Steven E. Aks

The diagnosis and management of poisoned patients presenting with alterations in mental status can be challenging, as patients are often unable (or unwilling) to provide an adequate history. Several toxidromes exist. Recognition hinges upon vital signs and the physical examination. Understanding these "toxic syndromes" may guide early therapy and management, providing insight into the patient's underlying medical problem. Despite toxidrome recognition guiding antidotal therapy, the fundamental aspect of managing these patients involves meticulous supportive care. The authors begin with a discussion of various toxidromes and then delve into the drugs responsible for each syndrome. They conclude with a discussion on drug-facilitated sexual assault ("date rape"), which is both an underrecognized problem in the emergency department (ED) and representative of the drug-related problems faced in a modern ED.

Twenty per Hour: Altered Mental State Due to Ethanol Abuse and Withdrawal **683**

Henry Z. Pitzele and Vaishal M. Tolia

This article discusses the physiology and clinical syndromes involved in ethanol absorption, intoxication, and withdrawal, with special emphasis on the evidentiary backing for common treatments, as well as some discussion of the medicolegal sequelae of treatment of ethanol abusers in the emergency department.

Index **707**

FORTHCOMING ISSUES

November 2010
Orthopaedic Emergencies
Michael C. Bond, MD,
Guest Editor

February 2011
Gastrointestinal Emergencies
Angela M. Mills, MD and
Anthony Dean, MD, *Guest Editors*

May 2011
Cardiovascular Emergencies
J. Stephen Bohan, MD and
Joshua M. Kosowsky, MD,
Guest Editors

RECENT ISSUES

May 2010
HIV in the Emergency Department
Mercedes Torres, MD and
Rachel L. Chin, MD,
Guest Editors

February 2010
High Risk Emergencies
Jeffrey Tabas, MD and
Teri Reynolds, MD, PhD,
Guest Editors

November 2009
Risk Management
Joseph H. Kahn, MD,
Brendan Magauran Jr, MD,
and Jonathan S. Olshaker, MD,
Guest Editors

RELATED INTEREST

Ultrasound Clinics, January 2008, Vol. 3, No. 1 (pages 1–178)
Emergency Ultrasound
Vikram S. Dogra, MD and Shweta Bhatt, MD, *Guest Editors*

GOAL STATEMENT

The goal of *Emergency Medicine Clinics of North America* is to keep practicing physicians up to date with current clinical practice in emergency medicine by providing timely articles reviewing the state of the art in patient care.

ACCREDITATION

The *Emergency Medical Clinics of North America* is planned and implemented in accordance with the Essential Areas and Policies of the Accreditation Council for Continuing Medical Education (ACCME) through the joint sponsorship of the University of Virginia School of Medicine and Elsevier. The University of Virginia School of Medicine is accredited by the ACCME to provide continuing medical education for physicians.

The University of Virginia School of Medicine designates this educational activity for a maximum of 15 *AMA PRA Category 1 Credits*™ for each issue, 60 credits per year. Physicians should only claim credit commensurate with the extent of their participation in the activity.

The American Medical Association has determined that physicians not licensed in the US who participate in this CME activity are eligible for a maximum of 15 *AMA PRA Category 1 Credits*™ for each issue, 60 credits per year.

The Emergency Medicine Clinics of North America CME program is approved by the American College of Emergency Physicians for 60 hours of ACEP Category I Credit per year.

Credit can be earned by reading the text material, taking the CME examination online at http://www.theclinics.com/home/cme, and completing the evaluation. After taking the test, you will be required to review any and all incorrect answers. Following completion of the test and evaluation, your credit will be awarded and you may print your certificate.

FACULTY DISCLOSURE/CONFLICT OF INTEREST

The University of Virginia School of Medicine, as an ACCME accredited provider, endorses and strives to comply with the Accreditation Council for Continuing Medical Education (ACCME) Standards of Commercial Support, Commonwealth of Virginia statutes, University of Virginia policies and procedures, and associated federal and private regulations and guidelines on the need for disclosure and monitoring of proprietary and financial interests that may affect the scientific integrity and balance of content delivered in continuing medical education activities under our auspices.

The University of Virginia School of Medicine requires that all CME activities accredited through this institution be developed independently and be scientifically rigorous, balanced and objective in the presentation/discussion of its content, theories and practices.

All authors/editors participating in an accredited CME activity are expected to disclose to the readers relevant financial relationships with commercial entities occurring within the past 12 months (such as grants or research support, employee, consultant, stock holder, member of speakers bureau, etc.). The University of Virginia School of Medicine will employ appropriate mechanisms to resolve potential conflicts of interest to maintain the standards of fair and balanced education to the reader. Questions about specific strategies can be directed to the Office of Continuing Medical Education, University of Virginia School of Medicine, Charlottesville, Virginia.

The faculty and staff of the University of Virginia Office of Continuing Medical Education have no financial affiliations to disclose.

The authors/editors listed below have identified no professional or financial affiliations for themselves or their spouse/partner:

Steven E. Aks, DO; Jeffrey J. Bazarian, MD, MPH; Brian J. Blyth, MD; Sean M. Bryant, MD; Jennifer J. Casaletto, MD; Christine S. Cho, MD, MPH; Jason WJ Fischer, MD, MSc; Jin H Han, MD, MSc; Blaine Hannafin, MD; Chad Kessler, MD (Guest Editor); Jasmine Koita, MD; Christine Kulstad, MD; Patrick Manley, (Acquisitions Editor); Amal Mattu, MD (Consulting Editor); Timothy J. Meehan, MD, MPH; Helen Ouyang, MD, MPH; Henry Z. Pitzele, MD; Sylvana Riggio, MD; Douglas Rund, MD; David E. Slattery, MD; Vaishal M Tolia, MD, MPH; Jenny M. Tristano, MD; Amanda Wilson, MD; Bill Woods, MD (Test Author); and James L. Young, MD.

The authors/editors listed below have identified the following professional or financial affiliations for themselves of their spouse/partner:

Robert De Lorenzo, MD, MSM receives royalties from Pearson Education.

E. Wesley Ely, MD, MPH is an industry funded research/investigator, is a consultant, and is the Speakers Bureau for Pfizer, Hospira, GSK, and Aspect.

Andy Jagoda, MD is on the Speakers' Bureau for Network Continuing Medical Education, and is a consultant for Banyan Biomarkers.

Sharon E. Mace, MD is an industry funded research/investigator and is on the Speakers' Bureau for Baxter Healthcare.

Charles V. Pollack, Jr., MA, MD is an industry funded research/investigator for Sanofi-Aventis, GSK, and The Medicines Company; and is a consultant and is the Speakers Bureau for Sanofi-Aventis.

James Quinn, MD, MS is on the Advisory Board/Committee for iRhythm.

Disclosure of Discussion of Non-FDA Approved Uses for Pharmaceutical Products and/or Medical Devices.

The University of Virginia School of Medicine, as an ACCME provider, requires that all faculty presenters identify and disclose any off-label uses for pharmaceutical and medical device products. The University of Virginia School of Medicine recommends that each physician fully review all the available data on new products or procedures prior to clinical use.

TO ENROLL

To enroll in the Emergency Medicine Clinics of North America Continuing Medical Education program, call customer service at 1-800-654-2452 or visit us online at www.theclinics.com/home/cme. The CME program is available to subscribers for an additional fee of $190.00.

Foreword

Alterations of Consciousness in the Emergency Department

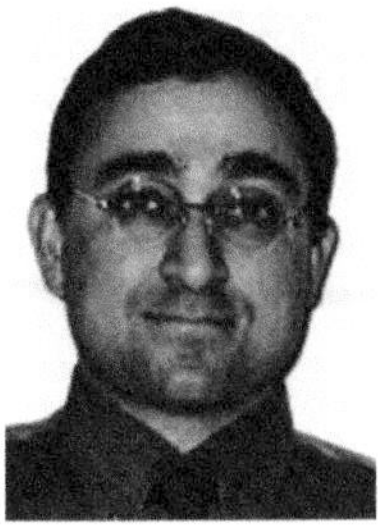

Amal Mattu, MD
Consulting Editor

Since the time of ancient civilizations, philosophers and scientists have tried to define and understand "consciousness." A simple internet search using this term reveals more than 47 *million* sites, many of them various definitions or quotes by philosophers, from Aristotle to Freud, about this term. A consistent description of consciousness that emerged from a cursory review of those sites was the description of consciousness as a sense of one's own identity. It is therefore arguable that an altered or loss of consciousness represents one of the most heinous medical presentations we encounter in emergency medicine—a loss of one's identity. Not surprisingly, one of the most basic and also most vital components of any medical student or resident curriculum in emergency medicine and one of the critical chapters in every major textbook of emergency medicine address the assessment and management of patients with altered levels of consciousness. This topic may be, in fact, the second thing students and residents in emergency medicine are taught, right after A-B-C.

In this issue of *Emergency Medicine Clinics of North America*, Guest Editor Dr Chad Kessler and an outstanding group of authors have done an excellent job of addressing the various causes and presentations associated with altered states of consciousness. An initial article addresses the mental status examination, after which an article addresses perhaps the most vexing of all emergency department presentations—the dizzy patient. Three articles are devoted to syncope in adults and pediatric patients. Other "bread-and-butter" causes of altered consciousness are addressed as well, including trauma, infections, psychiatric causes, metabolic causes, and drug toxicities. An entire article is devoted to the most common toxic cause of altered consciousness—ethanol, and an entire article is devoted to what is perhaps the most commonly overlooked, deadly cause of altered consciousness—delirium in the elderly patient.

This issue of *Emergency Medicine Clinics* is an invaluable addition to the library of emergency physicians and other health care providers that care for acutely ill patients.

Emerg Med Clin N Am 28 (2010) xiii–xiv
doi:10.1016/j.emc.2010.06.008
emed.theclinics.com

More importantly, this is must-reading for students and residents training in emergency medicine. Dr Kessler and colleagues have provided a comprehensive curriculum addressing the care of patients with altered consciousness. The contributors are to be commended for providing this outstanding resource to us all.

Amal Mattu, MD
Department of Emergency Medicine
University of Maryland School of Medicine
110 S. Paca Street, 6th Floor, Suite 200
Baltimore, MD 21201, USA

E-mail address:
amattu@smail.umaryland.edu

Preface
Alterations of Consciousness in the Emergency Department

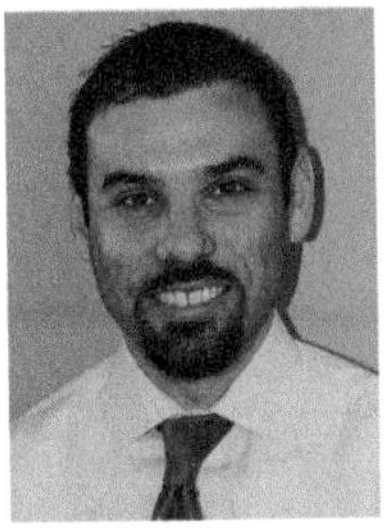

Chad Kessler, MD
Guest Editor

You know that awesome feeling, the one you get when you walk up to the rack (now computer tracking board) to find out who your next patient is? What disease process are you up against next? How can you use your detective skills to solve the next mystery, whether you are Inspector Clouseau or Inspector Gadget? That investigation might be one of the best parts of emergency medicine, unless the patient happens to have altered mental status, perhaps the most dreaded chief complaint. Now I could be wrong, but I do not recall hearing any of my colleagues or residents screaming for joy when they pick up that chart. What I do know is that altered mental status is an all too common presenting complaint in emergency departments (EDs) across the globe and for an astounding 25% of patients more than 70 years old.[1] I believe that much of emergency physicians' angst stems from uncertainty about these patients' presentations, our insecure diagnoses, and our tentative treatment plans. It is therefore vital that we have a firm grasp on all the different causes, presentations, and treatment options for any patient with altered mental status. After reading this issue of *Emergency Medicine Clinics of North America,* you will have a firmer grasp of this once fearful, now manageable, chief complaint.

This issue of *Emergency Medicine Clinics of North America* provides you with a framework for how to approach ED patients with a change in mental status. My goal as Guest Editor is to bring to you articles written and delivered by a team of expert authors, both master clinicians and original researchers. We present timely and novel content and current controversies into challenging and complex issues. These talented authors and researchers present their articles in a diverse format, ranging from case-based scenarios to in-depth analyses and literature reviews on 13 various topics. This amazing team draws its talent from across the country and truly represents national

Emerg Med Clin N Am 28 (2010) xv–xvi
doi:10.1016/j.emc.2010.06.007

and international leaders in their respective fields. We hope you find this material clinically relevant and easily translatable into everyday practice.

In this issue, we will walk you down the path to altered mental status enlightenment. It begins with a look at the mental status exam in emergency practice. Then we dive into the dizzy and confused patient. Following that, we present 3 articles on syncope: its diagnosis and evaluation, the ED approach to it, and cases involving children. Next, we look at seizures and central nervous system infections as causes of alterations of consciousness. An extensive review of traumatic brain injury in relation to change in mental status is followed by psychiatric considerations in patients with decreased levels of consciousness and an article on delerium. We round out the issue with metabolic and toxic causes of altered mental status, including a brilliant review of alcohol abuse and withdrawal.

This issue would not be complete if I did not take the time to thank so many wonderful people for making this a reality. First and foremost, to a mentor, a true idol in emergency medicine, and a friend, I would like to thank Dr Amal Mattu, the Consulting Editor for *Emergency Medicine Clinics of North America*, for the opportunity to share this issue with you. Patrick Manley and the entire Elsevier staff were absolutely amazing in organizing, preparing, editing, and walking everyone through the process seamlessly and effortlessly. It was a pleasure and honor to work with the best of the best in the preparation of these articles. All the authors, experts in their fields, were gracious in sharing their knowledge and expertise to bring this issue to life. The contributors made my job quite easy by delivering exceptional material, meeting deadlines, and putting an extraordinary amount of effort into each masterpiece. Their clever titles and writing styles along with the case-based writing truly give the reader a unique experience. Thank you all.

Finally, and most importantly, a few words to my family. My 2 little angels, Kiran and Shaan, were always there to put a huge smile on daddy's face, even when I became nauseated by the sight of the words "altered mental status." I dedicate this issue to my wife, Sonal, who must have been altered when she said, "I do," 6 years ago. She remains supportive of my craziness, and without her I could not do half the things I set out to do. Sonal is always there for a few words of editing wisdom or just a shoulder to lie on when my eyes will not open manually any longer. Thanks to my 2 sisters and my parents for the love and inspiration only the home team can provide. Finally, thank you, the readers. I hope you have as much fun reading this issue as I did, and as we did writing it.

Chad Kessler, MD
Jesse Brown VAMC
Department of Emergency Medicine
820 South Damen, M/C 111
Chicago, IL 60612, USA

E-mail address:
Chad.Kessler@va.gov

REFERENCE

1. Hustey F, Meldon S. The prevalence and documentation of impaired mental status in elderly emergency department patients. Ann Emerg Med 2002;39:248–53.

The Mental Status Examination in Emergency Practice

Jasmine Koita, MD[a,*], Sylvana Riggio, MD[b], Andy Jagoda, MD[b]

KEYWORDS

• Delirium • Altered mental status • Cognition • Dementia

An 84-year-old woman is sent to the emergency department by her private physician with a request for a psychiatric evaluation. According to the family, the patient has had a change in her behavior with intermittent periods of agitation and seeing strangers in her bedroom; she cannot rest, because she is afraid that the strangers will hurt her. The family had brought this to the primary physician's attention, who had prescribed risperdal for the paranoia and diphenhydramine for the agitation. The patient has a history of dementia, hypertension, diabetes, and arthritis; her medications include lisinopril, donepezil, metformin, and sulindac. On examination, the patient's blood pressure was 160/90, heart rate 110, respiratory rate 18, oxygen saturation 98%, tympanic temperature 98° F, blood sugar 140 mg/dL. Her skin was hot and dry. She appeared comfortable and in no distress and engaged in conversation with a smile. Her pupils were 5 mm but equally reactive. The rest of her examination was nonfocal. Because of the new-onset paranoia, a psychiatry consult is requested.

INTRODUCTION

A systematic approach to assessing mental status in the emergency department (ED) is key to identifying alterations in mental status, especially when subtle, and to directing diagnostic testing and management. In a prospective study performed by Hustey and Meldon[1] of 297 patients in a single center urban ED, approximately 25% of patients over 70 years of age had some change in their mental status. Often times, a medical illness may exacerbate an underlying neurobehavioral illness (eg, dementia), contributing to the challenge in ED diagnosis. Hustey and Meldon[1] reported that of the 78 ED patients with mental status changes, 62% had cognitive impairment without delirium, while the remaining 38% had delirium. Alterations in mental status also can be secondary to psychiatric illness. In a prospective, cross-sectional study at four urban EDs, Boudreaux and colleagues[2] reported that of 476 patients over 18

[a] Department of Emergency Medicine, Mount Sinai School of Medicine, One Gustave Levy Place, Box 1620, New York, NY 10029, USA
[b] Mount Sinai School of Medicine, New York, NY 10029, USA
* Corresponding author.
E-mail address: jasmine.koita@mssm.edu

Emerg Med Clin N Am 28 (2010) 439–451
doi:10.1016/j.emc.2010.03.008
emed.theclinics.com

years of age who were screened for mood disorders, approximately 4% of ED patients screened positive for manic mood, while approximately 30% screened positive for depression. Meldon and colleagues[3] also reported approximately 30% of ED patients over 65 suffer from some form of depression. Emergency physicians often are confronted with the diagnostic dilemma of deciding if the mental status changes are chronic, acute, medical, or psychiatric.

On superficial assessment, delirium, dementia, and psychiatric illnesses can seem similar, but management is significantly different; therefore, the emergency physician must be facile in conducting the neurologic and psychiatric mental status evaluation. A brief structured interview that focuses on a systematic testing of attention, memory, executive function, and/or visual–spatial testing may be helpful to the ED physician to identify the necessary treatment. In a study performed by Han and colleagues[4] at a single center tertiary care academic ED, it was found that emergency physicians missed the diagnosis of delirium in up to 75% of patients over 65; those patients were either misdiagnosed or discharged home. This is particularly alarming from both a quality-of-care and risk management point of view, because delirium in the elderly often is associated with high mortality.[5] In a retrospective review of ED patients admitted to a psychiatric service, Tintinalli and colleagues[6] reported that 4% had acute medical conditions requiring transfer out of the psychiatric ward. These two studies highlight potential pitfalls in ED evaluations of patients with altered behavior and suggest a need for improved assessment skills. Mental status evaluations are necessary and can guide the ED physician before making a decision regarding disposition plans.

The goal of this article is to provide a framework for understanding the need for a structured assessment of altered mental status to better understand underlying causes of the mental status changes and therefore potentially improve diagnostic skills and eventually management.

COGNITION, BEHAVIOR, AND CHANGES IN MENTAL STATUS

Alterations in mental status can include changes in alertness, cognition, or behavior. Cognition refers to one's ability to understand his or her environment, being able to integrate information and process information, while behavior refers to one's reaction to his or her environment. A patient's cognition and behavior are affected by his or her level of alertness.

Alertness

The first element that must be assessed when evaluating a patient with altered mental status is his or her level of consciousness. Consciousness is the ability of a person to be able to receive information, process that information, and then act upon it. To exhibit consciousness, one must have both alertness and awareness. Alertness refers to a person's ability to interact with his or her environment.[7] There are gradations describing levels of alertness ranging from fully alert to comatose. A person who is fully alert can interact freely with his or her environment. Someone who is stuporous may respond only partially to verbal or nonverbal stimuli. A person in a coma can at times respond to painful stimuli only with a reflex such as posturing or by withdrawing.[8]

Awareness refers to the person's ability to perceive his or her environment and is dependent on alertness. Attention refers to the person's ability to interact with his or her environment and is dependent on awareness.[7] A patient's level of consciousness, alertness, awareness and attention will affect the assessment of cognition and behavior on bedside examination.

Delirium is due to cognitive dysfunction of attention. The *Diagnostic and Statistical Manual of Mental Disorders* Fourth Edition, Text Revision *(DSM-IV-TR)* definition is *"a disturbance of consciousness that is accompanied by a change in cognition that cannot be better accounted for by a preexisting or evolving dementia. The disturbance develops over a short period of time, usually hours to days, and tends to fluctuate during the course of the day. There is evidence from the history, physical examination, or laboratory tests that the delirium is a direct physiologic consequence of a general medical condition, substance intoxication or withdrawal, use of a medication, or toxin exposure, or a combination of these factors."*[9]

Patients with delirium have difficulty focusing on a task and sustaining and shifting attention. Sleep–wake reversal is also seen. As a result of these cognitive deficits the patient may be confused or disoriented.

Cognition

An understanding of cognition is imperative as a foundation for the discussion of mental status in a fully alert patient. It is the faculty of being able to consider, evaluate, and make appropriate response to internal and external stimuli.[8] The main domains of cognition include orientation, attention, memory, and executive function. Orientation refers to the person's knowledge of who he or she is, the time, and his or her current location. Attention refers to the person's ability to focus on a given task such as naming the months forward and backward or spelling "world" forward and backward or doing calculations.[8] Of note, performing these tests backward is a reflection of executive function. Memory includes newly formed memories, such as a new phone number, as well as old memories, such as the patient's birthday.[8] In order for a patient to remember, he or she must be able to sustain attention, store information, and then retrieve the information. Executive function is the ability to judge a situation, shift parameters, plan, and appropriately take action.[8] A brief assessment of orientation, attention, memory, and executive function forms the foundation of the cognitive mental status examination.

Dementia can be secondary to cognitive deficits in different domains such as language, memory, visual–spatial or executive function. The *DSM IV-TR* definition is:

"the development of multiple cognitive deficits that include memory impairment and at least one of the following cognitive disturbances: aphasia, apraxia, or a disturbance in executive functioning. The cognitive deficits must be sufficiently severe to cause impairment in occupational or social functioning and must represent a decline from a previously higher level of functioning."[9]

Of note, in the presence of delirium and when no history is available, a diagnosis of a possible underlying dementia is difficult to make.

Psychiatric Disorders

Patients with mood disorders or psychotic disorders may present with a change in behavior, but these patients are usually oriented to person, place, and time, and their behavior is secondary to their primary psychiatric disorder (**Box 1**).

Of note dementia, delirium, and primary mental illness all coexist, and complex presentations may require the expertise of a neuropsychiatrist.

GENERAL APPROACH TO ASSESSING A PATIENT WITH ALTERED MENTAL STATUS

Triage

Upon entering a patient interaction in the ED, an immediate assessment of the patient's alertness should be made. Any decrease in alertness is a red flag for the potential of an underlying emergent condition. Every patient with altered mental status

Box 1
Axes diagnoses

Axis 1: Clinical disorders

- Delirium, dementia, amnestic, cognitive disorders
- Mental disorders caused by general medical conditions
- Substance-related disorders
- Psychotic disorders
- Mood disorders
- Anxiety disorders
- Somatoform disorders
- Dissociative disorder
- Adjustment disorders

Axis 2: Personality disorder

- Paranoid, schizoid, antisocial, borderline, histrionic, narcissistic, dependent, obsessive-compulsive

Axis 3: General medical conditions

Axis 4: Psychosocial and environmental problems

Axis 5: Global functioning

Adapted from Meyers J, Stein S. The psychiatric interview in the emergency department. Emerg Med Clin North Am 2000;18:174–5; with permission.

requires an immediate blood sugar determination and a complete set of vital signs including oxygen saturation.

Quick assessment tools have been developed to help initial evaluations and to provide baselines for sequential evaluations: Glasgow coma scale (GCS), AVPU, ACDU, and Simplified Motor Score (SMS). These assessment tools were not created to supplant the neuropsychiatric examination in patients with altered mental status.

The GCS score is the most commonly used tool for assessment of altered levels of consciousness. It was created in 1974 to facilitate communication in the neurocritical care unit for patients with head trauma (**Table 1**).[10]

Although the GCS was not developed as a metric in patients with altered mental status from medical causes, it has been tested on patients with nontraumatic coma, stroke, cardiac arrest, and toxic ingestions.[11] The GCS does not assess cognition and will not differentiate delirium from dementia or from psychiatric illness. Although the scale was not designed to differentiate severity of injury, the GCS score provides a useful guide for monitoring depth of coma and evolving brain herniation.

AVPU is an acronym used primarily in the triage of patients with neurologic impairment. It was created and promoted by the American College of Surgeons in the Advanced Trauma Life Support course.[12] The acronym stands for Alert, responsive to Verbal stimuli, responsive to Painful stimuli, and Unresponsive. In both the neurosurgical patient and the poisoned patient, AVPU scores roughly correlate to a GCS score of 15, 13, 8, and 6.[13,14] As with the GCS, the AVPU system does not differentiate etiologies of altered mental status.

ACDU is a reaction-level scale created in Sweden. The acronym stands for Alert, Confused, Drowsy, and Unresponsive.[12] In a study by McNarry and Godhill,[13]

Table 1
The Glasgow Coma Scale and the Glasgow Outcome Scale

Eye opening	
Spontaneous	4
To speech	3
To pain	2
No response	1
Verbal response	
Alert and oriented	5
Disoriented	4
Speaking but nonsensical	3
Moans	2
No response	1
Motor response	
Follows commands	6
Localizes pain	5
Withdraws to pain	4
Decorticate posture (flexion)	3
Decerebrate posture (extension)	2
No response	1
Grading of TBI[a]:	
Mild	13–15
Moderate	9–12
Severe	3–8

[a] A single Glasgow Coma Scale score in the emergency department is not diagnostic or prognostic.
From Teasdale G, Jennett B. Assessment of coma and impaired consciousness. A practical scale. Lancet 1974;2(7872):81–4; with permission.

ACDU scores roughly correlated to a GCS score of 15, 13, 10, and 6 in neurosurgical patients.

The SMS was created with the belief that the individual parts of the GCS score were as predictive in outcome as the GCS score as a whole. The SMS scale is: obeys commands (2), localizes pain (1), withdrawal to pain or less response (0).[12] The scale has been validated to be as predictive as the GCS score.[15] The SMS has shown to perform as well as the GCS for predicting outcomes in traumatic brain injury and is only marginally inferior than the GCS in predicting needs for intubation, neurosurgical intervention, significant brain injury, and death.[12,16] Furthermore, it has been found to have better inter-rater reliability than GCS, AVPU, and ACDU.[12]

Studies are conflicting on the best quick assessment tool for neurologic status. Any of the previously mentioned scales can be used to initially evaluate a patient for critical conditions such as impending airway compromise or brain herniation in a medically ill or trauma patient. Furthermore, these scales provide a baseline that is used for serial examinations and for communication with consultants.

Initial History and Physical Examination

Of primary importance in the management of patients with altered mental status is examiner and patient safety. In an agitated patient, the examiner should position himself or herself between the patient and the doorway. Sedation may be necessary in a patient who poses harm to him/herself or others.

The initial history and physical examination of the ED patient presenting with altered mental status must focus on stabilization and resuscitation. While examining a patient, a broad differential should be cast including toxic ingestions, infections, electrolyte disturbances, central nervous system lesions, seizure disorders, and endocrine disorders. Obtaining a clear history from emergency medical services, nursing homes, family members, and other caregivers can be critical. It is important to obtain a thorough medical review of symptoms including a psychiatric review of symptoms, such as changes in mood or memory.[17] Almost all patients, especially all elderly patients, should have an assessment of orientation to person, place, and time, and additional assessments as indicated.

The Neurologic Mental Status Examination

After assessing basic levels of alertness and orientation, select patients require a formal assessment of attention and memory. Assessing attention and memory in a structured way allows the practitioner to better differentiate between dementia versus delirium, thus facilitating the diagnostic evaluation and disposition (**Fig. 1**).

If the patient is not oriented to person, place, and time, the clinician should consider the possibility of delirium versus advanced dementia as one of the causes for impairment. The next step in the evaluation is giving the patient three objects to remember. If the patient's immediate recall is impaired, this is again suggestive of delirium versus advanced dementia. Next would be a test of attention and calculation such as having the patient perform serial 7s or alternatively spell world forward and backward or repeat the months of the year forward and backward. If the patient cannot perform these tests, the differential diagnosis again includes delirium versus dementia. If the patient has no impairment of attention but is not able to recall the three objects after 3 to 5 minutes, then the possibility of dementia as the cause for their change in mental status needs to be entertained and appropriate consultation obtained.

There are several types of examinations available to assess a patient's mental status. Given the chaotic environment and limited time available to an emergency physician, the mental status examination used in the ED ideally should be quick and easy to administer. Traditionally, the Mini-Mental State Examination (MMSE) has been recommended for formal cognitive evaluations. The MMSE tests orientation, registration recall, language, visual–spatial praxis, and attention.[18] The sensitivity and specificity for moderate-to-severe dementia is 71% to 92% and 56% to 96% respectively.[19] The examination has a total score of 30 and usually a cut-off score of less than 20 to 23 is used as the threshold for an abnormal result.[19] The cut-off score is adjusted for age and education level; for example, 25% of normal patients with less than an eighth grade level of education score less than 23 on the exam. Furthermore, there is a ceiling effect with those who are highly educated, thus potentially masking dementia. The 7 to 10 minutes needed to perform the MMSE and the copyright laws pose further barriers for easy ED use.[19]

Many other cognitive tests have been recommended over the last few decades (**Table 2**). The 1996 US Preventative Services Task Force literature review found the MMSE, Short Test of Mental Status, the Blessed Orientation Memory Concentration Test, and Functional Activities Questionnaire were all equivalent as a screening tool for detecting dementia.[19] These cognitive tests have not been studied in the ED setting, however, and do not have a defined role in the ED at this time.

Wilber and colleagues[20] performed a study in the ED setting comparing the MMSE, the Six-Item Screener, and the Mini-Cog. The Mini-Cog consists of three-item recall

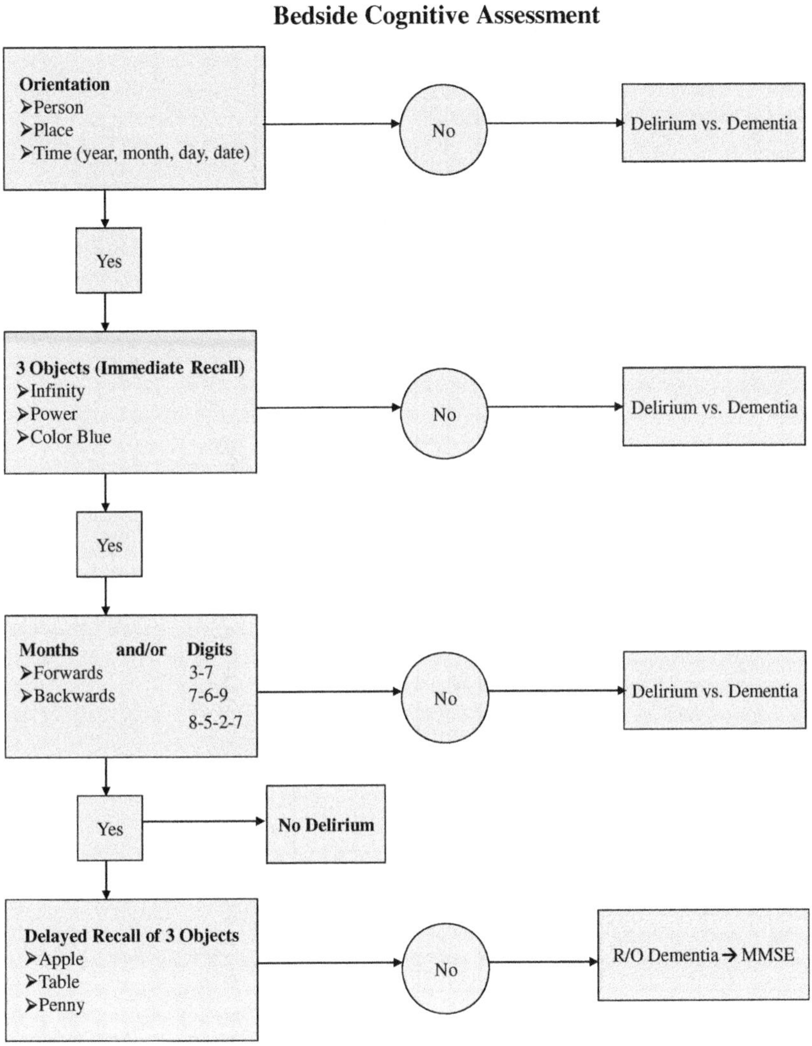

Fig. 1. The bedside cognitive assessment gives a systematic approach to the initial evaluation of a patient with mental status changes.

and clock drawing; the Six-Item Screener consists of three-item recall and three-item temporal orientation (ie, day of week, month, and year).[20,21] When using a cutoff score of less than or equal to 4 in the Six-Item Screener, the Six-Item Screener proved to be better than the Mini-Cog. In comparison to the MMSE, the Six-Item Screener had a sensitivity and specificity of 94% and 86%, respectively, while the Mini-Cog had a sensitivity and specificity of 75% and 85%, respectively.[20] Initially, Callahan and colleagues[21] found the Six-Item Screener to perform as well as the MMSE, but repeat studies have shown that the Six-Item Screener only had a sensitivity of 63% and specificity of 81%.[22] Cognitive assessment in the ED continues to be an area in need of research. Based on the best available evidence, assessment of orientation and memory followed by any of the previously mentioned tests when indicated is recommended.

Table 2
Comparison of cognitive tests

Scale	Time to Administer (Minutes)	Orientation	Registration Recall	Praxis, Visual–Spatial	Aphasia, Verbal Fluency	Attention
Six-Item Screener	1–2	X	X			
Clock drawing	1–3			X		X
Mini-Cog	3–4		X	X		
Memory impairment screen	4		X			
Brief Alzheimer screen	3–5	X	X		X	X
7-minute screen	7–9	X	X	X	X	
Mini-Mental State Examination	7–10	X	X	X	X	X

Data from Holsinger T, Deveau J, Boustani M, et al. Does this patient have dementia? JAMA 2007;297:2391–404.

The fluctuating course of delirium makes diagnosis in the ED setting difficult. For over a decade, the most common assessment used for delirium in both the research and clinical settings has been the Confusion Assessment Method (CAM) (**Box 2**).[4,23]

The CAM requires a few minutes to perform, and when tested in the ED by nonphyscians, it has a reported k = 0.91, sensitivity of 0.86, and specificity of 1.[4,24] The CAM for the Intensive Care Unit (CAM-ICU), which is a modification of the CAM, was created to assist with the diagnosis of delirium in ICU setting (**Box 3**).[25]

It has been suggested that the CAM-ICU may be a better test, because it only requires 2 to 3 minutes to perform, has been validated in mechanically and nonmechanically ventilated patients, and has a sensitivity of 93% to 100% and specificity of 98% to 100%. The CAM-ICU has yet to be validated in the ED setting.[4]

The Psychiatric Mental Status Examination

The final step in the formal evaluation of a patient's mental status is to assess his or her psychiatrics symptoms and to obtain a prior psychiatric and medical history when possible. Of utmost importance is verifying that a patient's symptoms are psychiatric and not medical. Predictors of medical conditions mimicking psychiatric symptoms are: acute onset, greater than 45 years of age, prior medical diseases, perceptual disturbances not including auditory hallucinations, neurologic symptoms, acute change in cognitive functions, no past psychiatric illness, new medications, abnormal vitals, and decreased level of consciousness.[26,27] Of those patients in whom the clinician is concerned for a possible psychiatric cause of the patient's change in mental status, the patient should be asked questions about mood disorders, anxiety disorders, psychotic disorders, and substance abuse disorders. Questions like: "Has your mood changed lately? Have you been upset, angry, or nervous? Has your thinking been different in any way? Have you used anything, like pills, to help you cope?" can be of help in the differential diagnosis. The emergency physician should pay attention to appearance, motor agitation or retardation, speech, affect/mood, thought content, and thought process (ie, how the patient thinks, perception, insight/judgment, impulse control/safety).[27] Always check for suicidal or homicidal ideation as well as for auditory and or visual hallucinations, and, when necessary, consult a psychiatrist.

PUTTING IT ALL TOGETHER

The assessment of mental status changes begins with a broad differential diagnosis that is narrowed by performing a systematic evaluation of the patient's cognitive

Box 2
Confusion Assessment Method (CAM) Diagnostic Algorithm[a]

Acute onset and fluctuating course

Inattention, distractibility

Disorganized thinking, illogical or unclear ideas

Alteration in consciousness

[a] The diagnosis of delirium requires the presence of both features 1 AND 2, plus EITHER feature 3 or 4.

Data from Inouye SK, van Dyck CH, Alessi CA, et al. Clarifying confusion: the confusion assessment method. A new method for detecting delirium. Ann Intern Med 1990;113:941–8.

Box 3
The CAM-ICU

Delirium is diagnosed when both feature 1 and 2 are positive, along with either feature 3 or feature 4.

Feature 1. Acute onset of mental status changes or fluctuating course

Is there evidence of an acute change in mental status from the baseline?

Did the (abnormal) behavior fluctuate during the past 24 hours (ie, tend to come and go or increase and decrease in severity?)

Sources of information: serial GCS or sedation score ratings or nursing and family input

Feature 2. Inattention

Did the patient have difficulty focusing attention?

Is there a reduced ability to maintain and shift attention?

Sources of information: attention screening examinations by using either picture recognition or Vigilance A random letter test. Neither of these tests requires verbal response, and thus they are ideally suited for mechanically ventilated patients.

Feature 3. Disorganized thinking

Was the patient's thinking disorganized or incoherent, such as rambling or irrelevant conversation, unclear or illogical flow of ideas, or unpredictable switching from subject to subject?

Was the patient able to follow questions and commands throughout the assessment?

" Are you having any unclear thinking?"

" Hold up this many fingers" (examiner holds two fingers in front of patient)

" Now, do the same thing with the other hand" (not repeating the number of fingers)

Feature 4. Altered level of consciousness

Any level of consciousness other than alert

Alert—normal, spontaneously fully aware of environment and interacts appropriately

Vigilant—hyperalert

Lethargic—drowsy but easily aroused, unaware of some elements in the environment, or not spontaneously interacting appropriately with the interviewer; becomes fully aware and appropriately interactive when prodded minimally

Stupor—difficult to arouse, unaware of some or all elements in the environment, or not spontaneously interacting with the interviewer; becomes incompletely aware and inappropriately interactive when prodded strongly

Coma—unarousable, unaware of all elements in the environment, with no spontaneous interaction or awareness of the interviewer, so that the interview is difficult or impossible even with maximal prodding

From Ely EW, Margolin R, Francis J, et al. Evaluation of delirium in critically ill patients: validation of the Confusion Assessment Method for the Intensive Care Unit (CAM-ICU). Critical Care Med 2001;29:1370–9; with permission.

function and behavior. In the ED, this assessment must be performed in a focused and efficient manner. The following are easily forgotten but important management suggestions:

Remember to obtain a finger stick glucose on all patients.

At a minimum, all patients should have an assessment of orientation.
Delirium can and does occur in patients with dementia; delirium can be distinguished from dementia using the CAM.
Err on medical management for those patients with unknown psychiatric histories.
Consult psychiatry early for suicidal ideation, homicidal ideation, or new/worsening of mood, anxiety, or psychotic symptoms.
Patients with persistent mental status changes even after management in the ED should be admitted to the hospital or have close follow-up. Do not assume dementia is being addressed as an outpatient. If the patient is being discharged, verify that his or her living situation is safe.

The mental status examination is an important part of emergency medicine. Knowing quick assessments of attention and memory that can be used to evaluate patients who present to the ED with a mental status change can be helpful in diagnosis as well as treatment, disposition, and ultimately better patient care.

SUMMARY

While waiting for psychiatry, the patient becomes mildly agitated and pulls out her intravenous line. A decision is made to discuss the sequence of events more carefully with the family and re-examine the patient. Despite being conversant, on directed mental status examination the patient is oriented only to person, and not oriented to place or time. The patient has difficulty spelling world forward and unable to spell it backward. The family is clear that for years the patient has had difficulty with planning and memory but generally she is oriented to person, place, and month (but not date); family members are also clear that she usually has good attention and can follow a conversation. On further questioning about recent medications, the family offers that the patient has insomnia and that they generally give her an over-the-counter sleep medication that the family has been doubling to ensure the patient gets a good nights rest. As the physician reflects on the new information, the recent addition of diphenhydramine and the physical examination, the decision for a psychiatry consult comes into question: tachycardia, dilated pupils, hot skin, fluctuating course with new onset visual hallucinations. The picture becomes clear and the patient is admitted to the medical unit: diagnosis—delirium due to anticholinergic overdose.

REFERENCES

1. Hustey F, Meldon S. The prevalence and documentation of impaired mental status in elderly emergency department patients. Ann Emerg Med 2002;39:248–53.
2. Boudreaux E, Clark S, Camargo C. Mood disorder screening among adult emergency department patients: a multicenter study of prevalence, associations, and interest in treatment. Gen Hosp Psychiatry 2008;30:4–13.
3. Meldon S, Emerman C, Schubert D, et al. Depression in geriatric ED patients: prevalence and Recognition. Ann Emerg Med 1997;30:141–5.
4. Han JH, Zimmerman EE, Cutler N, et al. Delerium in older emergency department patients: recognition, risk factors, and psychomotor subtypes. Acad Emerg Med 2009;16:193–200.
5. Kakuma R, Galbaud du Fort G, Larsenault L, et al. Delirium in older emergency department patients discharge home: effect on survival. J Am Geriatr Soc 2003;51:443–50.

6. Tintinalli J, Peacock F, Wright M. Emergency medical evaluation of psychiatric patients. Ann Emerg Med 1994;23:859–62.
7. Friedman J, Chou K. Mood, emotion, and thought. In: Goetz C, editor. Textbook of clinical neurology. 3rd edition. Philadelphia: WB Saunders; 2007. p. 43–4.
8. Pryse-Phillips W, Murray T. A concise textbook essential neurology. 4th edition. New York: Elsevier Science Publishing Company, Incorporated; 1992.
9. American Psychiatric Association. Diagnostic and statistical manual of mental disorders. Text Revision. 4th edition. Washington, DC: American Psychiatric Association; 2000.
10. Teasdale G, Jennett B. Assessment of coma and impaired consciousness. A practical scale. Lancet 1974;2(7872):81–4.
11. Gill MR, Reiley DG, Green SM. Interrater reliability of Glasgow Coma Scale scores in the Emergency Department. Ann Emerg Med 2004;43:215–23.
12. Gill M, Martens K, Lynch E, et al. Interrater reliability of 3 simplified neurologic scales applied to adults presenting to the emergency department with altered levels of consciousness. Ann Emerg Med 2007;49:403–7.
13. McNarry AF, Godhill DR. Simple bedside assessment of level of consciousness: comparison of two simple assessment scales with the Glasgow Coma scale. Anaesthesia 2004;54:34–7.
14. Kelly CA, Upex A, Bateman DN. Comparison of consciousness level assessment in the poisoned patient using the alert/verbal/painful/unresponsive scale and the Glasgow Coma Scale. Ann Emerg Med 2004;44:108–13.
15. Houkoos JS, Gill MR, Rabon RE, et al. Validation of the Simplified Motor Score for the prediction of brain injury outcomes after trauma. Ann Emerg Med 2007;50: 18–24.
16. Gill M, Windemuth R, Steele R, et al. A comparison of the Glasgow Coma Scale Score to Simplified Alternative Scores for the prediction of traumatic brain injury outcomes. Ann Emerg Med 2005;45:37–42.
17. Holsinger T, Jorm AF. Methods of screening for dementia: a meta-analysis of studies comparing an informant questionnaire with a brief cognitive test. Alzheimer Dis Assoc Disord 1997;11:158–62.
18. Folstein MF, Folstein SE, McHugh PR. Minimental state: a practical method for grading the cognitive state of patients for the clinician. J Psychiatr Res 1975; 12(3):189–98.
19. Holsinger T, Deveau J, Boustani M, et al. Does this patient have dementia? JAMA 2007;297:2391–404.
20. Wilber ST, Lofgren SD, Mager TG, et al. An evaluation of two screening tools for cognitive impairment in older emergency department patients. Acad Emerg Med 2005;12:612–6.
21. Callahan CM, Unverzagt FW, Hui SL, et al. Six-item screener to identify cognitive impairment among potential subjects for clinical research. Med Care 2002;40: 771–81.
22. Wilber ST, Carpenter CR, Hustey FM. The six-item screener to detect cognitive impairment in older emergency department patients. Acad Emerg Med 2008; 15:613–6.
23. Inouye SK, van Dyck CH, Alessi CA, et al. Clarifying confusion: the confusion assessment method. A new method for detection of delirium. Ann Intern Med 1990;113:941–8.
24. Monette J, du Fort GG, Fung SH, et al. Evaluation of the Confusion Assessment Method (CAM) as a screening tool for delirium in the emergency room. Gen Hosp Psychiatry 2001;23:20–5.

25. Ely EW, Margolin R, Francis J, et al. Evaluation of delirium in critically ill patients: validation of the Confusion Assessment Method for the Intensive Care Unit (CAM-ICU). Crit Care Med 2001;29:1370–9.
26. Karas S. Behavioral emergencies: differentiating medical from psychiatric disease. Emerg Med Pract 2002;4:1–26.
27. Meyers J, Stein S. The psychiatric interview in the emergency department. Emerg Med Clin North Am 2000;18:174–5.

Dizzy and Confused: A Step-by-Step Evaluation of the Clinician's Favorite Chief Complaint

Christine Kulstad, MD[a,*], Blaine Hannafin, MD[b]

KEYWORDS

• Dizziness • Vertigo • Altered mental status • Evaluation

Few chief complaints can provoke more of a sense of fear and loathing in the emergency physician than that of dizziness. The differential diagnosis is extensive and the symptoms and signs are frequently vague and hard to define. Moreover, life-threatening illnesses may masquerade as benign conditions and tests ordered to screen for such illness are often insensitive.[1] Dizziness ranks among the most frequent complaints leading to outpatient evaluation, and is the single most common complaint among patients older than 75 years of age.[2,3] Evaluating patients with a complaint of dizziness presents a significant challenge to the emergency physician, especially in the setting of patients with altered mentation. However, a systematic approach will produce good patient care and avoid considerable consternation on the part of the physician.

DEFINITIONS

Dizziness is an imprecise complaint that encompasses many and varied diagnoses, including syncope, pre-syncope, lightheadedness, gait instability, nausea, anxiety, or generalized weakness. Vertigo is a type of dizziness and has been defined as, "the sensation of motion when no motion is occurring relative to earth's gravity".[4] Vertigo occurs with asymmetric provocation of the vestibular system and is often described as a sensation of spinning relative to the patients' environment or vice-versa.[5] Vertigo can be further divided into central and peripheral depending on what part of the

Funding: The authors did not receive funding for this project and have no commercial disclosures.
[a] Department of Emergency Medicine, Advocate Christ Medical Center, 4440 West 95th Street, Oak Lawn, IL 60453, USA
[b] Department of Emergency Medicine, Chandler Regional Hospital, 475 South Dobson Road, Chandler, AZ 85224, USA
* Corresponding author.
E-mail address: ckulstad@gmail.com

Emerg Med Clin N Am 28 (2010) 453–469
doi:10.1016/j.emc.2010.03.004
0733-8627/10/$ – see front matter

vestibular system has triggered the patients' symptoms. The semicircular canals, otoliths, and vestibular nerve (cranial nerve eight) can all cause peripheral vertigo, whereas the vestibular nuclear complex, vestibulocerebellum, brainstem, spinal cord, and vestibular cortex are all potential causes of central vertigo. Even when patients describe their symptoms specifically as vertigo, it is advisable to clarify their complaint, because many patients are not familiar with the exact meaning of many medical terms.

EPIDEMIOLOGY

It is estimated that 7.5 million patients with dizziness are examined each year in ambulatory centers, and it is one of the most common chief complaints in the emergency department (ED).[5] The lifetime prevalence of vertigo in adults aged 18 to 79 years is 7.4%, with a clear increase in prevalence with age. With the advancing age of North America's population, dizzy and vertiginous patients will continue to be frequent visitors to our EDs.

APPROACH TO PATIENTS WITH DIZZINESS

Clarifying the nature of the complaint is critical because evaluation and management will differ dramatically depending on the history obtained. Generally, the approach to patients with dizziness begins with delineating whether or not patients have true vertigo. Such clarity will allow the physician to limit the scope of the workup and focus on conditions most relevant to the patients' presentation. Patients presenting with symptoms and signs of vertigo will need further evaluation to determine if it is central or peripheral in origin. To this end, a good history and physical examination are invaluable tools that will frequently lead clinicians to the correct diagnosis.[6,7] Alternatively, patients whose dizziness is not vertigo will need investigation into potential cardiovascular, infectious, toxicologic, or psychiatric etiologies of their symptoms.

HISTORY

Traditional teaching has recommended that the physician obtain clarification by asking patients to describe their symptoms without using the word dizziness. Although it is sometimes useful to get a good description with precise terms, patients' particular description can be unclear, inconsistent, or unreliable.[8] Therefore, while obtaining the history, the physician should encourage patients to focus on the timing, triggers, and progression of the symptoms.[8] Despite its limitations, a careful history is usually sufficient to distinguish between central and peripheral vertigo.[5] If the history is consistent with nonspecific dizziness, weakness, or gait instability, then evaluation should proceed in a manner most suitable to those complaints.

The onset of symptoms, whether abrupt or indolent, can be an important distinguishing feature. A slow indolent onset is characteristic of central vertigo. The duration of symptoms can be weeks to months and is characterized by the gradual progression of the overall disease process. Historically, much emphasis has been placed on whether the symptoms worsen with movement of the patients' head. However, most people experiencing dizziness or vertigo of any etiology will experience worsening symptoms with movement. The important distinction is whether the symptoms are *triggered* by head movement or merely worsened by it. Patients experiencing central vertigo may report worsening of their symptoms with head movement, but they should not report that symptoms are *triggered* by it. Finally, central vertigo is frequently associated with neurologic deficits, nystagmus, or visual field abnormalities.

In contrast, peripheral vertigo is characterized by the sudden onset of symptoms that are often severe. Symptoms are episodic and typically last from seconds to minutes with symptom-free intervals between attacks. Patients can frequently trigger attacks by movement of their heads, but can alleviate symptoms by lying still. Unlike central vertigo, peripheral vertigo is not associated with focal neurologic deficits or visual field abnormalities. Peripheral vertigo can be accompanied by a sensation of fullness in the affected ear. In some cases, hearing loss or tinnitus is reported. Careful history may localize the auditory symptoms to one ear, and usually the symptomatic ear is ipsilateral to the vestibular damage.[9] During an acute vertiginous attack, nausea and vomiting are quite common.

Inquiries into the patients' past medical history may be beneficial in determining the cause of the symptoms, especially if there is a history of cancer. Such a finding could heighten one's suspicion of a central nervous system (CNS) metastasis being the cause. Prior ear surgery, vestibular dysfunction, or recent trauma would also be pertinent history.

A social history can be illuminating, especially a history of significant alcohol intake. Chronic alcohol abuse can trigger peripheral neuropathy and resulting gait instability or foot drop that patients often describe as dizziness. Additionally, chronic alcohol abuse should raise the suspicion of vitamin deficiencies and Wernicke's encephalopathy, which classically presents with ophthalmoplegia, ataxia, and confusion. Review of patients' medications is also important because prescription medications can cause dizziness through direct ototoxicity or through a lowering of blood pressure, which may lead to diminished perfusion of the CNS. Though increasingly rare, tabes dorsalis (syphilitic myelopathy) can develop in untreated tertiary syphilis and cause gait instability secondary to proprioceptive abnormalities. Therefore, it is prudent to ask about prior exposure to sexually transmitted diseases. Finally, psychiatric illnesses, especially depression or anxiety, can manifest as almost any complaint, including dizziness, and should be considered as a potential cause of patients' symptoms.

PHYSICAL EXAMINATION

After obtaining a thorough history, the physical examination can often be used to confirm the suspected diagnosis. Patients' vital signs should not be overlooked because they may suggest infectious etiologies or cardiovascular instability as potential causes of dizziness and altered mentation.

Particular attention should be focused on the eye examination, where extraocular motion must be thoroughly tested. The presence of nystagmus is notable. If present, one must determine whether the nystagmus is vertical or horizontal, whether or not it is fatigable, and if it is triggered by a particular head movement. Nystagmus is characteristically vertical and indefatigable in central vertigo. Additionally, visual fields and conjugate gaze should be tested. Internuclear ophthalmoplegia, classically seen as unilateral nystagmus elicited by conjugate lateral gaze, can frequently be found in patients with CNS infarction or multiple sclerosis.[10] The ears should be examined for evidence of trauma or middle ear infection. If the history suggests hearing loss or tinnitus, a full auditory evaluation is prudent. The examination continues with the cranial nerves, with tests for symmetry and function. A deficit in ipsilateral cranial nerves VII and VIII is strongly suggestive of a central lesion.

Extremity strength, sensation, and deep tendon reflexes should be assessed. Gait should likewise be tested in patients who are able to stand. Pronator drift, finger-to-nose, and Romberg tests are useful for evaluating proprioceptive or cerebellar disorders. However, if patients are markedly symptomatic, these maneuvers may prove difficult and have questionable utility. Focal neurologic deficits discovered on the neurologic examination may be indicative of ischemic stroke or other central pathology. The cardiovascular system should be examined for carotid bruits or an irregular heart rhythm, which would raise the possibility of an embolic event.

Though no bedside examination maneuver is diagnostic, the head thrust maneuver deserves special mention. It assesses patients' vestibular ocular reflex (VOR) and can accurately distinguish cerebellar stroke from benign peripheral conditions, such as vestibular neuritis. The head thrust maneuver is performed by placing the examiner's hands on each side of the patients' head. Quick head movements are then made 20 to 30 degrees to the patients' left and right while attempting to focus on a fixed object (usually the examiner's nose). The response is abnormal if the patients' eyes move with their head and then snap back to the examiner's nose in a single corrective movement. Such an abnormal response is suggestive of a disruption of the VOR and implicates a peripheral cause of the vertigo, such as vestibular neuritis. A normal response to this maneuver is for patients' eyes to remain fixed on the object despite the head movements and suggests a normal intact VOR. Patients with cerebellar infarction give a normal response because the VOR bypasses the cerebellum. Therefore, in acutely vertiginous patients, a normal response is strongly suggestive of cerebellar stroke even in the presence of normal neuroimaging. In cases of suspected vestibular neuritis, an abnormal head thrust test, horizontal nystagmus, and the absence of vertical ocular misalignment can exclude 91% of acute strokes.[1]

Table 1 summarizes the characteristics of central and peripheral vertigo. Although each characteristic generally pertains to one or the other type of vertigo, no characteristic is diagnostic or exclusionary for either type. A thorough history should touch on each of these characteristics and more often than not, a clear trend will become apparent and the differential diagnosis will be narrowed considerably.[6] Although most conditions causing peripheral vertigo are benign and do not require emergent treatment or stabilization in the ED, patients with altered mentation and vertigo are not typical of this disease process and require careful evaluation.

VERTIGO

Vertigo is a symptom that generally has a benign underlying cause. However, in patients presenting with altered mental status, vertigo should never be assumed to have a trivial cause. The type of vertigo, along with other neurological deficits or signs, can be important clues for physicians investigating patients' illness.

A 62-year-old man with hypertension and diabetes presents complaining of dizziness and gait instability. He has no history of these symptoms and notes that they are present

Table 1
Characteristics of central and peripheral vertigo

Characteristic	Central	Peripheral
Onset	Slow	Sudden
Frequency	Constant, progressive	Episodic, recurrent
Duration	Weeks to months	Seconds to minutes
Changes in head position triggers?	No, symptoms may worsen but are not triggered by motion	Yes, symptoms triggered by motion and alleviated by being motionless
Nystagmus	Vertical	Horizontal
Associated symptoms	Neurologic or visual deficits	Tinnitus, nausea
Fatigable	No	Yes

at rest or with movements of his head. His wife reports he has fallen at home several times and is concerned. On examination he is noted to have indefatigable horizontal nystagmus, a normal head thrust maneuver, and a positive Romberg sign.

CEREBELLAR STROKE

Although many strokes located in the anterior or middle circulations do not present a diagnostic dilemma, diagnosing an acute cerebellar infarction can be quite challenging. The most common symptoms, dizziness, vertigo, and gait instability, are nonspecific and frequently have benign underlying causes.[1] Moreover, CT of the brain frequently does not detect acute infarctions in the posterior fossa. Misdiagnosis can be problematic when and if clinicians fail to recognize this limitation.[1] Once again, clinicians must rely on a thorough history and physical examination to help guide the evaluation and ultimate disposition of patients.[1,11]

Approximately 20,000 new cerebellar strokes are diagnosed in the United States each year.[1] In nine studies of consecutive subjects with ischemic strokes, cerebellar infarction accounted for approximately 3% of strokes. General risk factors for ischemic stroke, including hypertension, diabetes, tobacco usage, dyslipidemia, atrial fibrillation, and history of ischemic stroke or transient ischemic attack (TIA), likewise apply to cerebellar stroke.

Patients often present with nonspecific symptoms, such as dizziness, nausea, vomiting, unsteady gait, or headache, when acute infarction is limited to the cerebellum. Neurologic signs, such as dysarthria, ataxia, or nystagmus, may be subtle or absent. Although dizziness or vertigo occurs in nearly three quarters of patients with cerebellar infarction, they are also common complaints in many benign disorders. Indeed, an isolated complaint of dizziness is a poor predictor of stroke of any kind. In a retrospective study of 1660 subjects presenting to the ED with a chief complaint of dizziness, only 3% had a stroke or TIA; and of subjects presenting with an isolated complaint of dizziness, less than 1% were found to have had an ischemic stroke or TIA.[12]

Signs of cerebellar stroke can include limb or truncal ataxia, dysarthria, and nystagmus. Though confusion can be present, it has been noted in only about one third of patients with cerebellar stroke.[1] Coma is even less likely to be present, and usually indicates basilar artery occlusion or secondary complications, such as brainstem compression or herniation. In patients experiencing vertigo, the VOR can be assessed rapidly at the bedside by using the head thrust maneuver (described earlier). A normal response is strongly suggestive of cerebellar stroke, whereas an abnormal response implicates a peripheral cause of vertigo. No one feature is diagnostic, and it is incumbent upon the clinician to interpret each feature in the context of the entire clinical encounter.

Neuroimaging is crucial in the evaluation of suspected cerebellar stroke. Head CT is the most readily available form of neuroimaging for emergency physicians, but has significant limitations. It is uncommon to visualize acute stokes in the posterior cranial fossa with CT. Therefore, in patients with suspected cerebellar or brainstem stroke, CT scan should not be used to exclude this diagnosis.[1,11,13] One study suggests that misdiagnosis occurs more frequently in junior physicians who place too much emphasis on the role of CT in excluding acute stroke.[14] MRI has greater sensitivity than CT, especially when diffusion weighted imaging is used, but is not readily available to many emergency physicians. Given these constraints, CT scan is the preferred initial screening test.[11,13]

In patients with suspected acute brainstem or cerebellar stroke, admission and neurologic consultation is warranted for definitive neuroimaging and treatment, even in the presence of negative head CT scan. Antiplatelet agents should be withheld until neuroimaging has been completed and the physician is satisfied that no hemorrhage is present.

An 80-year-old women presents by ambulance to the emergency department with report of sudden onset left-sided facial weakness, disorientation, and right-sided extremity weakness. Family members note abnormal slurred speech and disorientation. On examination, the patient is noted to have nystagmus and ataxic limb movements.

VERTEBROBASILAR STROKE

Vertebrobasilar strokes usually cause more neurologic abnormalities than isolated cerebellar infarctions because a larger area of the brain is affected by occlusions of the posterior circulation. Headache, dizziness, vertigo, or confusion are all possible presenting complaints.[15] Physical examination findings include, but are not limited to, pupillary abnormalities, abnormal ocular movements, facial palsy, and hemiplegia or quadriplegia.[15]

Evaluation and workup should follow the same basic guidelines outlined previously with respect to history and physical examination, followed by appropriate neuroimaging and admission for suspected acute infarction. Again, physicians should be cognizant of the limitations of CT for diagnosis of acute infarctions in the posterior cranial fossa.

An infrequent but notable link between cervical manipulative therapy (CMT) in chiropractic practice and vertebral artery dissection has been demonstrated.[16,17] History of antecedent CMT in the face of neurologic findings should raise suspicion for this entity. Diagnosis can be made with CT angiography, conventional angiography, or MRI angiography.

A 75-year-old man presents with gradual onset of disorientation, worsening dizziness, and falling over the past several months. His family noted these symptoms were subtle at first and thought they were caused by the patient's advancing age. However, the family notes increasing difficulty walking and a broad based shuffling gait. He has a history of being treated for urinary incontinence and recently had a Foley catheter placed.

IDIOPATHIC ADULT HYDROCEPHALUS SYNDROME (NORMAL PRESSURE HYDROCEPHALUS)

Normal pressure hydrocephalus (NPH) is a syndrome of gait dysfunction and enlarged cerebral ventricles in the absence of another cause. Contrary to its traditional name, however, intracranial pressure is not always normal and a more accurate name is idiopathic adult hydrocephalus syndrome.[18] The more familiar term, NPH, is used in the following discussion. NPH usually presents in the sixth or seventh decade of life, and although the incidence increases with age it is still considered a rare diagnosis.[18,19]

The classic triad of abnormal gait, dementia, and urinary incontinence is well described. However, because NPH generally occurs in the elderly population, these findings are not uncommon in patients with other illnesses. Patients will frequently use the terms dizziness or weakness to describe gait instability or inability to ambulate normally. Abnormal gait is characteristically the first and most prominent finding and occurs in 89% of people diagnosed with NPH.[19] The gait is typically wide based with reduced step height and stride length, along with reduced velocity and imbalance or unsteadiness. With time, gait impairment progresses so that patients find it difficult to initiate walking. This condition is described as a "magnetic gait" because patients' feet seem stuck to the floor as if magnetized.[18,19] Other conditions common in this age group, such as peripheral neuropathy, parkinsonism, and lumbar canal stenosis, can also cause gait abnormalities and should be considered when evaluating patients with a complaint of dizziness or abnormal gait.

An estimated 45% to 90% of patients with NPH experience urinary incontinence.[19] Urinary frequency and urgency are the earliest manifestations of NPH, and are caused by stretching of the periventricular nerve fibers that control the urinary bladder. This stretching leads to partial loss of bladder contraction inhibition and progressive urge incontinence.[19] Other causes of urinary incontinence should be considered, such as prostatic hypertrophy, stress incontinence, neuropathy, or anticholinergic effects of medications.

Up to 77% of patients with NPH develop dementia, which is described as subcortical.[19] Typical findings are memory impairment, with decreased attention, alertness, and speed of mental processing. Cortical deficits of aphasia, apraxia, and agnosia are typically absent in NPH and may point to an alternative diagnosis,[19] such as depression with pseudodementia, Alzheimer's disease, or vascular dementia.

The diagnosis of NPH can be made by the astute examiner with the aid of either CT or MRI of the brain. Neuroimaging reveals ventriculomegaly, which is distinct from hydrocephalus ex vacuo, a common normal finding in elderly patients. Patients admitted with suspected NPH benefit from neurologic and especially neurosurgical consultation for assessment of potential shunt placement. NPH has variable resolution with shunt placement, but is one of the few reversible causes of dementia in those patients who do respond to treatment.

A 25-year-old woman presents to the emergency department with 2 years of intermittent motor and sensory complaints. In her most recent episode, she experienced frank vertigo. She has been seen by several physicians for complaints ranging from foot drop and dizziness to paresthesias and generalized fatigue. Several laboratory and diagnostic tests have been run and her primary care physician suggested she start treatment for anxiety and stress. On examination, she is noted to have internuclear ophthalmoplegia.

MULTIPLE SCLEROSIS

Multiple sclerosis (MS) is a chronic inflammatory disorder affecting the brain, spinal cord, and optic nerve that typically presents in young adults aged between 20 to 45 years.[20–22] By definition, MS is characterized as having multiple episodes of inflammation disseminated in time and space.[20,21] Because MS can affect nearly any part of the CNS, presenting symptoms are highly variable and are often confused with other disease processes.[21]

Vertigo is the initial symptom in approximately 5% of patients diagnosed with MS and affects 50% of patients with MS at some point during the course of their disease.[5] Other prominent presenting symptoms are sensory complaints, such as frank numbness, or paresthesias. Sensory symptoms are typically vague and patients will often have a normal sensory examination. The discordance between the history and physical examination can lead to falsely attributing patients' symptoms to anxiety or emotional distress.[21]

Motor symptoms typically involve weakness or spasticity, but can also involve complaints of diminished hand dexterity or gait instability. Gait abnormalities can develop from weakness, dizziness, incoordination, sensory loss, or a combination of these problems.[20] Finally, fatigue is reported in up to 90% of patients with MS and may refer specifically to exertional muscle fatigue or general lassitude.[21]

MRI is an important tool that assists with the diagnosis of MS. Images of the brain can demonstrate multiple T2 signal abnormalities in the cerebral white matter.

Although other modalities, such as spinal fluid analysis, serologic testing, and evoked potentials, can be helpful to the neurologist, they are not available during a single ED encounter. Because MRI is not routinely available in many EDs, it is recommended that the clinician evaluate patients for other disease processes that could mimic MS and arrange follow-up for definitive testing.

A 35-year-old man presents with complaints of gradually worsening vertigo for the last several months. Although his symptoms wax and wane in intensity, they have recently worsened and he notes no symptom-free intervals. He also notes a painful occipital headache. His wife notes hearing loss specifically to the right ear. On physical examination, signs of cerebellar ataxia are noted when testing the patient's gait and coordination.

SPACE OCCUPYING LESIONS

Dizziness may be one of a variety of signs and symptoms of a CNS tumor, depending on the size and location of the tumor within the brain. Typically, the onset of symptoms is insidious, gradually worsening with tumor growth as adjacent structures are compromised. However, it can be more acute if the tumor undergoes acute infarction or bleeding.

Tumors of the cerebellopontine angle and posterior fossa are characterized by the accumulation and augmentation of neurologic signs and symptoms over weeks to months.[5] Symptoms include vertigo, dizziness, hearing loss, tinnitus, or facial weakness or numbness. Occipital headache is the most common symptom with cerebellar tumors.[5] Ataxia, nystagmus, or hearing loss can also be seen on examination. Late in the course of disease, cranial nerve palsies or vomiting when recumbent can develop. With progression, intracranial pressure may increase causing papilledema and changes in mental status. When patients present with vertigo of central origin, or focal neurologic deficits as described above, neuroimaging is indicated.

POOR PERFUSION STATES

Because many patients have difficulty describing exactly what their symptoms of dizziness are, disease processes that might cause lightheadedness or unsteadiness should also be considered. Causes of dizziness in patients with altered mental status include any disease state that leads to decreased cerebral perfusion or any of the various causes of shock. Although most patients with shock demonstrate tachycardia and hypotension along with altered mental status, patients with chronic hypertension may have a 50 mmHg drop in blood pressure with a normal reading and a resulting altered mental status.[23] Additionally, patients on beta-blockers or calcium channel blockers may not manifest tachycardia.

COMMON CAUSES OF SHOCK PRESENTING WITH DIZZINESS AND ALTERED MENTAL STATUS

A 78-year-old woman arrives at your ED with her family who reports that she seems more confused today. The patient complains of generalized weakness, dizziness, and nausea, but denies any pain. Her vital signs from triage show a heart rate of 108, blood pressure of 106/58, and temperature of 36°C.

Septic Shock

Classic septic shock is not difficult to diagnose in patients with fever, infection, and hypotension, but may not be considered as a differential diagnosis in this patient with altered mental status and dizziness. However, in the early stages of the disease process, sepsis is often difficult to diagnose. Alterations in CNS function occur at higher blood pressures in septic shock compared to other types of shock because of the influence of inflammatory mediators.[23] Familiarity with the components of the systemic inflammatory response syndrome (SIRS), the first stage of the sepsis syndrome, can lead clinicians in the right direction. The diagnosis of SIRS requires two of the following criteria: temperature greater than 38°C or less than 36°C; heart rate greater than 90 beats/min; a respiratory rate greater than 20 breaths/min or a PaCO2 of less than 32 mm Hg; or a white blood cell count greater than 12,000 cells/μL or less than 4000 cells/μL.[24] Sepsis is then defined by the addition of infection, severe sepsis with the addition of end organ dysfunction, and septic shock with the addition of hypotension despite adequate fluid resuscitation.[25] Mortality rates for sepsis range from 25% to 80%,[26] with the incidence of sepsis and the mortality rate increasing with increasing patient age.[27] The presence of encephalopathy, as measured by changes in the Glasgow Coma Score, has also been associated with increased mortality.[28] It is therefore important for this patient complaining of dizziness to be evaluated for the presence of severe sepsis as the cause of her symptoms.

Aside from having a routine complete blood count (CBC), patients with suspected sepsis should have blood drawn for cultures (preferably before antibiotics are started), a lactate level measured, and prompt imaging to confirm clinically suspected sources of infection.[29] A complete metabolic panel and arterial blood gas analysis are useful to determine organ dysfunction and to calculate a severity of illness score. Once severe sepsis or septic shock is identified, rapid resuscitation dramatically decreases mortality.[30–33] Key components of early resuscitation include timely, broad spectrum antibiotics; adequate fluid resuscitation to restore circulating volume; the use of vasopressors when required to maintain a mean arterial pressure of greater than or equal to 65 mm Hg; and the addition of dobutamine when adequate cardiac output is not achieved with fluid resuscitation and vasopressors.[29] If patients are intubated, low tidal volumes and inspiratory plateau pressures reduce the risk for developing acute respiratory distress syndrome.[29] Less strongly recommended are the use of recombinant activated protein C and steroids.[29]

A 54-year-old man presents with lightheadedness and epigastric pain. He tells you he has had epigastric pain for years, but it seems to be getting worse over the last few months. He has felt lightheaded for the last few weeks. When questioned, he does report that his stool is dark, but he attributes the color to his frequent use of bismuth subsalicylate (Pepto-Bismol). He seems to have trouble concentrating and answering complex questions.

Hemorrhagic Shock

Although hemorrhagic states are generally not a diagnostic dilemma, patients with occult gastrointestinal (GI) bleeds may complain only of dizziness or near syncope. As the disease progresses undiagnosed and untreated, patients may develop altered mental status caused by relative hypotension and poor cerebral perfusion. Physical examination should check for pallor of mucus membranes and for the presence of blood or melena in the stool. Laboratory testing should include a CBC, type and screen, a basic metabolic profile, and coagulation studies. An elevated blood urea nitrogen (BUN)/Cr ratio (>30 or 36) may suggest an upper GI source of bleeding,[34,35] although the degree of overlap between upper and lower bleeds is significant.[36] All patients in whom GI bleeding is suspected of being the cause of their dizziness and altered mental status should have two, large bore needles intravenously (IV) placed, IV fluids administered, and cardiac monitoring started. Oxygen should be given to elderly patients and those with preexisting cardiac disease to supplement the oxygen-carrying capacity of blood.[37] The patient previously described developed hypotension while in the ED, had new anemia and a BUN/Cr ratio of 38, confirming your suspected diagnosis of bleeding peptic ulcer. He, and most other patients with symptomatic GI bleeding, requires admission to an ICU.

A 45-year-old man complains of dizziness and groin pain. He was seen in your ED 3 days ago with chest pain, had a coronary CT with a 70% stenosis, and was then admitted for a coronary angiogram. He had no lesion requiring intervention and was discharged later that day on aspirin, clopidogrel, metoprolol, and lovastatin. Shortly after returning home, he started to have increasing pain in his groin, noted swelling at the catheterization site, and now feels dizzy. He appears restless and slightly agitated, unusual for him according to his wife.

Patients with recent invasive procedures involving access to femoral vessels or retroperitoneal surgery are at risk for developing retroperitoneal hemorrhage. Patients with bleeding disorders are at risk for spontaneous bleeding into the retroperitoneal space, most commonly as a result of anticoagulant use and less commonly as a result of antiplatelet medications or hemophilia. As the number of patients on anticoagulants increases, the number of patients at risk for bleeding complications also grows. Somewhere between one half and two thirds of patients with retroperitoneal hematomas are not over-anticoagulated, and mortality rates for all patients with retroperitoneal hematomas are as high as 20%.[38]

A classic presentation of retroperitoneal hematoma begins, like the case previously mentioned, with patients reporting pain in the groin, lower back, or abdomen. As the bleeding persists, paresthesias, paresis, and a palpable mass may develop. Large hematomas may lead to abdominal compartment syndrome. Patients may have dizziness and altered mental status from hypotension, and may describe unsteadiness or difficulty walking because of leg weakness stemming from nerve compression caused by the hematoma. Diagnosis is commonly made by CT, but ultrasound may also be helpful. However, ultrasound provides limited information about the extent of the hematoma or the presence of ongoing bleeding. Treatment includes standard resuscitative measures, such as IV fluids, blood transfusion as needed, and reversal of anticoagulation. More invasive therapies are of unproven benefit. The published literature investigating the treatment of retroperitoneal hematomas consists mostly of case reports or limited case series. Embolization by interventional radiology seems to be effective when a bleeding source can be identified.[39] Percutaneous drainage may provide only temporary benefits, but may also prevent permanent nerve damage by relieving compression from the hematoma.[40] Early surgery is advocated by some to ensure that permanent nerve compression does not occur,[41] whereas other authors suggest that surgery should only be used in patients who cannot be treated with less invasive means or in patients who remain unstable or who develop abdominal compartment syndrome. Conservative therapy is usually sufficient in stable patients who do not demonstrate mass effect from a large hematoma, such as paresthesias or paresis, abdominal compartment syndrome, or other signs of end organ damage.[39] In the previous case, the patient should be admitted for close monitoring, transfusion of red blood cells as needed, and stopping further doses of aspirin and clopidogrel. If the hematoma increases in size, more invasive measures would be appropriate.

A 78-year-old woman is brought to the ED by ambulance. She called for an ambulance because she felt too dizzy to get out of bed, but hasn't been able to provide much other history. She arouses to loud questions, but is unable to respond to anything but brief, simple questions. Her vital signs show a heart rate of 116, respiratory rate of 24, and blood pressure of 98/52. She denies chest pain, but does admit that she is short of breath and nauseated. Her electrocardiogram shows ST elevation in inferior leads.

ACUTE CORONARY SYNDROMES

Decreased perfusion from a primary cardiac cause is a grave complication of acute coronary syndromes (ACS), affecting roughly 2% of unstable angina or non-ST elevation myocardial infarctions and 7% of ST-elevation myocardial infarctions.[42] Patients, such as in the previous case, present with signs of decreased perfusion despite having adequate circulating volume because of decreased cardiac output. In addition to the typical signs and symptoms of ACS, most patients will be hypotensive and have cool skin, dyspnea, and rales. Dizziness and altered mental status result from decreased cerebral perfusion. In the elderly, the classic signs of chest pain and ECG changes may be absent and confusion, altered mental status, or dizziness may be the chief complaint, as seen in the previous case.[43,44]

Left heart failure from a large left ventricular infarction is the most common cause of cardiogenic shock.[42] Right heart failure, likely the cause of the symptoms in the case described here, is less common and will show some improvement with volume resuscitation. Mechanical causes of cardiogenic shock complicating infarction, such as ventricular septal defect, acute valvular regurgitation, myocardial wall rupture, and tamponade, are uncommon, occurring in 2.8% to 10.7% of patients in the Global Utilization of Streptokinase and Tissue Plasminogen Activator to Treat Occluded Arteries (GUSTO) trial.[45] Failure to consider a mechanical cause, however, could delay lifesaving surgical repair.

TOXICOLOGIC CAUSES OF DIZZINESS AND ALTERED MENTAL STATUS

There are several toxicologic causes of altered mental status that also produce ataxia and nystagmus, which are often perceived by patients as dizziness. Many also have dizziness as a presenting symptom. Although ethanol is the most common intoxicant that produces these symptoms, it is not discussed here, but is covered in another section of this issue. Cases are described in the following discussion to illustrate some typical presentations.

A 14-year-old boy was found by his brother to have passed out in the garage. By the time you examine him, he complains of dizziness, being tired, and nausea. You note that he has an erythematous rash around his mouth, his speech is slurred, and he has nystagmus. As you lean closer to examine his heart, you note a chemical aroma.

INHALANTS

Inhalants used as drugs of abuse are a diverse group of compounds that are all volatile, and provide a quick-onset high followed by a rapid dissolution of symptoms. Most abused inhalants are available as legal substances, such as paints and solvents, fuels, aerosolized room deodorizers, and nitrous oxide in spray whipping cream, and are abused by adolescents.[46] Inhalants are absorbed through the lungs, cause intoxication in seconds to minutes, and then are excreted through the lungs or rapidly metabolized in the liver, or both.[47] The intoxication produced generally resembles that produced by alcohol, with euphoria, ataxia, slurred speech, and diplopia. Higher levels of intoxication may produce hallucinations, seizures, or coma.

The diagnosis of inhalant abuse is clinical because there are no specific diagnostic tests. Staining of the skin or clothing from pigments and characteristic odors may suggest the diagnosis. Wheezing from pulmonary irritation and a perioral rash may also be seen. Treatment is generally supportive, with attention to the usual ABCs of resuscitation (ie, airway, breathing, circulation) and no treatment other than substance abuse counseling would be required for the case described previously. In the more serious overdose, cardiac effects are the most critical complication. The myocardium of patients who have abused inhalants becomes more sensitive to circulating catecholamines, provoking arrhythmias that are often not successfully resuscitated.[48] Standard treatment with advanced cardiac life support should be instituted, with the exception that further sympathomimetic medications are avoided and beta-blockers are added to blunt the effects of catecholamine sensitization.[49]

A 42-year-old woman presents to your ED with dizziness, headache, and decreased responsiveness. Her aunt reports that she went to her house today and found her to be confused and complaining of the previously mentioned symptoms. The patient is HIV positive with a recent CD4 count in her medical records of 198. Her aunt reports that she recently had some new medications added to her regimen to protect her from developing infections, but she is not sure what they are. You note that the patient is tachycardic, hypoxic, cyanotic, and confused.

METHEMOGLOBINEMIA

Methemoglobinemia is yet another potential cause of altered mental status and dizziness. Patients present with cyanosis, nausea, tachycardia, and headache at lower methemoglobin levels. Dizziness and altered mental status may occur as methemoglobin levels reach 30% to 50% of normal hemoglobin.[50] Above 50% to 60%, patients become lethargic and then comatose, and are prone to arrhythmias and seizures. Death usually occurs at levels above 70%.[50]

Methemoglobinemia is most commonly drug induced, with dietary and genetic conditions being the next most common causes.[50] Methemoglobinemia can also complicate the sequelae of nitrite abuse. The drugs that most commonly cause methemoglobinemia are local anesthetics, antimalarial drugs, and dapsone. In the case described previously, dapsone had been added to the patient's regimen for pneumocystis carinii pneumonia prophylaxis.[51] Nitroglycerin, phenazopyridine, and sulfonamides are other medications commonly used in the ED that may trigger methemoglobinemia.

A diagnosis of methemoglobinemia should be suspected in patients who are cyanotic with normal pulse oximetry whose cyanosis does not respond to oxygen therapy. Blood drawn from patients will classically appear chocolate brown. An arterial blood gas with co-oximetry should be drawn if the diagnosis is suspected. The partial pressure of O2 and CO2 will be normal, and metabolic acidosis may be present. Because the oxygen saturation of hemoglobin reported on the blood gas is calculated rather than measured, it will be normal. Co-oximetry directly measures the amount of methemoglobin and will confirm the diagnosis.[52] If co-oximetry is unavailable or will be delayed, a drop of the patients' blood can be placed on a piece of filter paper next to a drop of normal blood. The normal blood will appear dark red, but brighten with exposure to oxygen. The methemoglobinemic blood will stay chocolate brown.[50]

The patient described previously should be treated with high flow oxygen to increase the oxygen-carrying capacity of the blood. Healthy patients with methemoglobin levels below 30% do not need other treatment.[50] Methylene blue will convert methemoglobin to hemoglobin, and should be given to patients with methemoglobin levels higher than 30% or to more symptomatic patients, including the one described here. The dosage given should be proportionate to the symptoms and methemoglobin levels, with 1 mg/kg used for levels around 30% in patients with milder symptoms and

2 mg/kg used for patients with more severe symptoms or with methemoglobin levels near 50%.[52] Patients who do not respond to methylene blue treatment may require treatment with p450 inhibitors, such as cimetidine or ketoconazole; exchange transfusion; or treatment with n-acteylcysteine.[50,52,53]

A 38-year-old woman is sent from the rehabilitation center for evaluation of confusion. She is in rehabilitation because of a seizure disorder that led to a motor vehicle accident 2 months ago with significant injuries. Her husband reports that she had been complaining of feeling off balance and nauseated the day before. Her medications are phenytoin, fentanyl patch, cimetidine, and ibuprofen as needed.

PHENYTOIN

Antiepileptic medications can cause altered mental status and dizziness at supratherapeutic or toxic levels. Although acute phenytoin toxicity is most commonly seen in overdose, chronic toxicity can result after small dosage changes or after the addition of another medication that either alters its binding to serum proteins or its hepatic metabolism.[54] The patient discussed previously may have increased phenytoin concentrations in her blood as a result of her taking cimetidine, or she may have decreased concentrations of serum proteins as a result of her prolonged debilitated state. Supratherapeutic levels of phenytoin cause nausea, confusion, ataxia, and nystagmus.[55] Higher levels produce lethargy and coma. Toxicity is difficult to predict from the total concentration in the blood, especially in patients who are critically ill or hypoalbuminemic, because free serum phenytoin is the pharmacologically active component, and routine blood tests measure bound and free serum concentrations.[56]

Treatment is generally supportive, with focus on fall prevention for milder toxicity, although intubation for airway protection may be required in more severe toxicity. Because phenytoin is mainly protein bound, extra-corporeal methods of elimination are generally not effective. Multidose activated charcoal (MDAC) has been reported to lower the levels of phenytoin,[57–59] but the American Academy of Clinical Toxicology and European Association of Poisons Centres and Clinical Toxicologists do not recommend its use in phenytoin overdose.[60]

CARBAMAZEPINE

Carbamazepine is another widely used antiepileptic medication that can cause altered mental status and dizziness, but has more severe effects in overdose. Most patients will have a decreased level of consciousness, many develop changes in muscle tone, ataxia, vertigo, and nystagmus, and up to 24% will have seizures.[61] Cardiac conduction effects, such as atrioventricular block, ventricular arrhythmias, and QRS widening, are also commonly seen.[62] Many of the toxic effects result from the sodium channel blocking and anticholinergic effects. The severity of presentation appears to correlate with serum level, with a cutoff of 170 μmol/L or 40 mg/L indicating increased risk.[62]

Seizures should be treated with benzodiazepines, and close attention should be paid to the patients' ability to protect their airway because intubation is usually necessary with serious overdoses.[63] Telemetry monitoring should be continued until the serum carbamazepine levels have returned to the therapeutic range,[64] with the understanding that absorption of the drug is often delayed and erratic. Electrocardiogram, complete metabolic profile, and a CBC should be ordered to evaluate for the hyponatremia and cardiac conduction effects that are seen in acute toxicity, and for the hepatic toxicity and blood dyscrasias that can occur with chronic use of the medication.

Decontamination and elimination of carbamazepine will speed recovery. Activated charcoal should be given immediately to patients who are alert and to those with secured airways. The American Academy of Clinical Toxicology and European Association of Poisons Centres and Clinical Toxicologists recommend the use of MDAC for life-threatening carbamazepine overdoses.[60] One recent, small study of 12 subjects did show decreased time of mechanical ventilation requirements and decreased time comatose after the use of MDAC.[65] If a patient has ileus, or if MDAC is not felt to be appropriate for other reasons, charcoal hemoperfusion is also effective at reducing serum concentrations of carbamazepine.[66]

SUMMARY

The causes of vertigo and dizziness in patients with altered mental status are varied and broad. A careful history and physical examination will guide the clinician's further evaluation and testing. Patients who have vertigo require imaging, CT and often MRI, and most patients will be admitted for further evaluation. Patients with other forms of dizziness require a more broad differential diagnosis. Careful review of vital signs and components of the history and physical examination may suggest decreased perfusion from early cardiogenic, septic, or hemorrhagic shock. Patients with confusion and nystagmus or unsteadiness require a careful review of the medications they have received, because a toxicological cause may explain their symptoms. Careful and systematic evaluation of patients will alleviate the distress associated with the evaluation of dizzy and confused patients.

REFERENCES

1. Edlow JA, Newman-Toker DE, Savitz SI. Diagnosis and initial management of cerebellar infarction. Lancet Neurol 2008;7(10):951–64.
2. Burt CW, Schappert SM. Ambulatory care visits to physician offices, hospital outpatient departments, and emergency departments: United States, 1999–2000. Vital Health Stat 13 2004;157:1–70.
3. Kroenke K, Mangelsdorff AD. Common symptoms in ambulatory care: incidence, evaluation, therapy, and outcome. Am J Med 1989;86(3):262–6.
4. Neuhauser HK. Epidemiology of vertigo. Curr Opin Neurol 2007;20(1):40–6.
5. Karatas M. Central vertigo and dizziness: epidemiology, differential diagnosis, and common causes. Neurologist 2008;14(6):355–64.
6. Agrup C, Gleeson M, Rudge P. The inner ear and the neurologist. J Neurol Neurosurg Psychiatr 2007;78(2):114–22.
7. Delémont C, Rutschmann O. [Vertigo: it all revolves around the physical exam]. Rev Med Suisse 2007;3(121):1826–8 1830–2 [in French].
8. Newman-Toker DE, Cannon LM, Stofferahn ME, et al. Imprecision in patient reports of dizziness symptom quality: a cross-sectional study conducted in an acute care setting. Mayo Clin Proc 2007;82(11):1329–40.
9. Chawla N, Olshaker JS. Diagnosis and management of dizziness and vertigo. Med Clin North Am 2006;90(2):291–304.
10. Keane JR. Internuclear ophthalmoplegia: unusual causes in 114 of 410 patients. Arch Neurol 2005;62(5):714–7.
11. Goldstein LB, Simel DL. Is this patient having a stroke? JAMA 2005;293(19):2391–402.
12. Kerber KA, Brown DL, Lisabeth LD, et al. Stroke among patients with dizziness, vertigo, and imbalance in the emergency department: a population-based study. Stroke 2006;37(10):2484–7.
13. Kerber KA. Vertigo and dizziness in the emergency department. Emerg Med Clin North Am 2009;27(1):39–50, viii.

14. Savitz SI, Caplan LR, Edlow JA. Pitfalls in the diagnosis of cerebellar infarction. Acad Emerg Med 2007;14(1):63–8.
15. Idicula TT, Joseph LN. Neurological complications and aspects of basilar artery occlusive disease. Neurologist 2007;13(6):363–8.
16. Chen W, Chern C, Wu Y, et al. Vertebral artery dissection and cerebellar infarction following chiropractic manipulation. Emerg Med J 2006;23(1):e1.
17. Miley ML, Wellik KE, Wingerchuk DM, et al. Does cervical manipulative therapy cause vertebral artery dissection and stroke? Neurologist 2008;14(1):66–73.
18. Shprecher D, Schwalb J, Kurlan R. Normal pressure hydrocephalus: diagnosis and treatment. Curr Neurol Neurosci Rep 2008;8(5):371–6.
19. Factora R. When do common symptoms indicate normal pressure hydrocephalus? Cleve Clin J Med 2006;73(5):447–50, 452, 455–6 passim.
20. Calabresi PA. Diagnosis and management of multiple sclerosis. Am Fam Physician 2004;70(10):1935–44.
21. Fox RJ, Bethoux F, Goldman MD, et al. Multiple sclerosis: advances in understanding, diagnosing, and treating the underlying disease. Cleve Clin J Med 2006;73(1):91–102.
22. Leary SM, Porter B, Thompson AJ. Multiple sclerosis: diagnosis and the management of acute relapses. Postgrad Med J 2005;81(955):302–8.
23. Parrillo J. Approach to the patient with shock. In: Goldman L, Ausiello D, editors. Cecil medicine. 23rd edition. Philadelphia: Saunders Elsevier; 2008. p. 742–50.
24. American College of Chest Physicians/Society of Critical Care Medicine Consensus Conference: definitions for sepsis and organ failure and guidelines for the use of innovative therapies in sepsis. Crit Care Med 1992;20(6):864–74.
25. Levy MM, Fink MP, Marshall JC, et al. 2001 SCCM/ESICM/ACCP/ATS/SIS International Sepsis Definitions Conference. Crit Care Med 2003;31(4):1250–6.
26. Angus DC, Wax RS. Epidemiology of sepsis: an update. Crit Care Med 2001;29(7 Suppl):S109–16.
27. Angus DC, Linde-Zwirble WT, Lidicker J, et al. Epidemiology of severe sepsis in the United States: analysis of incidence, outcome, and associated costs of care. Crit Care Med 2001;29(7):1303–10.
28. Eidelman LA, Putterman D, Putterman C, et al. The spectrum of septic encephalopathy: definitions, etiologies, and mortalities. JAMA 1996;275(6):470–3.
29. Dellinger RP, Levy MM, Carlet JM, et al. Surviving sepsis campaign: international guidelines for management of severe sepsis and septic shock: 2008. Crit Care Med 2008;36(1):296–327.
30. Micek ST, Roubinian N, Heuring T, et al. Before-after study of a standardized hospital order set for the management of septic shock. Crit Care Med 2006; 34(11):2707–13.
31. Rivers E, Nguyen B, Havstad S, et al. Early goal-directed therapy in the treatment of severe sepsis and septic shock. N Engl J Med 2001;345(19):1368–77.
32. Nguyen HB, Corbett SW, Menes K, et al. Early goal-directed therapy, corticosteroid, and recombinant human activated protein C for the treatment of severe sepsis and septic shock in the emergency department. Acad Emerg Med 2006;13(1):109–13.
33. Jones AE, Focht A, Horton JM, et al. Prospective external validation of the clinical effectiveness of an emergency department-based early goal-directed therapy protocol for severe sepsis and septic shock. Chest 2007;132(2):425–32.
34. Witting MD, Magder L, Heins AE, et al. ED predictors of upper gastrointestinal tract bleeding in patients without hematemesis. Am J Emerg Med 2006;24(3): 280–5.

35. Ernst AA, Haynes ML, Nick TG, et al. Usefulness of the blood urea nitrogen/creatinine ratio in gastrointestinal bleeding. Am J Emerg Med 1999;17(1):70–2.
36. Chalasani N, Clark WS, Wilcox CM. Blood urea nitrogen to creatinine concentration in gastrointestinal bleeding: a reappraisal. Am J Gastroenterol 1997;92(10):1796–9.
37. Gralnek IM, Barkun AN, Bardou M. Management of acute bleeding from a peptic ulcer. N Engl J Med 2008;359(9):928–37.
38. González C, Penado S, Llata L, et al. The clinical spectrum of retroperitoneal hematoma in anticoagulated patients. Medicine (Baltimore) 2003;82(4):257–62.
39. Chan YC, Morales JP, Reidy JF, et al. Management of spontaneous and iatrogenic retroperitoneal haemorrhage: conservative management, endovascular intervention or open surgery? Int J Clin Pract 2008;62(10):1604–13.
40. Merrick HW, Zeiss J, Woldenberg LS. Percutaneous decompression for femoral neuropathy secondary to heparin-induced retroperitoneal hematoma: case report and review of the literature. Am Surg 1991;57(11):706–11.
41. Parmer SS, Carpenter JP, Fairman RM, et al. Femoral neuropathy following retroperitoneal hemorrhage: case series and review of the literature. Ann Vasc Surg 2006;20(4):536–40.
42. Menon V, Hochman JS. Management of cardiogenic shock complicating acute myocardial infarction. Heart 2002;88(5):531–7.
43. Rich MW. Epidemiology, clinical features, and prognosis of acute myocardial infarction in the elderly. Am J Geriatr Cardiol 2006;15(1):7–11, [quiz 12].
44. Gregoratos G. Clinical manifestations of acute myocardial infarction in older patients. Am J Geriatr Cardiol 2001;10(6):345–7.
45. Hasdai D, Topol EJ, Califf RM, et al. Cardiogenic shock complicating acute coronary syndromes. Lancet 2000;356(9231):749–56.
46. Williams JF, Storck M. Inhalant abuse. Pediatrics 2007;119(5):1009–17.
47. Brouette T, Anton R. Clinical review of inhalants. Am J Addict 2001;10(1):79–94.
48. Shepherd RT. Mechanism of sudden death associated with volatile substance abuse. Hum Toxicol 1989;8(4):287–91.
49. Adgey AA, Johnston PW, McMechan S. Sudden cardiac death and substance abuse. Resuscitation 1995;29(3):219–21.
50. Wright RO, Lewander WJ, Woolf AD. Methemoglobinemia: etiology, pharmacology, and clinical management. Ann Emerg Med 1999;34(5):646–56.
51. Rehman HU. Methemoglobinemia. West J Med 2001;175(3):193–6.
52. Bradberry SM. Occupational methaemoglobinaemia. Mechanisms of production, features, diagnosis and management including the use of methylene blue. Toxicol Rev 2003;22(1):13–27.
53. Coleman MD, Coleman NA. Drug-induced methaemoglobinaemia. Treatment issues. Drug Saf 1996;14(6):394–405.
54. Seger D. Anticonvulsants. In: Shannon MW, Borron SW, Burns MJ, editors. Haddad and Winchester's clinical management of poisoning and drug overdose. 4th edition. Philadelphia: Saunders; 2007. p. 736–7.
55. Craig S. Phenytoin poisoning. Neurocrit Care 2005;3(2):161–70.
56. von Winckelmann SL, Spriet I, Willems L. Therapeutic drug monitoring of phenytoin in critically ill patients. Pharmacotherapy 2008;28(11):1391–400.
57. Howard CE, Roberts RS, Ely DS, et al. Use of multiple-dose activated charcoal in phenytoin toxicity. Ann Pharmacother 1994;28(2):201–3.
58. Mauro LS, Mauro VF, Brown DL, et al. Enhancement of phenytoin elimination by multiple-dose activated charcoal. Ann Emerg Med 1987;16(10):1132–5.
59. Weichbrodt GD, Elliott DP. Treatment of phenytoin toxicity with repeated doses of activated charcoal. Ann Emerg Med 1987;16(12):1387–9.

60. Position statement and practice guidelines on the use of multi-dose activated charcoal in the treatment of acute poisoning. American Academy of Clinical Toxicology; European Association of Poisons Centres and Clinical Toxicologists. J Toxicol Clin Toxicol 1999;37(6):731–51.
61. Seymour JF. Carbamazepine overdose. Features of 33 cases. Drug Saf 1993; 8(1):81–8.
62. Hojer J, Malmlund HO, Berg A. Clinical features in 28 consecutive cases of laboratory confirmed massive poisoning with carbamazepine alone. J Toxicol Clin Toxicol 1993;31(3):449–58.
63. Spiller HA. Management of carbamazepine overdose. Pediatr Emerg Care 2001; 17(6):452–6.
64. May DC. Acute carbamazepine intoxication: clinical spectrum and management. South Med J 1984;77(1):24–6.
65. Brahmi N, Kouraichi N, Thabet H, et al. Influence of activated charcoal on the pharmacokinetics and the clinical features of carbamazepine poisoning. Am J Emerg Med 2006;24(4):440–3.
66. Cameron RJ, Hungerford P, Dawson AH. Efficacy of charcoal hemoperfusion in massive carbamazepine poisoning. J Toxicol Clin Toxicol 2002;40(4):507–12.

Diagnosis and Evaluation of Syncope in the Emergency Department

Helen Ouyang, MD, MPH[a,b,*], James Quinn, MD, MS[c]

KEYWORDS

• Syncope • Diagnosis • Evaluation • Prognosis

Syncope accounts for approximately 1.3% of all presentations to the emergency department (ED). Determining the exact cause remains a diagnostic challenge, even with an in-patient admission and comprehensive work-up. Studies have shown that the cause of syncope is diagnosed with variable degrees of certainty in only about 50% of patients after an initial ED evaluation,[1,2] and about 30% of patients remain undiagnosed on discharge from a hospital admission.[3–5]

However, with a careful history and physical examination and select diagnostic studies, the differential diagnosis can be narrowed, and physicians can effectively risk stratify patients to determine whether an in-patient admission is necessary. One group of investigators concluded that a reasonable diagnosis can be made in about 80% of ED patients with a more focused history and physical examination and directed investigations.[3] For those without a clear diagnosis, physicians can effectively risk stratify patients to determine whether in-patient admission is necessary. This article reviews the diagnosis and ED work-up of syncope, the different classifications of syncope, and prognosis. The use of specific decision rules in risk stratification and syncope in the pediatric population are discussed in another article.

CLASSIFICATION AND DIFFERENTIAL DIAGNOSIS

Common Classifications

There are 5 major classifications of syncope. Their frequencies from the Framingham Heart Study of nearly 8000 patients are[6]:

- Reflex-mediated (21%)
- Orthostatic (9%)

[a] Department of Emergency Medicine, Brigham and Women's Hospital, 75 Francis Street, Neville House, Boston, MA 02115, USA
[b] Massachusetts General Hospital, Department of Emergency Medicine, 55 Fruit Street, Boston, MA 02114, USA
[c] Division of Emergency Medicine, Stanford University, 701 Welch Road, Suite A1126, Palo Alto, CA 94304, USA
* Corresponding author. Department of Emergency Medicine, Brigham and Women's Hospital, 75 Francis Street, Neville House, Boston, MA 02115.
E-mail address: houyang@partners.org

Emerg Med Clin N Am 28 (2010) 471–485
doi:10.1016/j.emc.2010.03.007 emed.theclinics.com

- Neurologic (4%)
- Unknown (including psychiatric causes) (37%).

While it may not be possible to determine the cause of syncope in the ED, it is useful to divide the differential diagnoses into benign and dangerous to guide diagnostic work-up and disposition, as shown in **Table 1**.

Benign Causes

Reflex-mediated and orthostatic causes are usually benign causes of syncope. After initial evaluation, these patients rarely require admission. The exception is the elderly patient who may require admission to rule out more malignant mechanisms. However, repeat benign episodes that are very similar to past contexts by history usually do not require extensive work-up and admission.

Reflex-mediated syncope

Reflex-mediated syncope is considered the same as the term "neurally mediated syncope." The mechanism is an inappropriate neural control over the circulation resulting in vasodilation, with or without bradycardia. Under the classification of reflex-mediated syncope, there are several types, including vasovagal, situational, and carotid sinus hypersensitivity.

Vasovagal syncope is induced by emotion or pain. It is sometimes termed "neuro-cardiogenic," and it is sometimes used as a synonym for reflex-mediated syncope. Situational syncope is also in this category and is induced by such physiologic mechanisms as cough, micturition, or defecation. Patients diagnosed with vasovagal syncope have excellent prognosis.[3] Patients believed to have vasovagal syncope in the Framingham study had a lower long-term mortality compared with those patients followed who never had syncope. However, it is problematic that vagal symptoms tend to be subjective and vague, and physicians do not always agree on their diagnosis or presence.[7] Nonetheless, those given the diagnosis are clearly at low risk for mortality or significant morbidity.[3]

Carotid sinus hypersensitivity is a reflex-mediated syncope and should be considered in patients who are older and have syncope in the context of stimulation of their carotid arteries. Some examples include wearing a tight necktie, shaving the neck, or a history of neck malignancy. Carotid sinus hypersensitivity is more common in the elderly, men, and those with structural heart disease.[8,9]

Table 1
Benign versus malignant causes of syncope

Benign	Dangerous
Reflex-mediated (neurally mediated)	Cardiac
Vasovagal	Arrhythmias
Situational	Ischemia
Carotid sinus hypersensitivity	Structural cardiopulmonary abnormalities
Orthostatic (autonomic failure)	Neurologic
Medications	TIA
Postprandial hypotension	Subarachnoid hemorrhage
Intravascular volume loss	Subclavian steal
	Migraines

Even though syncope from carotid sinus hypersensitivity is usually benign, cardiac pacing can be useful in at-risk patients.[10,11]

Orthostatic syncope

Orthostatic syncope is the same as autonomic failure. The mechanism in orthostatic syncope is an insufficient autonomic response to counter a drop in cardiac output. The cardinal difference between orthostatic and reflex-mediated syncope is that in orthostatic syncope, the autonomic nervous system attempts to control blood pressure with increased heart rate but fails, whereas in reflex-mediated syncope the autonomic nervous system acts inappropriately resulting in reflex bradycardia and vasodilation.

Most causes of orthostatic syncope are benign. Orthostasis can be caused by medications such as antihypertensives, diuretics, and antidepressants. It can be triggered by postprandial hypotension, which is thought to be secondary to various causes such as impaired baroreflex compensation for splanchnic blood pooling during digestion, inadequate postprandial increases in cardiac output, insulin-induced vasodilation, and release of vasodilatory gastrointestinal peptides.[12]

Orthostatic syncope may also be caused by intravascular volume depletion such as in dehydration or blood loss. This type of syncope is often considered benign, as the treatment may involve simple repletion of intravascular volume. However, orthostatic syncope can also result from life-threatening hemorrhage, such as from trauma, gastrointestinal bleeding, retroperitoneal bleeding, a ruptured spleen, a ruptured aortic aneurysm, a ruptured ectopic pregnancy, or a ruptured ovarian cyst.

Psychiatric causes of syncope

Nearly 40% of patients presenting with syncope may not have a determinable organic cause for their presentation. Psychiatric causes are often by default classified under this category. In one study, the most frequent psychiatric diagnoses were generalized anxiety disorder and major depressive disorder.[13] However, patients with hypoxia and poor cerebral confusion may also appear similarly confused or anxious.

Dangerous Causes

The physician must recognize the potential for cardiac or neurologic syncope, as both are considered dangerous causes and should be reasonably excluded before discharge.

Cardiac syncope

Cardiac syncope is the most dangerous cause of syncope and is the reason for most syncope admissions. Without intervention, the 6-month mortality associated with cardiac causes of syncope is greater than 10%.[3,14] Fortunately, most of these can be identified by risk stratifying patients in the ED with a thorough history, physical examination, and an electrocardiogram (ECG).

The basic mechanism underlying cardiac syncope is the inadequacy of cardiac output to maintain cerebral perfusion. Often, an underlying structural abnormality or preexisting heart condition is the primary cause or contributing cause of cardiac syncope. These abnormalities include dysrhythmias, ischemia, and structural cardiopulmonary lesions. Dysrhythmias are clearly the most common and the most dangerous cause of cardiac syncope, although most lethal arrhythmias such as ventricular tachycardias arise from structural heart lesions. Ischemia is an infrequent cause of syncope (<3% of all presentations)[15] and rarely occurs alone without concomitant chest pain, and ECG findings. Primary structural lesions with reduced cardiac output such as valvular disease and cardiomyopathies are yet another important cause. Pulmonary embolism can be included here as a rare but serious cause of syncope when cardiac output is significantly obstructed.

Neurologic syncope

True syncope is defined as a transient loss of consciousness (LOC) with return to baseline neurologic function. Although older patients are often admitted to rule out cerebrovascular accidents or transient ischemic attacks (TIA) as the cause of their syncope, isolated LOC without accompanying neurologic signs or symptoms is actually a rare cause of syncope, usually reported as 1% to 3%.[16] For syncope to occur, transient interruption of blood flow to the brain stem or cerebral cortex must take place. Subarachnoid hemorrhage is another perilous cause of syncope. These patients almost always complain of headache or have other focal neurologic findings on examination. In addition, because many syncope patients sustain a head injury related to falling, there is a tendency to associate subarachnoid hemorrhage with syncope, when in fact syncope may be posttraumatic and not primary.

Subclavian steal may also cause syncope. In this syndrome, stenosis of the subclavian artery results in the poststenotic portion of the artery receiving additional blood supply through the ipsilateral vertebral artery, causing blood in that artery to flow inferiorly, and drawing blood away from the brainstem. These patients usually present with different blood pressures in each arm. They can also experience a LOC after using their arm on the affected side, usually the left.

Migraine headache is a benign cause of neurologic syncope and often presents with an aura.[17] It is a diagnosis of exclusion in the correct clinical context and requires ruling out other, more malignant causes. Furthermore, there is likely an orthostatic, reflex-mediated, or situational component to the root cause of syncope in patients with migraine.[18]

DIAGNOSIS

Nearly half of syncope patients can be diagnosed on the grounds of history and physical examination alone. Recent studies suggest that yield can be increased with better and more focused and detailed history and physical examination in the ED.[19]

History

The most important first step in evaluating a patient with LOC or near LOC is to establish whether this is true syncope. Syncope is a symptom complex that is composed of a brief LOC associated with an inability to maintain postural tone that spontaneously and completely resolves to baseline neurologic function without resuscitation. It is, by definition, transient. Syncope is distinct from vertigo, seizures, stroke, coma, and other states of altered consciousness.[20] Near syncope has the same implications as syncope and deserves the same work-up.

Syncope can be an extremely broad symptom. When patients present with the chief complaint of passing out or fainting, that might be very different from a physician's idea of syncope. Thus, it is imperative to elicit a comprehensive history. The circumstances surrounding a syncopal event are most important and even minute details may be significant. Any witnesses to the incident should be interviewed. The most important aspects of a patient's history are listed in **Box 1**.

Syncope versus other altered mental states

The first branch point for the physician approaching a patient who presents with LOC is to establish whether this is truly syncope or not. One of the biggest challenges facing clinicians is discerning between syncope and seizure. In several studies, 20% to 30%

Box 1
Detailed history

Age

Position

Prodrome

Triggers

Associated symptoms

Associated injury

Duration of symptoms

Previous episodes

Family history

of patients initially diagnosed with seizures were subsequently diagnosed with syncope.[21,22] These patients can present with sudden cardiac death when cardiac syncope is not initially considered. Furthermore, some seizure conditions are associated with prolonged QT and sudden death.[23,24] In general, cardiac abnormalities should be considered in patients with seizure with the minimum of a history, physical examination, and ECG.[25] **Table 2** lists important clues when trying to differentiate the 2 entities.

Aside from seizures, other neurologic conditions such as strokes, metabolic disorders such as hypoglycemia, and toxic causes such as alcohol can lead to LOC and mimic syncope. Further diagnostic strategies are discussed later in this article and other articles in this issue. However, these conditions are not transient and usually present with persistent altered mental status and should not, by proper definition, be termed syncope.

Age

Younger patients are more likely to have a benign cause of syncope but can still have rare life-threatening causes. One should consider arrhythmias in young patients, such as the athlete who presents after a syncopal event while exercising or the young patient with a question of a first-time seizure. At the opposite end of the age spectrum, elderly patients tend to have more risk factors and comorbidities categorizing them as higher risk, but using a discrete age cut-off for high and low risk is nonspecific and

Table 2
Syncope versus seizure

Syncope	Seizure
No aura	Aura
Post-LOC jerks	Pre-LOC jerks
Asynchronous jerks	Synchronous jerks
Tongue bite at tip	Tongue bite lateral
Flaccid	Stiff
Quick recovery	Postictal
No anion gap acidosis	Transient anion gap acidosis

difficult. Several studies have suggested using 60 or 70 years of age as the upper limit of low risk.[26,27] Another study assessed 1 month outcomes in syncope patients older than 50 years of age, and showed no significant short-term outcomes in patients with unremarkable ED work-ups.[16] Given the variation in studies, it is safe to say that age alone is a marker for increased morbidity and mortality regardless of the patient's presentation, and it may be more helpful to use age as a gradual continuum in risk stratification associated with other factors, rather than choosing a specific cut-off.

Position

The position the patient was in when the event occurred can often provide an important clue to the cause. Syncope while lying supine may be more likely caused by an arrhythmogenic trigger. Positional changes, such as from sitting to standing, may be indicative of orthostasis. The position the patient assumed on recovery that improved the symptoms may also be helpful. In pregnant women, inferior vena cava compression is not an uncommon cause of syncope. However, position is only a small part of the overall history; that is, a patient may still have a malignant cardiogenic cause for the syncope, even if the event occurred while changing positions.

Prodrome

Any prodrome must be elicited from the patient's history. This includes any auras, which may distinguish syncope from seizure. Other clues in the history that may aid in differentiating syncope from seizure are shown in **Table 2**. A sudden LOC without preceding symptoms, is more suggestive of arrhythmia.[28,29] One study evaluating patients with implantable loop recorders found that arrhythmia was the cause in 64% of patients experiencing a sudden LOC without prodrome.[30] In another study, two-thirds of patients with benign vasovagal syncope had prodromal symptoms elicited from their history, most often a feeling of warmth, diaphoresis, or nausea.[31]

Triggers

Asking the patient about circumstances surrounding the syncopal event may be helpful, especially in determining whether it was neurally mediated. Important hints include an emotional stimulus, pain, or fear. Situational triggers such as cough, micturition, or defecation are common in reflex-mediated syncope. Carotid sinus hypersensitivity can often be elicited by asking the patient about neckties, tight collars, or turning their head while driving a vehicle in reverse.

Patients experiencing syncope while exerting themselves are a concern for an arrhythmia or significant outflow tract obstruction from hypertrophic cardiomyopathy.[32,33] This is a consideration in the classic example of the young athlete who has a syncopal event while playing basketball, such as the well-documented cases of Hank Gathers and Reggie Lewis.

Associated symptoms

Often patients are so startled and distressed by the LOC that they may neglect to give a complete history; the physician needs to perform a complete review of systems, with emphasis on palpitations, chest pain, shortness of breath, headache, paresthesias, slurred speech, aphasia, and focal weakness. The review of neurologic symptoms helps separate syncope from other forms of altered consciousness such as stroke. Although TIA that present with isolated LOC are technically considered syncope, as the patient returns to neurologic baseline without resuscitation, it is important to note that TIA presenting without any other neurologic deficits is exceedingly rare (<1%).[34]

In addition, chest pain accompanying syncope may indicate an acute coronary syndrome. Shortness of breath may suggest pulmonary embolus. Headache, in the appropriate context, may prompt one to investigate for subarachnoid hemorrhage. Tongue biting and incontinence may indicate seizure rather than syncope, as shown in **Table 2**. By extracting these details from the history, the physician will be able to narrow the differential diagnosis and pursue a directed diagnostic work-up. The work-up of lone syncope is very different from the work-up of syncope with associated symptoms.

Determining the duration of altered consciousness will again help the physician decide if the event was truly syncope or another altered mental state. True syncope exists only when patients' symptoms are transient and self-limited. Any patient who presents in a postictal state or with persistent neurologic symptoms did not, by definition, have a syncopal event. Patients who present with symptoms of near syncope should be treated as if they had syncope. Near syncope and true syncope are on a spectrum, with similar underlying causes resulting in decreased blood flow to the brain.

Associated injury during a syncopal event

Contrary to common belief, injuries suffered from syncope do not help in determining whether the inciting mechanism is dangerous or benign. It is often thought that those without prodrome are more likely to be cardiac and would therefore be more likely to have associated injuries. However, those with prodrome who ignore their prodrome can also incur significant injury. In one study of patients in whom the diagnosis of vasovagal syncope was established, 10% suffered injury severe enough to require hospitalization and nearly 30% reported at least one traumatic injury.[35] Another study looking at associated injuries among consecutive ED patients found no significant differences between those with serious and benign outcomes.[36]

Although injury may not necessarily signify a malignant cause, patients may still require hospitalization for their specific injury and to prevent further injury from future syncopal events.

Previous episodes

Patients' previous episodes of syncope, and the context in which they occurred, are especially helpful in determining cause and the need for admission. If patients have had complete work-ups in the past demonstrating a benign cause of syncope, they can often be discharged without additional extensive work-ups.

The number of previous episodes and duration between episodes may also help differentiate benign and malignant causes. Several episodes over a short period of time in a patient without a past history may suggest a more significant underlying disorder. In contrast, a single episode or multiple episodes over many years may be more suggestive of a benign cause.

Family history

A family history of sudden cardiac death is an important historical feature to elicit and document. A positive family history, especially in younger patients should lead to further cardiac work-up.[37] Family history can be particularly important in determining inherited cardiac disorders that may often be fatal. Classic examples of this include hypertrophic cardiomyopathy and prolonged or short QT syndromes.[38–40]

Physical Examination

Although the history is of tremendous value, especially because patients are at their neurologic baseline by the time of ED presentation, a thorough physical examination can be useful and sometimes diagnostic. A physical examination, like the history, can help the physician distinguish between true syncope and other altered states of consciousness.

Abnormal vital signs

Transient hypotension and an abnormal heart rate are the most common and immediate causes of many syncopal events. Abnormal vital signs during the event will often normalize on presentation to the ED; however, persistently abnormal vital signs should be of concern. For example, a low oxygen saturation rate or tachypnea may be signs of congestive heart failure (CHF) or pulmonary embolism.

In order for orthostatic vital signs to be helpful, patients who are orthostatic by number ought to have associated symptoms and a supporting history. These signs should be used to supplement and confirm decision making, as opposed to existing as a sole diagnostic tool. Multiples studies have confirmed that orthostatic vital signs are neither sensitive nor specific. Up to 40% of asymptomatic outpatients older than 70 years of age have positive orthostatic vital signs.[41,42] In another study, 16% of 2500 people of all ages in a population-based study had orthostatic changes in vital signs.[43] Thirty-one percent of syncope patients of all ages have orthostatic vital signs, regardless of the cause of the syncope.[41,42] In a recent retrospective review, orthostatic vital signs were found to be cost-effective from an inpatient perspective after other more expensive tests were negative, but again, orthostatic vital signs cannot stand alone to confirm a diagnosis in medium- and high-risk patients to justify discharge without further testing in the ED.[44]

Head-to-toe physical examination

Any bleeding or lacerations in the mouth suggestive of tongue biting should be investigated. Tongue biting on the lateral side may indicate seizure activity rather than a syncopal event. Although tongue biting is neither sensitive nor specific for seizure activity, it rarely occurs in syncope, and if it does, it is most often at the tip.[45]

Carotid artery stenosis can be found with careful auscultation of the neck, although severe stenosis may not produce a bruit. Carotid murmurs radiating from the precordium are usually caused by aortic stenosis. Increased jugular venous pressure may suggest CHF.

In the appropriate context, as suggested by age and history, carotid sinus massage can be attempted in certain patients, as shown in **Fig. 1**. Carotid sinus massage should not be performed in patients with or suspected to have had a myocardial infarction, stroke, or TIA in the past 3 months. Relative contraindications include older age, carotid bruit heard on examination, or history of ventricular tachycardia or

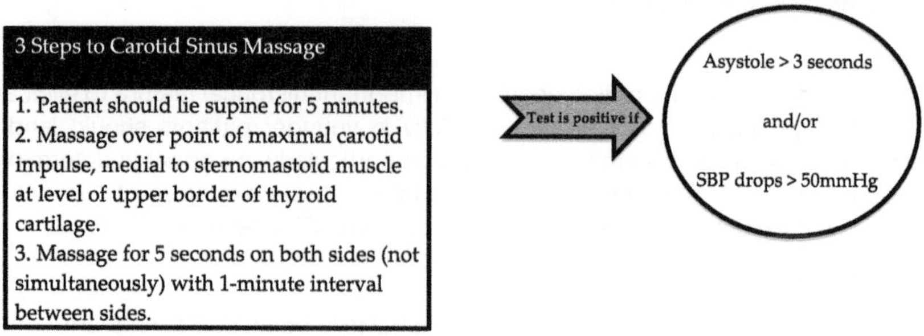

Fig. 1. Carotid sinus massage.

fibrillation.[46] The maneuver should be performed by an experienced physician, with careful cardiac and respiratory monitoring.

Any findings on the cardiac examination suggestive of structural heart disease or CHF deserve special attention. Patients with hypertrophic cardiomyopathy can have a laterally displaced and abnormally forceful, apical precordial impulse. They may also have an S_3 and S_4.

Murmurs are especially important to identify structural or valvular heart disease. About 30% to 40% of patients with hypertrophic cardiomyopathy have midsystolic ejection murmurs, thought to be secondary to the systolic anterior motion of the mitral valve on the thickened interventricular septum, producing high-velocity flow. These murmurs are best appreciated over the left second or third intercostal space along the sternal border.[47] Aortic stenosis is yet another urgent diagnosis that can be easily diagnosed in the ED with a careful cardiac examination. Classically, aortic stenosis produces a harsh crescendo-decrescendo murmur heard loudest at the right upper sternal border, which increases with squatting and radiates to both carotid arteries. In addition, these patients tend to present with narrow pulse pressures.

Patients with CHF can have an S_3 or S_4 that is best heard in the lateral decubitus position. These findings, especially if associated with crackles or increased jugular venous pressure suggest CHF. Although wheezes are not a sign of CHF, new wheezes could be concerning for pulmonary embolism. All findings on cardiac examination suggesting structural heart disease or CHF require further investigation. An echocardiogram is usually the best test to determine the significance of any of these findings.

The abdominal examination can also be useful in diagnosing any orthostatic causes of syncope resulting from hemorrhage. These include ruptured abdominal aortic aneurysm, ruptured spleen, gastrointestinal bleeding, and retroperitoneal bleeding. Any abnormalities in the examination should prompt the physician to do a rectal examination.

Patients with syncope, by definition, return to baseline neurologic function. A thorough neurologic examination should be performed to identify any focal abnormalities that may suggest stroke, TIA, or other neurologic diagnoses.

The physician must screen for any traumatic injury. Although this may not differentiate between benign and more malignant causes of syncope, related traumatic injuries may require admission. Common injuries include facial fractures, hip fractures, wrist fractures, and subdural hematomas from syncope-related falls.[3] Special consideration should be given to even minor head injuries in elderly patients on anticoagulation and antiplatelet agents.

Diagnostic Tests

ECG

Level A recommendations are generally accepted principles for patient management that reflect a high degree of clinical certainty (ie, based on strength of evidence Class I or overwhelming evidence from strength of evidence Class II studies that directly address all of the issues.) The American College of Emergency Physicians recommends obtaining a 12-lead ECG in all patients presenting to the ED with syncope.[48] Although the yield may be low (estimated to be $< 5\%$),[49–51] it is a noninvasive, inexpensive, and quick test that can detect life-threatening conditions. It is also the most consistent test used in risk stratification rules and guidelines.

There are many definitions about what constitutes an abnormal ECG in syncope, and all abnormalities are not of equal risk. For example, up to 45% of bundle branch blocks may be associated with cardiac causes of syncope, whereas nonspecific changes are less likely to be problematic.[7,52] The primary reason why such variability exists in the effectiveness of clinical decision rules is because there is such a wide spectrum of abnormal ECG definitions, resulting in the subjectivity of ECG interpretation.[53–55]

Laboratory data

Laboratory tests should only be ordered based on the history, physical examination, and ECG. Multiple studies have concluded that routine, unguided laboratory tests are not valuable.[31,36,37,56] Measuring serum electrolytes can be useful in the correct clinical context. For example, a serum chemistry panel can help further validate dehydration as a likely cause of syncope. Furthermore, a hematocrit less than 30% has been shown to be a predictor of adverse events.[7]

Qualitative urine human chorionic gonadotropin (HCG) should be performed on all women of childbearing age. This inexpensive and relatively quick test may help detect normal or ectopic pregnancy, either of which can present with true syncope.[57,58] If the urine HCG is positive, the physician should have a low threshold for ruling out an ectopic pregnancy with a pelvic ultrasound.

Although many lone syncope patients are admitted to rule out cardiac ischemia, studies have shown this to be very low yield. Cardiac enzymes are positive in less than 3% of patients with syncope. Moreover, nearly all of these patients with a significant cardiac cause related to their syncope present with chest pain or ECG changes.[15] One study demonstrated that of more than 300 syncope patients (65 years and older), 50% had cardiac enzymes drawn; of those patients, only 3 were positive. Furthermore, of those 3 patients, 2 presented with chest pain and ECG changes, and the third patient had dementia preventing a through history but did have a new left bundle branch block.[59] In another study, ED management was only affected in 1% of 2000 patients admitted with syncope who had their cardiac enzymes cycled.[32] Therefore, cardiac enzymes should be ordered only if deemed necessary after a careful history, physical examination, and an ECG. Thus, it is not recommended to admit lone syncope patients without chest pain to complete two sets of cardiac enzymes when they otherwise would have been discharged.

Further diagnostic studies

Echocardiography can be a useful test in the evaluation of patients with syncope because people with structural heart disease and/or impaired ejection fraction are at serious risk. However it is not recommended as a routine test and is unlikely to identify patients at risk that could not be identified by history examination and ECG.[4,60] If a patient is at risk or needs further investigation for suspected structural or valvular heart disease or CHF, an echo can be a very useful next test.

Any neuroimaging or investigation should not be used routinely in patients with syncope unless indicated and guided after a history and physical examination. Computed tomography and magnetic resonance imaging scans of the head are generally low-yield tests in the context of a normal physical examination.[61] Should the history suggest that head imaging may be necessary secondary to trauma or anticoagulation, the Canadian or the New Orleans head CT rules can provide guidance.[62] Likewise, if a TIA is suspected based on history and physical examination, then neuroimaging may be appropriate.

Similarly, neurovascular ultrasound such as transcranial Doppler and carotid ultrasound have also been found to be nondiagnostic with a normal physical examination. In 1 study of 140 syncope patients in a stroke-age population, 95% of those with positive neurovascular ultrasound results had marked findings on physical examination.

Only 1% of those with findings on imaging had lesions that could have been contributing to syncope, but none of the lesions were concluded to be the primary cause.[63]

As indicated in **Fig. 2**, there are many signs and symptoms that can help the physician differentiate syncope from seizure. However, at times, the two can be challenging

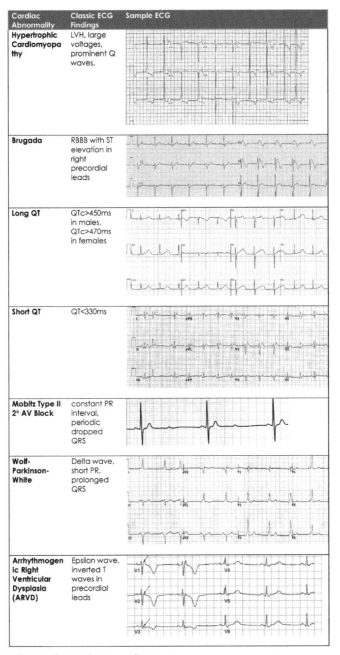

Cardiac Abnormality	Classic ECG Findings	Sample ECG
Hypertrophic Cardiomyopathy	LVH, large voltages, prominent Q waves,	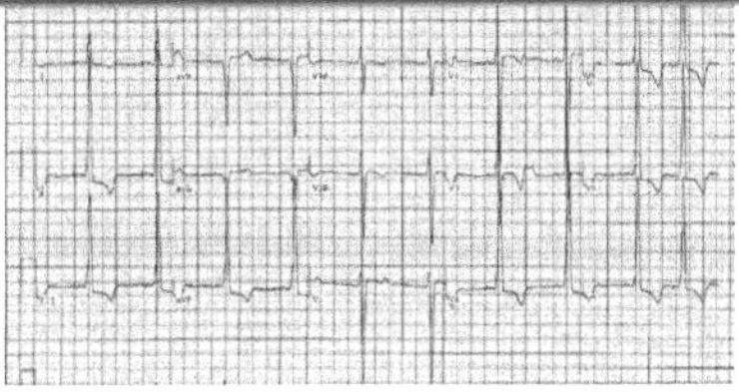
Brugada	RBBB with ST elevation in right precordial leads	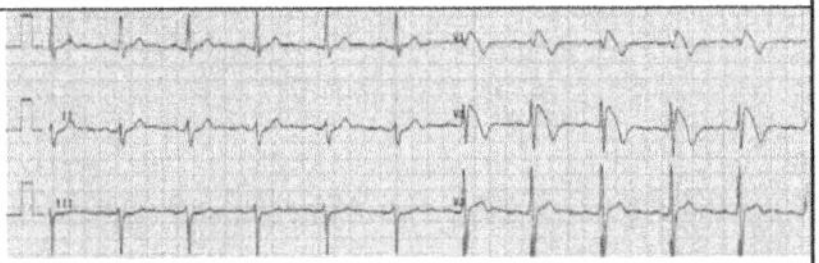
Long QT	QTc>450ms in males, QTc>470ms in females	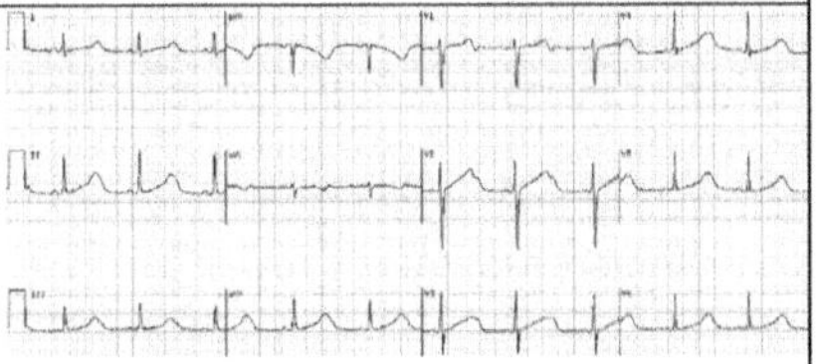
Short QT	QT<330ms	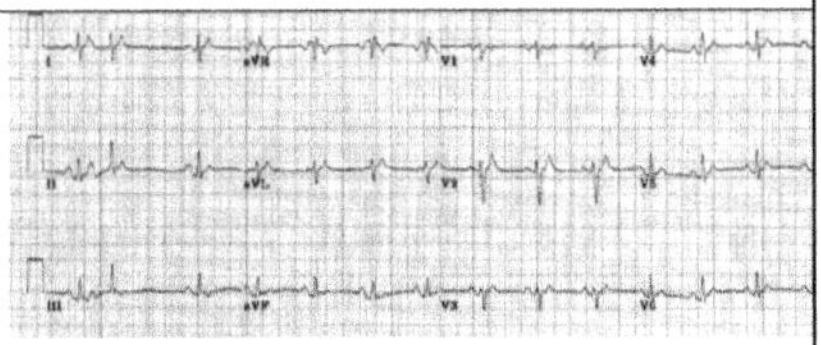
Mobitz Type II 2° AV Block	constant PR interval, periodic dropped QRS	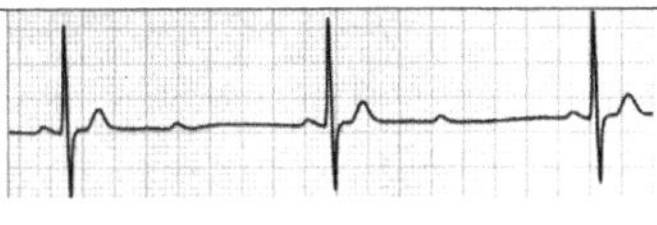
Wolf-Parkinson-White	Delta wave, short PR, prolonged QRS	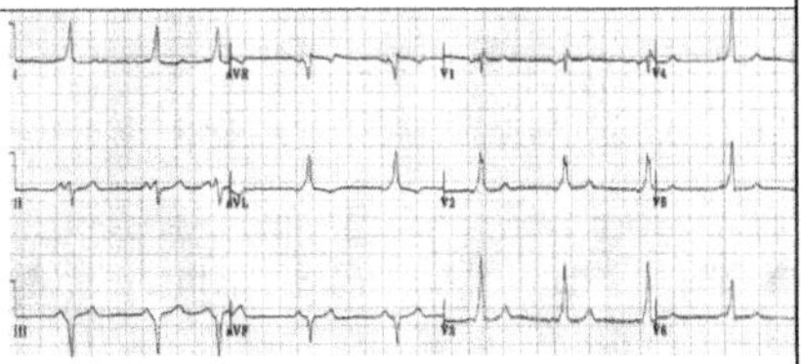
Arrhythmogenic Right Ventricular Dysplasia (ARVD)	Epsilon wave, inverted T waves in precordial leads	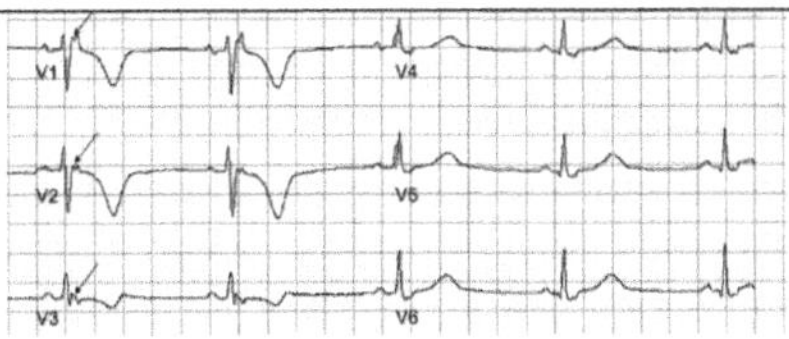

Fig. 2. Clinically significant electrocardiograms.

to distinguish. In these rare cases, an electroencephalogram may be helpful,[64] but in general they are low yield.[44]

Admission for telemetry

While in the ED, all syncope patients should be placed on continuous cardiac monitoring. Patients, especially the elderly, are often admitted for cardiac monitoring, searching for arrhythmias, bradycardia, or pauses on telemetry. Most patients should have some high-risk finding on history, examination, or ECG to warrant admission. For low-risk patients, physicians can arrange outpatient Holter monitoring, when practical.[65] This includes younger patients with normal ECGs and palpitations who are suspected of having nonmalignant rhythms such as supraventricular tachycardia or paroxysmal atrial fibrillation. For those with suspected vagal syncope, telemetry is very low yield (<1%).[66]

MANAGEMENT

Management of syncope patients is guided by diagnosis. Those with malignant rhythms need admission for urgent placement of pacemakers or implantable defibrillators. These patients need to be stabilized in the ED with medications, defibrillation, and temporary pacemaking, as indicated. Similarly those with pulmonary embolism or strokes need anticoagulation and thrombolysis as indicated. In general, those with a clear diagnosis have clear management pathways. Those without a clear diagnosis have less defined management pathways. Risk stratification of these patients into high and low risk to guide further investigation and admission seems to be the best way to manage these patients efficiently.

SUMMARY

With a careful history, physical examination, and directed investigation, physicians can determine the likely cause of syncope in more than 50% and perhaps up to 80% of patients. Understanding the cause of syncope allows clinicians to determine the disposition of high- and low-risk patients. Patients with a potential malignant cause, such as a cardiac or neurologic condition, should be treated and admitted. Those with benign causes can be safely discharged. Those remaining patients with an unclear cause should be accurately risk stratified, and their disposition determined by their risk factors as discussed in the next article.

REFERENCES

1. Blanc JJ, L'Her C, Touiza A, et al. Prospective evaluation and outcome of patients admitted for syncope over a 1 year period. Eur Heart J 2002;23(10):815–20.
2. Crane SD. Risk stratification of patients with syncope in an accident and emergency department. Emerg Med J 2002;19(1):23–7.
3. Alboni P, Brignole M, Menozzi C, et al. Diagnostic value of history in patients with syncope with or without heart disease. J Am Coll Cardiol 2001;37(7):1921–8.
4. Sarasin FP, Luis-Simonet M, Carball D, et al. Prospective evaluation of patients with syncope: a population-based study. Am J Med 2001;111(3):177–84.
5. Ammirati F, Colivicchi F, Santini M. Diagnosing syncope in clinical practice. Implementation of a simplified diagnostic algorithm in a multicentre prospective trial—the OESIL 2 study (Osservatorio Epidemiologico della Sincope nel Lazio). Eur Heart J 2000;21(11):935–40.

6. Soteriades ES, Evans JC, Larson MG, et al. Incidence and prognosis of syncope. N Engl J Med 2002;347(12):878–85.
7. Quinn JV, Stiell IG, McDermott DA, et al. Derivation of the San Francisco Syncope Rule to predict patients with short-term serious outcomes. Ann Emerg Med 2004; 43(2):224–32.
8. Tan MP, Newton JL, Reeve P, et al. Results of carotid sinus massage in a tertiary referral unit–is carotid sinus syndrome still relevant? Age Ageing 2009;38(6):680–6.
9. Tan MP, Newton JL, Chadwick TJ, et al. The relationship between carotid sinus hypersensitivity, orthostatic hypotension, and vasovagal syncope: a case-control study. Europace 2008;10(12):1400–5.
10. Kenny RA, Richardson DA, Steen N, et al. Carotid sinus syndrome: a modifiable risk factor for nonaccidental falls in older adults (SAFE PACE). J Am Coll Cardiol 2001;38:1491–6.
11. Brignole M, Menozzi C, Lolli G, et al. Long-term outcome of paced and non paced patients with severe carotid sinus syndrome. Am J Cardiol 1992;69:1039–43.
12. Jansen RW, Lipsitz LA. Postprandial hypotension: epidemiology, pathophysiology, and clinical management. Ann Intern Med 1995;122(4):286–95.
13. Kapoor WN, Fortunato M, Hanusa BH, et al. Psychiatric illnesses in patients with syncope. Am J Med 1995;99(5):505–12.
14. Maisel WH, Stevenson WG. Syncope—getting to the heart of the matter. N Engl J Med 2002;347(12):931–3.
15. McDermott D, Quinn JV, Murphy CE. Acute myocardial infarction in patients with syncope. CJEM 2009;11(2):156–60.
16. Morag RM, Murdock LF, Khan ZA, et al. Do patients with a negative Emergency Department evaluation for syncope require hospital admission? J Emerg Med 2004;27(4):339–43.
17. Vuković V, Plavec D, Galinović I, et al. Prevalence of vertigo, dizziness, and migrainous vertigo in patients with migraine. Headache 2007;47(10):1427–35.
18. Thijs RD, Kruit MC, van Buchem MA, et al. Syncope in migraine: the population-based CAMERA study. Neurology 2006;66(7):1034–7.
19. Oh JH, Hanusa BH, Kapoor WN. Do symptoms predict cardiac arrhythmias and mortality in patients with syncope? Arch Intern Med 1999;159(4):375–80.
20. Quinn JV, McDermott D. Syncope. Tintinalli Chapter. 7th edition. 2010, in press.
21. Smith D, Defalla BA, Chadwick DW. The misdiagnosis of epilepsy and the management of refractory epilepsy in a specialist clinic. QJM 1999;92(1):15–23.
22. Scheepers B, Clough P, Pickles C. The misdiagnosis of epilepsy: findings of a population study. Seizure 1998;7(5):403–6.
23. Johnson JN, Hofman N, Haglund CM, et al. Identification of a possible pathogenic link between congenital long QT syndrome and epilepsy. Neurology 2009;72(3):224–31.
24. Carinci V, Barbato G, Baldrati A. Asystole induced by partial seizures: a rare cause of syncope. Pacing Clin Electrophysiol 2007;30(11):1416–9.
25. McKeon A, Vaughan C, Delanty N. Seizure versus syncope. Lancet Neurol 2006; 5(2):171–80.
26. Linzer M, Yang EH, Estes NA 3rd, et al. Diagnosing syncope. Part 1: value of history, physical examination, and electrocardiography. Clinical Efficacy Assessment Project of the American College of Physicians. Ann Intern Med 1997; 126(12):989–96.
27. Huff JS, Decker WW, Quinn JV, et al. Clinical policy: critical issues in the evaluation and management of patients presenting with syncope. Ann Emerg Med 2001;37(6):771–6.

28. Calkins H, Shyr Y, Frumin H, et al. The value of the clinical history in the differentiation of syncope due to ventricular tachycardia, atrioventricular block, and neurocardiogenic syncope. Am J Med 1995;98(4):365–73.
29. Sud S, Klein GJ, Skanes AC, et al. Predicting the cause of syncope from clinical history in patients undergoing prolonged monitoring. Heart Rhythm 2009;6(2): 238–43.
30. Krahn AD, Klein GJ, Yee R, et al. Predictive value of presyncope in patients monitored for assessment of syncope. Am Heart J 2001;141(5):817–21.
31. Graham LA, Kenny RA. Clinical characteristics of patients with vasovagal reactions presenting as unexplained syncope. Europace 2001;3(2):141–6.
32. McKenna WJ, Franklin RC, Nihoyannopoulos P, et al. Arrhythmia and prognosis I infants, children and adolescents with hypertrophic cardiomyopathy. J Am Coll Cardiol 1988;11:147–53.
33. Sadoul N, Prasad K, Elliott PM, et al. Prospective prognostic assessment of blood pressure response during exercise in patients with hypertrophic cardiomyopathy. Circulation 1997;96(9):2987–91.
34. Savitz SI, Caplan LR. Vertebrobasilar disease. N Engl J Med 2005;352(25): 2618–26.
35. Ammirati F, Colivicchi F, Velardi A, et al. Prevalence and correlates of syncope-related traumatic injuries in tilt-induced vasovagal syncope. Ital Heart J 2001; 2(1):38–41.
36. Bartoletti A, Fabiani P, Bagnoli L, et al. Physical injuries caused by a transient loss of consciousness: main clinical characteristics of patients and diagnostic contribution of carotid sinus massage. Eur Heart J 2008;29(5):618–24.
37. Grossman SA, Fischer C, Lipsitz LA, et al. Predicting adverse outcomes in syncope. J Emerg Med 2007;33(3):233–9.
38. Autore C, Quarta G, Spirito P. Risk stratification and prevention of sudden death in hypertrophic cardiomyopathy. Curr Treat Options Cardiovasc Med 2007;9(6):431–5.
39. Zareba W, Cygankiewicz I. Long QT syndrome and short QT syndrome. Prog Cardiovasc Dis 2008;51(3):264–78.
40. McKenna WJ, Thiene G, Nava A, et al. Diagnosis of arrhythmogenic right ventricular dysplasia/cardiomyopathy. Task Force of the Working Group Myocardial and Pericardial Disease of the European Society of Cardiology and of the Scientific Council on Cardiomyopathies of the International Society and Federation of Cardiology. Br Heart J 1994;71:215–8.
41. Lipsitz LA, Storch HA, Minaker KL, et al. Intra-individual variability in postural blood pressure in the elderly. Clin Sci (Lond) 1985;69(3):337–41.
42. Atkins D, Hanusa B, Sefcik T, et al. Syncope and orthostatic hypotension. Am J Med 1991;91(2):179–85.
43. Wu JS, Yang YC, Lu FH, et al. Population-based study on the prevalence and correlates of orthostatic hypotension/hypertension and orthostatic dizziness. Hypertens Res 2008;31(5):897–904.
44. Mendu ML, McAvay G, Lampert R, et al. Yield of diagnostic tests in evaluating syncopal episodes in older patients. Arch Intern Med 2009;169(14):1299–305.
45. Benbadis SR, Wolgamuth BR, Goren H, et al. Value of tongue biting in the diagnosis of seizures. Arch Intern Med 1995;155(21):2346–9.
46. Wijetunga MN, Schatz IJ. Carotid sinus hypersensitivity: differential diagnoses & workup. eMedicine 2009. Available at: http://emedicine.medscape.com/article/153312-diagnosis. Accessed December 15, 2009.
47. Chatterjee K. Physical examination. In: Topol EJ, editor. Textbook of cardiovascular medicine. 3rd edition. Philadelphia: Lippincott; 2007. p. 193–226.

48. Huff JS, Decker WW, Quinn JV, et al. Clinical policy: critical issues in the evaluation and management of adult patients presenting to the ED with syncope. Ann Emerg Med 2007;49(4):431–44.
49. Eagle KA, Black HR. The impact of diagnostic tests in evaluating patients with syncope. Yale J Biol Med 1983;56:1–8.
50. Martin GJ, Adams SL, Martin HG, et al. Prospective evaluation of syncope. Ann Emerg Med 1984;13:499–504.
51. Kapoor WN, Karpf M, Wieand S, et al. A prospective evaluation and follow-up of patients with syncope. N Engl J Med 1983;309(4):197–204.
52. Donateo P, Brignole M, Alboni P, et al. A standardized conventional evaluation of the mechanism of syncope in patients with bundle branch block. Europace 2002; 4(4):357–60.
53. Sun BC, Mangione CM, Merchant G, et al. External validation of the San Francisco Syncope Rule. Ann Emerg Med 2007;49(4):420–7.
54. Birnbaum A, Esses D, Bijur P, et al. Failure to validate the San Francisco Syncope Rule in an independent emergency department population. Ann Emerg Med 2008;52(2):151–9.
55. McDermott D, Quinn J. Response to "failure to validate the San Francisco Syncope Rule in an independent emergency department population". Ann Emerg Med 2009;53(5):693 [author reply: 693–4].
56. European Society of Cardiology. Guidelines for the diagnosis and management of syncope (version 2009): the Task Force for the Diagnosis and Management of Syncope of the European Society of Cardiology (ESC). Eur Heart J 2009; 30(21):2631–71.
57. Dussoix P, Hagelberg T, Vermeulen B. An unusual case of syncope. Eur J Emerg Med 2004;11(1):59.
58. Wong E, Suat SO. Ectopic pregnancy—a diagnostic challenge in the emergency department. Eur J Emerg Med 2000;7(3):189–94.
59. Grossman SA, Van Epp S, Arnold R, et al. The value of cardiac enzymes in elderly patients presenting to the emergency department with syncope. J Gerontol A Biol Sci Med Sci 2003;58(11):1055–8.
60. Sarasin FP, Junod AF, Carballo D, et al. Role of echocardiography in the evaluation of syncope: a prospective study. Heart 2002;88(4):363–7.
61. Goyal N, Donnino MW, Vachhani R, et al. The utility of head computed tomography in the emergency department evaluation of syncope. Intern Emerg Med 2006;1(2):148–50.
62. Stiell IG, Clement CM, Rowe BH, et al. Comparison of the Canadian CT Head Rule and the New Orleans Criteria in patients with minor head injury. JAMA 2005;294(12):1511–8.
63. Schnipper JL, Ackerman RH, Krier JB, et al. Diagnostic yield and utility of neurovascular ultrasonography in the evaluation of patients with syncope. Mayo Clin Proc 2005;80(4):480–8.
64. Britton JW, Benarroch E. Seizures and syncope: anatomic basis and diagnostic considerations. Clin Auton Res 2006;16(1):18–28.
65. Sarasin FP, Carballo D, Slama S, et al. Usefulness of 24-h Holter monitoring in patients with unexplained syncope and a high likelihood of arrhythmias. Int J Cardiol 2005;101(2):203–7.
66. Suzuki T, Matsunaga N, Kohsaka S. Diagnostic patterns in the evaluation of patients hospitalized with syncope. Pacing Clin Electrophysiol 2006;29(11): 1240–4.

The Emergency Department Approach to Syncope: Evidence-based Guidelines and Prediction Rules

Chad Kessler, MD[a,b,c,d,*], Jenny M. Tristano, MD[e], Robert De Lorenzo, MD, MSM[f,g]

KEYWORDS

- Syncope • Emergency department • Guidelines
- San Francisco Syncope Rule

There are many admissions for syncope because of concern that this generally benign condition can occasionally be an ominous sign of a life-threatening disease process. Although the need for admission is obvious when a cardiac cause of syncope is diagnosed in an emergency department (ED), a large percentage of patients have undiagnosed causes of syncope after the standard evaluation. Admissions for syncope are costly[1] and often return an unrevealing work-up.

[a] Department of Emergency Medicine, Jesse Brown VA Hospital, 820 South Damen Avenue, MC 111, Chicago, IL 60612, USA
[b] Department of Internal Medicine, The University of Illinois School of Medicine at Chicago, 840 South Wood Street (M/C 718), Chicago, IL 60612-7315, USA
[c] Department of Emergency Medicine, The University of Illinois School of Medicine at Chicago, 808 South Wood Street, M/C 724, Chicago, IL 60612, USA
[d] Combined Internal Medicine/Emergency Medicine Residency, The University of Illinois School of Medicine at Chicago, 808 South Wood Street, M/C 724, Chicago, IL 60612, USA
[e] Departments of Internal Medicine and Emergency Medicine Residency Program, University of Illinois-Chicago, 808 South Wood Street, M/C 724, Chicago, IL 60612, USA
[f] Uniformed Services University of the Health Sciences, 4301 Jones Bridge Road, Bethesda, MD 20814-4799, USA
[g] Department of Clinical Investigation, MCHE-CI, Brooke Army Medical Center, 3851 Roger Brooke Drive, Fort Sam Houston, TX 78234-6200, USA
* Corresponding author. Emergency Medicine, Jesse Brown VA Hospital, 820 South Damen Avenue, MC 111, Chicago, IL 60612.
E-mail address: Chad.Kessler@va.gov

Emerg Med Clin N Am 28 (2010) 487–500
doi:10.1016/j.emc.2010.03.014
0733-8627/10/$ – see front matter. Published by Elsevier Inc.
emed.theclinics.com

In the past two decades, many researchers have attempted to develop clinical decision criteria that emergency physicians (EPs) may use to categorize patients into high versus low risk for serious outcomes. Because syncope is a presentation with a broad differential diagnosis, these risk stratification guidelines have historically been problematic in 2 ways:

- They ensure identification of all patients who might benefit from acute intervention but increase the number of unnecessary and costly admissions.
- They decrease the number of unwarranted admissions but miss identification of at least a few patients who are predicted to have serious outcomes soon after ED presentation.

This clinical review focuses on current studies and recommendations that outline risk stratification and treatment guidelines for patients who present with syncope. It also briefly discusses the management of syncope, patient outcomes in various syncope causes, and the survival benefit accrued from acute hospitalization.

METHODS

Every attempt was made to include the most recent and relevant articles. To conduct a current and thorough review of the literature, OvidMEDLINE and PubMedMEDLINE searches were performed, including but not limited to the following queries: "Syncope," "Syncope AND emergency," "Syncope AND risk," "Syncope AND outcomes," "Syncope and Prognosis," and "Syncope AND presyncope." Articles were limited to those written in English and published after 1980. Articles were reviewed for relevance to the topic of risk stratification in the ED as well as patient disposition and outcomes. PubMed-suggested related articles and bibliographies of chosen articles were also reviewed for additional sources.

WHAT IS SYNCOPE?

Syncope is characterized by a sudden, transient loss of consciousness associated with an inability to maintain postural tone.[2–7] The presentation is sometimes confused with other conditions that lead to loss of consciousness, such as seizure, vertigo, dizziness, drop attacks, coma, or shock and cannot be the result of trauma, ethanol, or other toxic substances. By definition, patients with syncope have regained consciousness and baseline neurologic status spontaneously, promptly, and independently, in other words, without the aid of electrical or chemical cardioversion.[8] Syncope is most accurately categorized as a syndrome rather than a discrete medical entity.[9] Symptom combinations vary significantly and have a broad differential diagnosis. There is variability between investigators as to whether or not "presyncope" is considered a variation of the syncope syndrome as it does not include a loss of consciousness.

WHAT IS THE PREVALENCE OF SYNCOPE IN THE ED AND IN HOSPITAL ADMISSIONS?

Syncope is responsible for 1.2% to 1.5% of ED visits and up to 6% of hospital admissions.[3,10–12] In 2000, an estimated 460,000 patients were hospitalized with discharge diagnoses that included syncope, 230,000 of whom had primary diagnoses of syncope.[1] The incidence of syncope increases with advancing age.[13,14] With the United States population growing older, the number of syncope admissions will increase and contribute to the growth of health care expenditures.

Of patients who present to the ED with syncope, from 39% to 50% of patients do not have the cause of syncope established after the initial ED evaluation.[13,15–17]

This leads to syncope admission rates upwards of 60%,[11] with most undergoing a hospital admission that is nondiagnostic.[3,8]

WHAT IS THE COST OF SYNCOPE ADMISSIONS?

In 2005, Sun and colleagues[1] estimated the total annual cost for syncope-related hospitalizations was $2.4 billion (95% CI, 2.2 to 2.6 billion) with a mean cost of $5,400 (95% CI, 5100 to 5600) per hospitalization. A more recent study by Alshekhlee and colleagues[18] estimates a more modest but still significant $1.7 billion annually. These costs were similar to that of asthma, HIV, and chronic obstructive pulmonary disease–related diagnoses. It is this high cost coupled with low diagnostic yield of inpatient syncope work-ups that has largely driven the development of ED-focused clinical guidelines.

WHAT IS THE STANDARD SYNCOPE WORK-UP IN THE ED?

The standard syncope work-up for a patient presenting to the ED includes a detailed history, physical examination, and 12-lead ECG. These are the only level A recommendations put forth by the American College of Emergency Physicians (ACEP) updated 2007 guidelines.[19,20] The history and physical examination reveals the cause of syncope in 32% to 74% of patients with an additional 1% to 11% of patients diagnosed by ECG.[17,21,22] The most common diagnoses established by this evaluation include vasovagal syncope, orthostatic hypotension, arrhythmia, and acute coronary syndrome.[17] The history should be detailed and include preceding events, a description of and the duration of any prodrome, events after regaining consciousness, and current medications. Past medical history should focus on the cardiac history and any family history of sudden cardiac death.[15,23,24] Witnesses to the event should be questioned. The physical examination should include detailed vital signs, orthostatic blood pressures, abdominal and rectal examinations, and detailed neurologic and cardiac examinations.[25] Although history and physical are helpful during syncope evaluation, a commonly encountered difficulty is patients who are often unable to provide accurate historical information.[20]

Compared with the history and physical examination, the yield of the ECG is low. The test, however, is low risk and inexpensive and continues to be recommended in almost all patients as it contributes to decisions regarding immediate therapy and future testing.[5,10,21,22] There is limited evidence to guide the use of other tests, and a complete blood cell count, blood chemistries, urine pregnancy, and other laboratory tests are ordered only if indicated by a history and physical examination. Specific tests, such as urine toxicology screens and cardiac enzymes, should be performed as directed by pertinent history and physical examination findings. Other potentially diagnostic studies include CT, MRI, stress testing, and electrophysiologic studies. These are not part of the routine initial ED syncope evaluation and should only be performed when indicated by the individual patient presentation.[4,5,21,26–28]

WHAT IS THE PROGNOSIS AFTER A SYNCOPAL EPISODE?

Most syncopal episodes have less ominous origins, but syncope can reflect serious conditions. Serious morbidity or mortality occurs in 4% to 6% in the period after presentation to the ED. For unknown causes of syncope, this rate approaches 30% for patients diagnosed with high-risk causes of syncope.[6,10,11]

It has long been known that patients with cardiac syncope have lower survival rates than those without syncope.[13,16,26,29] It has been less clear, however, whether or not the syncopal episode or the cardiac history was related to the decreased survival. In 1996, Kapoor and Hanusa[16] compared all-cause mortality, cardiac mortality, and other cardiovascular outcomes in patients with syncope to a matched group of patients without syncope. There were no significant differences in mortality attributed to cardiac and noncardiac comorbidities when syncope patients were compared with their nonsyncope counterparts. After successfully matching 470 pairs of patients with and without syncope, they found that the overall 1-year mortality in patients with cardiac syncope was 22% (cardiac mortality 12%) compared with 20% in the matched nonsyncope group (cardiac mortality 11%). They found no significant difference in survival rates when patients with syncope were compared with matched patients without syncope. Age, congestive heart failure, and coronary artery disease were all predictors of cardiac and overall mortality in both groups of patients, but syncope alone was not a risk factor. In the end, they concluded prognosis was primarily determined by patients' underlying cardiac conditions. Currently, the guidelines from ACEP and the European Society of Cardiology strongly recommend admission for any potential cardiac or neurologic etiology of syncope.[4,19,20,30–32]

WHAT ARE THE GUIDELINES TO RISK STRATIFY PATIENTS WITH SYNCOPE?

Before the San Francisco Syncope Rule

The first modern syncope risk stratification rule was developed in an original article by Martin and colleagues.[2] These researchers performed a prospective cohort study that identified 4 predictors of arrhythmia and mortality within the first year for patients presenting to the ED with syncope. A second prospective cohort evaluated the validity of those predictors as a clinical prediction rule that could stratify ED patients into low- and high-risk groups (**Table 1**). Findings in the validation study were consistent with the derivation cohort, and it was shown that an increasing number of risk factors corresponded to increasing mortality rates at 1 year.

In 2003, Italy produced the Osservatorio Epidemiologico della Sincope nel Lazio (OESIL) study, a prospective cohort study that included patients as young as 12 years, did not include presyncopal patients, and defined the primary endpoint as death from any cause within 12 months of the initial ED.[33] Significant multivariate predictors were identified and a score was calculated by assigning each risk factor a value of 1. The mortality rate at 12 months increased with increasing OESIL score (see **Table 1**). This article was the first to make recommendations for management based on the results of risk stratification. The investigators suggested discharging patients with 0 to 1 risk factors and admitting patients with 2 to 4 risk factors. A follow-up study showed that measuring the serum troponin added little to the score's usability and was not recommended for risk stratification.[34]

Also in 2003, Sarasin and colleagues[35] developed a risk score that looked at an even more specific outcome, the risk of significant arrhythmia. Again, derivation and validation cohorts were used to develop a risk score predicting arrhythmias in patients with syncope still unexplained after performing clinical history, physical examination, and 12-lead ECG. Consistent with previous studies looking at all potential for all serious outcomes, significant predictors of arrhythmia were an abnormal ECG, age greater than 65, a history of congestive heart failure, a history of myocardial infarction, and history of any type of cardiac disease. An increasing number of risk factors corresponded with an increasing risk for arrhythmia. The study focusrf on only those patients in whom the cause of syncope after traditional evaluation was still unknown. It answered only one question, however: whether or not the cause of syncope was likely or unlikely due to an arrhythmia.

Table 1
Commonalities of Syncope Risk Stratification Rules[a]

Risk Stratification of Patients with Syncope (Martin et al[2])[a]	OESIL Risk Score (Colivicchi et al[33])[a]	Derivation of the SFSR (Quinn et al[36])[b]	Boston Syncope Criteria (Grossman et al[44])[c]	EGSYS scoring system (Del Rosso et al[45])[d]	
				Risk Factor	**Points**
Abnormal ECG	Abnormal ECG	Congestive heart failure history	Signs and Symptoms of Acute Coronary Syndrome	Palpitations preceding syncope	+ 4
Age >45years	Age >65years	Hematocrit < 30%	Signs of Conduction Disease	Heart Disease and/or abnormal ECG	+ 3
History of Ventricular Arrhythmia	Cardiovascular disease in clinical history	Abnormal ECG	Worrisome Cardiac History	Syncope during effort	+ 3
History of CHF	Syncope without prodrome	Shortness of Breath	Valvular heart disease by history or by physical exam	Syncope while supine	+ 2
		Systolic Blood Pressure <90 mmHg at triage	Family history of sudden death	Presence of Precipitating and/or predisposing factors	-1
			Persistent abnormal vital signs in the ED	Presence of Autonomic Prodromes	-1
			Volume depletion such as persistent dehydration, GI bleeding, or hematocrit<30		
			Primary CNS event		

Key:
- ECG
- Age
- Past Med Hx
- Phys Exam findings
- Labs
- HPI/symptoms

[a] Increasing number of risk factors indicates increased risk of mortality.
[b] The presence of any one of these risk factors signifies patient is high risk.
[c] Patients considered at risk for serious outcomes if they fall into one of the 8 symptom categories.
[d] A total point score greater than or equal to 3 is considered an indicator that admission is required.

Derivation of the San Francisco Syncope Rule

In a prospective cohort study by Quinn and colleagues,[36] the goal was to derive a clinical decision rule that could be used to risk stratify patients based on potential short-term (7-day) serious outcomes and determine admission necessity. Syncopal and presyncopal events were included. Unlike previous studies that focused on death and arrhythmias as serious outcomes, the San Francisco Syncope Rule (SFSR) had several serious outcomes that were used as endpoints:

1. Death
2. Myocardial infarction
3. Arrhythmia
4. Pulmonary embolism
5. Stroke

6. Subarachnoid hemorrhage
7. Significant hemorrhage (tied to syncope and requiring transfusion)
8. Any condition causing return to ED and hospitalization for related event, including being readmitted for the same or similar symptoms related to the initial syncopal event
9. Patients admitted who required an acute intervention during their stay that would have caused them to return if they were discharged. Acute intervention was defined as any procedure required to treat a condition related to a patient's symptom of syncope, including pacemaker, use of vasopressors, surgery for abdominal aortic aneurysm, ruptured spleen, ectopic pregnancy, and endoscopic treatment of esophageal varices.

Through multivariate analysis, 5 predictive variables were elicited to make the San Francisco Syncope Rule (**Table 2**).

When applied to the derivation cohort in this study, the CHESS factors (history of *C*ongestive heart failure, *H*ematocrit <30%, *E*CG abnormality, *S*hortness of breath, and *S*ystolic blood pressure <90) were found to have a sensitivity and specificity of 96.2% (95% CI, 92% to 100%) and 61.9% (95% CI, 58% to 66%), respectively. The rule categorized 45% of cohort patients as high risk, yielding a potential 10% absolute reduction from the actual study admission rate of 55%. Including "age older than 75" as another risk factor would have achieved 100% sensitivity, identifying the 3 patients not predicted by the rule but decreasing specificity to 44%. This would have caused an additional 108 patients without serious outcomes to be classified as high risk and admitted.[36]

The SFSR made several contributions to syncope risk evaluation. It was the first study that derived a major clinical prediction rule based on short-term serious outcomes, with previous studies evaluating outcomes 1 year. It is currently unclear how long after ED presentation serious outcomes can be considered temporally related to the initial syncopal episode. It was also the first study to include multiple serious outcomes, recognizing that syncope may be a sentinel of other types of preventable morbidity.

The study also garnered several criticisms. First, the rule was intended to be applied to all ED patients with syncope, not just those with unexplained syncope after work-up. Theoretically, when the cause of syncope is identified, the diagnosis provides sufficient information to determine admission necessity. Age, historically considered an important factor in admission decisions, was not included as risk criterion. The investigators believed that although age could have been part of the rule, it would have been difficult to determine an appropriate cutoff, and other risk factors were found better discriminators. Lastly, because the rule did not have 100% sensitivity, it could only be used as a guideline and not as a definitive tool in directing admission decisions. The SFSR is

Table 2
San Francisco Syncope Rule[a]

C	Congestive heart failure history
H	Hematocrit <30%
E	ECG abnormal (nonsinus rhythm or new changes compared with old ECG)
S	Shortness of breath
S	Systolic blood pressure <90 mm Hg at triage

[a] The presence of any one of these risk factors signifies patient is high risk.
Data from Quinn JV, et al. Derivation of the San Francisco Syncope Rule to predict patients with short term serious outcomes. Ann Emerg Med 2004;43(2):224–32.

a collection of risk factors that help to determine high- and low-risk presentations, thereby augmenting physician judgment and guiding decision making.

Of the syncope risk stratification systems currently published, the SFSR has undergone the most rigorous evaluation. In the first of a series of follow-up studies by Quinn and colleagues,[37] the SFSR was compared with the ability of physician judgment to identify patients at greater than 2% risk for a serious outcome (**Table 3**).

The investigators found that there was no significant difference in the sensitivities of the SFSR and physician judgment. The specificity of the SFSR at 61.9% was significantly higher compared with the specificity of physician judgment at 52%. It was predicted that the SFSR could potentially lower the study's admission rate from 55% to 45%. Quinn and colleagues[38] then attempted to prospectively validate the SFSR. In this study, patient follow-up continued until 30 days after the ED visit although in the original study follow-up was limited to 7 days. Validation sensitivity and specificity for predicting serious outcomes were consistent with those of the original derivation study. Application of the rule would have decreased this study's admission rate by 7%, but the rule still did not meet 100% sensitivity. Quinn and colleagues[39] then examined the incidence of death in consecutive ED patients presenting with syncope to determine whether or not the risk factors from SFSR could predict death up to 1 year after the initial ED visit. At 6 months, the SFSR had a sensitivity of 100% for predicting deaths possibly related to syncope and 89% sensitivity for predicting all-cause mortality. At 1 year, the rule's sensitivity and specificity decreased for both categories.[39]

Independent Evaluation of SFSR

In an external validation study of the San Francisco Syncope Rule performed by Sun and colleagues,[40] the SFSR was shown less sensitive than in previous study populations. The primary outcome was all 7-day serious events, and the secondary outcome was 7-day events diagnosed only after the ED visit (see **Table 3**). The decision by the managing physicians to admit was 100% sensitive and 30% specific for all 7-day outcomes, but the SFSR demonstrated poor sensitivity for identifying patients with a serious event first diagnosed after the initial ED visit. It would have decreased admissions by 12% but missed 10% of patients with a 7-day serious outcome. Age greater than 60 accounted for a majority of the serious outcomes missed by the SFSR,[40] indicating a need to re-evaluate the importance of age as a risk factor. They also made an distinction by specifically evaluating the rule's ability to identify serious events that would be found only after the ED visit, suggesting a need to focus on predicting the risk of those short-term events. The investigators concluded that the SFSR required further validation before safe application in all patient populations.

Recently, Birnbaum and colleagues[41] attempted to validate the ability of SFSR to identify serious outcomes within 7 days of an ED visit in another independent patient population. Again, the SFSR had decreased sensitivity compared with previously published studies and failed to identify 26% of patients with serious outcomes.The study, however, used different ECG criteria than the SFSR study and admitted more patients. A different, retrospective study of the SFSR in patients older than 65 also found similarly low sensitivity and specificity in this more at risk patient population.[42]

As promising as the SFSR was as a clinical prediction system, it has never been shown 100% sensitive by those who developed it or by those who have attempted external validations. It appears sensitive if applied appropriately but can only be used as a risk stratification tool and not something to replace physician judgment. Several independent researchers have been unable to validate the rule in an external independent study population.

Table 3
Sensitivities and specificities of various risk stratification systems for syncope

Study	System	Derivation Sensitivity	Derivation Specificity	Validation Sensitivity	Validation Specificity
Quinn et al 2004	Derivation SFSR	96.2% (95% CI, 92%–100%)	61.9% (95% CI, 58%–66%)	—	—
Quinn et al 2005	Physician judgment	94% (95% CI, 86%–94%)	52% (95% CI, 51%–53%)	—	—
Quinn et al 2006	Validation SFSR	—	—	98% (95% CI, 89%–100%)	56% (95% CI, 52%–60%)
Sun et al	External validation SFSR All 7-day outcomes	—	—	89% (95% CI, 81%–97%)	42% (95% CI, 37%–48%)
	External validation SFSR Delayed 7-day outcomes	—	—	69% (95% CI, 46%–92%)	42% (95% CI, 37%–48%)
Birnbaum et al	Failure to validate SFSR	—	—	74% (95% CI, 61%–84%)	57% (95% CI, 53%–61%)
Schladenhaufen et al	Application SFSR in Elderly ED patients	—	—	76.5% (95% CI, 66.7%–84.3%)	36.8% (95% CI, 32.2%–41.6%)
Reed et al	ROSE pilot high risk only	0.636 (*P* value .035)	0.716 (*P* value .035)	—	—
Reed et al	ROSE pilot high/medium risk	1.000 (*P* value .203)	0.182 (*P* value .203)	—	—
Grossman et al	Boston Syncope criteria	—	—	97% (95% CI, 93%–100%)	62% (95% CI, 56%–69%)
Del Rosso et al	EGSYS	95% (CI, 84.4–99.4)	61% (CI, 54.3–76.6%)	92% (CI, 76.9–98.2)	69% (CI, 62.7–75.2)

Since the SFSR

In the United Kingdom, a pilot study evaluated a particular hospital's current departmental syncope guidelines to predict serious outcomes of syncope at various time points.[43] The hospital's guidelines were derived from those published by the European Society of Cardiology, the American College of Physicians, and the ACEP and were, therefore, extremely detailed, complex, and not meant for easy memorization and use. Risk stratification was performed to compare 3 scoring systems: the SFSR, the OESIL scoring system, and the hospital's ED guidelines. The most interesting finding was that the OESIL risk factor, "age > 65," alone performed better than the SFSR and the ED guidelines, with a sensitivity and specificity of 1.000 and 0.466, respectively (*P* value .002, significant).[43]

In Boston, a prospective observational cohort study was performed to validate a decision rule created from existing published recommendations and evidence.[44] Presyncopal events were excluded and patients were considered at risk for adverse outcomes or clinical intervention if they had any of 8 symptom categories (see **Table 1**) The primary outcome was any critical intervention or adverse outcome noted during the ED stay, hospitalization, or 30-day follow-up period (see **Table 3**). Admitting those identified by the Boston Syncope Criteria would have reduced admissions by 48% but with a sensitivity of 97%, 2 adverse outcomes would not have been identified.

Again from Italy, the Evaluation of Guidelines in Syncope Study (EGSYS) study by Del Rosso and colleagues[45] developed a diagnostic score to identify those patients presenting to the ED with syncope of a cardiac cause. A derivation cohort was used identify independent predictors of cardiac syncope and assign point scores based on regression coefficients. The system was then validated by a separate cohort (see **Table 1**). A point score greater than or equal to 3 was considered the best discriminator for a diagnosis of cardiac syncope and no patients in the study with an EGSYS score less than 3 died within the first month of follow-up. The investigators concluded a score greater than or equal to 3 indicated high risk for cardiac syncope/mortality and necessitated admission. The EGSYS rule was the first to account for different aspects of the syncope presentation increasing or decreasing the likelihood of cardiac etiology. The rule could not meet 100% sensitivity, however, for discerning cardiac syncope without having a specificity that was worse than previously published physician judgment specificities.

WHAT ROLE DOES AGE FULFILL AS A RISK FACTOR FOR SYNCOPE?

In 2007, Sun and colleagues[46] specifically looked at age as a risk factor for short-term, serious events after a syncopal episode. The study included patients with syncopal or presyncopal events. The primary outcome was any serious clinical event that occurred during the 14 days after presentation to the ED. The secondary outcome was any 14-day serious clinical event that was not identified until after the initial ED evaluation. The majority of patients who experienced a primary (76%) or secondary (83%) outcome were greater than or equal to 60 years of age. They found that serious 14-day events increase with advancing age and that a majority of events happen in patients 60 and older. Sun and colleagues[47] then described the diagnostic yield and predictive accuracy of ECG testing as a function of age. Specifically, they explored the frequency at which the initial ED ECG identified a cardiac cause of syncope and how often abnormalities correlated with patients' risks of a 14-day cardiac event. They found ECG testing was diagnostic for a cardiac cause of syncope in 4% of all patients in the study.The ECG, however, did not identify any cardiac causes of syncope in patients younger than 40 years of age. Moreover, in patients under 40,

ECG testing was associated with a 10% frequency of incidental findings leading to additional unnecessary cardiac evaluations and hospitalizations. The investigators concluded it may be reasonable to defer ECG testing in young patients whose presentation, medical history, and physical examination are consistent with a benign cause of syncope. The ECG, however, is relatively easy to perform, inexpensive, and many to most practitioners still perform ECG on young patients.

WHAT ARE THE EFFECTS OF ADMISSION ON PATIENT OUTCOMES IN UNDIAGNOSED SYNCOPE?

Morag and colleagues[48] sought to determine whether or not immediate hospitalization is beneficial to syncope patients who have a nondiagnostic ED evaluation. A nondiagnostic ED evaluation was defined as

1. History of present illness devoid of cardiopulmonary, abdominal, or focal neurologic symptoms
2. Physical examination with vital signs within a predetermined acceptable range
3. No clinical evidence of congestive heart failure
4. No new neurologic deficits
5. Normal blood glucose
6. Benign 12-lead ECG.

From a group of 45 patients greater than or equal to 50 years of age who presented to the ED with syncope and had a nondiagnostic ED evaluation, 76% (34/45) were admitted to the hospital. None of the hospitalizations established a diagnosis that was missed in the ED. Furthermore, complete follow-up at 1 month showed that 1 patient had an adverse event—a repeat syncopal episode. This yielded an overall morbidity rate of 2.2%, with no deaths occurring in this nondiagnostic group at 1 month.[48] Although this study was limited by a small number of patients with a small number of adverse outcomes, it acknowledged that hospitalizing patients who undergo a negative ED evaluation may have no actual affect on short-term morbidity and mortality.

Recently, Constantino and colleagues[49] assessed the short-term and long-term prognosis of patients who presented with syncope and the predictors of adverse advents at 10 days and 1 year from the visit to the ED. They also compared the rate of severe outcomes in admitted and discharged patients. They did not include in their evaluation anyone who had a clinical condition primarily confirmed in the ED that would have required hospitalization independent of the syncope. Multivariate analysis showed abnormal ECG at presentation, a concomitant trauma, absence of previous symptoms preceding the syncope, and male gender were all independent risk factors for the development of severe adverse outcomes in the short term, and the rate of severe outcomes was significantly greater in admitted (14.7%) than in discharged (2.0%) patients. One-year mortality was also greater in those admitted compared with those discharged. Risk factors affecting long-term prognosis included age greater than 65, coexistence of neoplasms at presentation, cerebrovascular disease, structural heart disease, and ventricular arrhythmias.

The study was helpful in that it showed risk factors affecting short-term prognosis were significantly different than risk factors affecting long-term prognosis. It also illustrated that there was a significant difference in short-term outcomes between admitted and discharged patients, with admitted patients having a worse short-term prognosis. In other words, hospital admission after syncope did not significantly improve long-term prognosis.

SUMMARY

The evaluation and disposition of syncope presenting to the ED is a complex and costly problem. As the size and average age of the population increases, its share of resources will parallel in growth. Currently at minimum, every patient with syncope receives a thorough interview, physical examination, and ECG. It has been demonstrated, however, that it is not the isolated syncopal episode but the underlying cause that has the impact on future prognosis. With the number of possible serious and elusive causes, the additional work-up continues to be variable but significant in time and monetary expense.

As yet, there is still no single set of rules or guidelines that the EP can completely rely on. All current prediction rules (1) sacrifice risk stratification of a few patients to decrease overall admission rates, thereby missing patients with potentially serious outcomes, or (2) recognize all patients with potential for serious outcomes but require a large number of unnecessary admissions as a result of the decreased specificity (see **Table 3**). The relatively high sensitivity and simplicity of the SFSR has made it one of the most referenced clinical prediction rules. Lack of sufficient sensitivity, however, and an inability to validate the rule in an independent patient population continues to limit its clinical usefulness. There have been attempts to derive other clinical prediction rules. These recent studies continue to have problems creating a set of guidelines that sufficiently balance the concern for patient safety with cost reduction. The most interesting conclusion derived from the many studies is that physicians were highly sensitive and tended to admit patients that eventually developed a serious outcome, including those missed by the risk stratification systems. This increased sensitivity, however, came at the price of many excessive admissions (low specificity).

There are many studies about syncope, most of which focus on sorting patients into categories of high versus low risk for serious outcomes. There are certain criteria that are consistently present in every stratification system derived:

- Abnormal ECG, whatever the definition may be
- History of structural or arrhythmic heart disease, often clinically represented by shortness of breath or other symptoms of heart failure
- Persistently abnormal vital signs in the ED
- Older age, especially in combination with any of the other criteria.

Those with high risk should be admitted and undergo further immediate work-up. Those who look well and do not have any of the complaints are usually low risk and can likely be safely discharged with appropriate follow-up. Even low risk does not signify no risk. To that effect, these studies have not really developed rules but have ascertained specific factors that can guide decision making. An absolute clinical decision rule to direct syncope admissions is not currently feasible, and no rule should ever override physician judgment.

There are many questions that still need to be answered. The optimal follow-up interval must be determined. It is still unclear for how long an episode of syncope can truly be considered an indicator of future morbidity and mortality. After a certain length of time, other aspects of patients' interval health status likely develop a stronger predictive relationship than a previous syncopal episode. It is not ever certain what constitutes appropriate follow-up. Is a primary care physician check for symptom resolution and routine cardiac risk stratification sufficient or should follow-up patients undergo more in-depth evaluation? It should also be clarified as to whether or not "presyncope" should be included or studied as its own unique presentation. Future studies might try to determine if presyncope and syncope convey the same concern for prognosis.

A question for EPs is what disposition is appropriate to patients without a specified cause of syncope after ED evaluation. It is these patients that provide the most difficulty during clinical decision making. Future research should attempt to address the following questions. For those patients with no definite syncopal cause after ED work-up, does hospitalization affect short- or long-term outcomes? Does hospitalization affect outcomes in those with a specific syncope diagnosis? Is there a way to stratify risk for patients with an undiagnosed cause? Addressing these questions may help determine what a clinical decision rule must accomplish to achieve maximal sensitivity and specificity. Moreover, the answer to these questions may lie outside of a clinical prediction rule.

ACKNOWLEDGMENTS

The authors would very much like to thank Dr James Quinn for taking the time to review and critique this article.

REFERENCES

1. Sun BC, Emond JA, Camargo CA Jr. Direct medical costs of syncope-related hospitalizations in the United States. Am J Cardiol 2005;95(5):668–71.
2. Martin TP, Hanusa BH, Kapoor WN. Risk stratification of patients with syncope. Ann Emerg Med 1997;29(4):459–66.
3. Kapoor WN. Evaluation and management of the patient with syncope. JAMA 1992;268(18):2553–60.
4. Brignole M, Alboni P, Benditt DG, et al. Guidelines on management (diagnosis and treatment) of syncope–update 2004. Europace 2004;6(6):467–537.
5. Kapoor WN. Syncope. N Engl J Med 2000;343(25):1856–62.
6. Kapoor WN, Karpf M, Wieand S, et al. A prospective evaluation and follow-up of patients with syncope. N Engl J Med 1983;309(4):197–204.
7. Thijs RD, Wieling W, Kaufmann H, et al. Defining and classifying syncope. Clin Auton Res 2004;14(Suppl 1):4–8.
8. Kapoor WN. Current evaluation and management of syncope. Circulation 2002; 106(13):1606–9.
9. Harrigan RA. Syncope: emergency department evaluation and disposition. AAEM; 2007. Available at: http://www.medscape.com/viewarticle/557901. Accessed March 30, 2010.
10. Day SC, Cook EF, Funkenstein H, et al. Evaluation and outcome of emergency room patients with transient loss of consciousness. Am J Med 1982;73(1):15–23.
11. Blanc JJ, L'Her C, Touiza A, et al. Prospective evaluation and outcome of patients admitted for syncope over a 1 year period. Eur Heart J 2002;23(10):815–20.
12. Olde Nordkamp LR, van Dijk N, Ganzeboom KS, et al. Syncope prevalence in the ED compared to general practice and population: a strong selection process. Am J Emerg Med 2009;27(3):271–9.
13. Soteriades ES, Evans JC, Larson MG, et al. Incidence and prognosis of syncope. N Engl J Med 2002;347(12):878–85.
14. Grossman SA, Shapiro NI, Van Epp S, et al. Sex differences in the emergency department evaluation of elderly patients with syncope. J Gerontol A Biol Sci Med Sci 2005;60(9):1202–5.
15. Martin GJ, Adams SL, Martin HG, et al. Prospective evaluation of syncope. Ann Emerg Med 1984;13(7):499–504.
16. Kapoor WN, Hanusa BH. Is syncope a risk factor for poor outcomes? Comparison of patients with and without syncope. Am J Med 1996;100(6):646–55.

17. Sarasin FP, Pruvot E, Louis-Simonet M, et al. Stepwise evaluation of syncope: a prospective population-based controlled study. Int J Cardiol 2008;127(1): 103–11.
18. Alshekhlee A, Shen WK, Mackall J, et al. Incidence and mortality rates of syncope in the United States. Am J Med 2009;122(2):181–8.
19. American College of Emergency Physicians. Clinical policy: critical issues in the evaluation and management of patients presenting with syncope. Ann Emerg Med 2001;37(6):771–6.
20. Huff JS, Decker WW, Quinn JV, et al. Clinical policy: critical issues in the evaluation and management of adult patients presenting to the emergency department with syncope. Ann Emerg Med 2007;49(4):431–44.
21. Linzer M, Yang EH, Estes NA 3rd, et al. Diagnosing syncope. Part 1: value of history, physical examination, and electrocardiography. Clinical Efficacy Assessment Project of the American College of Physicians. Ann Intern Med 1997; 126(12):989–96.
22. Sarasin FP, Louis-Simonet M, Carballo D, et al. Prospective evaluation of patients with syncope: a population-based study. Am J Med 2001;111(3):177–84.
23. Martin GJ. Syncope: evaluation and general considerations. In: Schwartz GR, Hanke BK, Mayer TA, et al. Principles and practice of emergency medicine, section part V: evaluation and management of selected common presentations. 4th edition. Lippincott Williams & Wilkins; 1999. ISBN-13:9780683076462. p. 331–6.
24. Alboni P, Brignole M, Menozzi C, et al. Diagnostic value of history in patients with syncope with or without heart disease. J Am Coll Cardiol 2001;37(7): 1921–8.
25. Sarasin FP, Louis-Simonet M, Carballo D, et al. Prevalence of orthostatic hypotension among patients presenting with syncope in the ED. Am J Emerg Med 2002; 20(6):497–501.
26. Kapoor WN. Evaluation and outcome of patients with syncope. Medicine (Baltimore) 1990;69(3):160–75.
27. Strickberger SA, Benson DW, Biaggioni I, et al. AHA/ACCF Scientific Statement on the evaluation of syncope: from the American Heart Association Councils on Clinical Cardiology, Cardiovascular Nursing, Cardiovascular Disease in the Young, and Stroke, and the Quality of Care and Outcomes Research Interdisciplinary Working Group; and the American College of Cardiology Foundation: in collaboration with the Heart Rhythm Society: endorsed by the American Autonomic Society. Circulation 2006;113(2):316–27.
28. Reed MJ, Newby DE, Coull AJ, et al. Role of brain natriuretic peptide (BNP) in risk stratification of adult syncope. Emerg Med J 2007;24(11):769–73.
29. Linzer M, Newby DE, Coull AJ, et al. Diagnosing syncope. Part 2: unexplained syncope. Clinical Efficacy Assessment Project of the American College of Physicians. Ann Intern Med 1997;127(1):76–86.
30. Elesber AA, Decker WW, Smars PA, et al. Impact of the application of the American College of Emergency Physicians recommendations for the admission of patients with syncope on a retrospectively studied population presenting to the emergency department. Am Heart J 2005;149(5):826–31.
31. Brignole M, Alboni P, Benditt D, et al. Guidelines on management (diagnosis and treatment) of syncope. Eur Heart J 2001;22(15):1256–306.
32. Brignole M, Alboni P, Benditt DG, et al. Guidelines on management (diagnosis and treatment) of syncope-update 2004. Executive summary. Eur Heart J 2004; 25(22):2054–72.

33. Colivicchi F, Ammirati F, Melina D, et al. Development and prospective validation of a risk stratification system for patients with syncope in the emergency department: the OESIL risk score. Eur Heart J 2003;24(9):811–9.
34. Hing R, Harris R. Relative utility of serum troponin and the OESIL score in syncope. Emerg Med Australas 2005;17(1):31–8.
35. Sarasin FP, Hanusa BH, Perneger T, et al. A risk score to predict arrhythmias in patients with unexplained syncope. Acad Emerg Med 2003;10(12):1312–7.
36. Quinn JV, Stiell IG, McDermott DA, et al. Derivation of the San Francisco Syncope Rule to predict patients with short-term serious outcomes. Ann Emerg Med 2004; 43(2):224–32.
37. Quinn JV, Stiell IG, McDermott DA, et al. The San Francisco Syncope Rule vs physician judgment and decision making. Am J Emerg Med 2005;23(6):782–6.
38. Quinn J, McDermott D, Stiell I, et al. Prospective validation of the San Francisco Syncope Rule to predict patients with serious outcomes. Ann Emerg Med 2006; 47(5):448–54.
39. Quinn J, McDermott D, Kramer N, et al. Death after emergency department visits for syncope: how common and can it be predicted? Ann Emerg Med 2008;51(5): 585–90.
40. Sun BC, Mangione CM, Merchant G, et al. External validation of the San Francisco Syncope Rule. Ann Emerg Med 2007;49(4):420–7 [427 e1–4].
41. Birnbaum A, Esses D, Bijur P, et al. Failure to validate the San Francisco Syncope Rule in an independent emergency department population. Ann Emerg Med 2008;52(2):151–9.
42. Schladenhaufen R, et al. Application of San Francisco Syncope Rule in elderly ED patients. Am J Emerg Med 2008;26(7):773–8.
43. Reed MJ, Newby DE, Coull AJ, et al. The Risk stratification Of Syncope in the Emergency department (ROSE) pilot study: a comparison of existing syncope guidelines. Emerg Med J 2007;24(4):270–5.
44. Grossman SA, Fischer C, Lipsitz LA, et al. Predicting adverse outcomes in syncope. J Emerg Med 2007;33(3):233–9.
45. Del Rosso A, Ungar A, Maggi R, et al. Clinical predictors of cardiac syncope at initial evaluation in patients referred urgently to general hospital: the EGSYS score. Heart 2008;94(12):1620–6.
46. Sun BC, Hoffman JR, Mangione CM, et al. Older age predicts short-term, serious events after syncope. J Am Geriatr Soc 2007;55(6):907–12.
47. Sun BC, Hoffman JR, Mower WR, et al. Low diagnostic yield of electrocardiogram testing in younger patients with syncope. Ann Emerg Med 2008;51(3): 240–6 [246 e1].
48. Morag RM, Murdock LF, Khan ZA, et al. Do patients with a negative Emergency Department evaluation for syncope require hospital admission? J Emerg Med 2004;27(4):339–43.
49. Costantino G, Perego F, Dipaola F, et al. Short- and long-term prognosis of syncope, risk factors, and role of hospital admission: results from the STePS (Short-Term Prognosis of Syncope) study. J Am Coll Cardiol 2008;51(3):276–83.

Pediatric Syncope: Cases from the Emergency Department

Jason W.J. Fischer, MD, MSc[a,b,*], Christine S. Cho, MD, MPH[b,c]

KEYWORDS

• Syncope • Pediatric • Emergency • Cardiac
• Vasodepressor • Dysrhythmia

Pediatric syncope is a common presentation in the emergency department (ED).[1] The emergency physician (EP) must handle the complaint with finesse, as an abrupt loss of consciousness can be dramatic and alarming to patients, family, friends, and caregivers. The EP should perform a thorough evaluation of cause, care for any resulting injury and emotional reassurance in a focused and resource-effective manner.

Syncope is defined as the sudden loss of consciousness and postural tone with spontaneous and complete recovery after a brief duration. *Pre-syncope* is the feeling that one is about to pass out but remains conscious with a transient loss of postural tone. Pre-syncope may or may not reflect the same pathology as syncope but the approach should be the same.[1]

Syncope follows a common pathophysiologic pathway with many potential inciting stimuli. Cerebral perfusion is compromised by a transient decrease in cardiac output caused by vasomotor changes decreasing venous return, a primary dysrhythmia, or impairment of vascular tone.[1,2] Frank syncope occurs when cerebral blood flow decreases to less than 30% to 50% of baseline.[3]

The incidence of pediatric syncope is common with 15% to 25% of children and adolescents experiencing at least one episode of syncope before adulthood.[4–6] Incidence peaks between the ages of 15 and 19 years for both sexes. There appears to be a female predominance.[7] Before age 6, syncope is unusual except in the setting of

[a] Department of Emergency Medicine, Alameda County Medical Center, 1411 East 31st Street, Oakland, CA 94602, USA
[b] Division of Emergency Medicine, Children's Hospital and Research Center Oakland, 747 52nd Street, Oakland, CA 94609, USA
[c] Department of Pediatrics, University of California, 505 Parnassus Avenue, San Francisco, CA 94143, USA
* Corresponding author. Department of Emergency Medicine, Alameda County Medical Center, 1411 East 31st Street, Oakland, CA 94602.
E-mail address: fischerjwj@mac.com

Emerg Med Clin N Am 28 (2010) 501–516
doi:10.1016/j.emc.2010.03.009
emed.theclinics.com

seizure disorders, breath holding, and cardiac arrhythmias. Pediatric syncope may account for as high as 3% of ED visits.[8]

Most causes of pediatric syncope are benign, but an evaluation must exclude rare life-threatening disorders. In contrast to adults, vasodepressor syncope is the most frequent cause of pediatric syncope (61%–80%).[9] Other causes include neuropsychiatric, cardiac, pregnancy, and metabolic disorders (**Table 1**).[9–11] Cardiac disorders represent 2% to 6% of pediatric cases.[7] Although the annual incidence of nontraumatic sudden death in the pediatric population is very low (less than 4/100,000), underlying cardiac disease is very common among these cases.[12]

WHY IS THE HISTORY SO IMPORTANT IN PEDIATRIC SYNCOPE?

The lack of objective findings in pediatric syncope can pose a challenge for the EP. An accurate and detailed history becomes essential for clinical decision making (**Fig. 1**). However, pediatric patients may not be able to provide a complete or specific history.

Table 1
Causes of pediatric syncope

Noncardiac	Cardiac
Vasodepressor syncope	Arrhythmias
Orthostatic hypotension	Ventricular tachycardia
Postural orthostatic tachycardia syndrome	No congenital heart disease
Exercise-related syncope	Postoperative congenital heart disease
Breath-holding syncope	Supraventricular tachycardia (ie, Wolff-Parkinson-White syndrome)
Tussive syncope	Ion channel abnormalities
Situational syncope	Long-QT syndrome
Dysautonomia	Congenital
Carotid sinus hypersensitivity	Drug induced
Neuropsychiatric	Brugada syndrome
Seizure	Atrioventricular block
Migraine	Congenital
Hyperventilation	Acquired (ie, Lyme disease)
Conversion syncope	Arrhythmogenic right ventricular disease
Intracranial tumors	Pacemaker malfunction
Metabolic	Sick sinus syndrome
Hypoglycemia	Commotio cordis
Electrolyte disorder	Obstructive Lesions
Malnutrition	Hypertrophic cardiomyopathy
Endocrine disease	Valvular aortic stenosis
Drugs and toxins	Primary pulmonary hypertension
Carbon monoxide poisoning	Eisenmenger syndrome
Pregnancy	Myocardial dysfunction
Normal pregnancy	Primary ventricular dysfunction
Ectopic pregnancy	Dilated cardiomyopathy
Pulmonary embolism	Neuromuscular disorders
Pregnancy-related cardiac disease	Secondary ventricular dysfunction
	Inflammatory disease
	Acute myocarditis
	Kawasaki disease
	Ischemia
	Anomalous coronary artery
	Kawasaki disease
	Cardiac tumors

Data from Refs.[8–11]

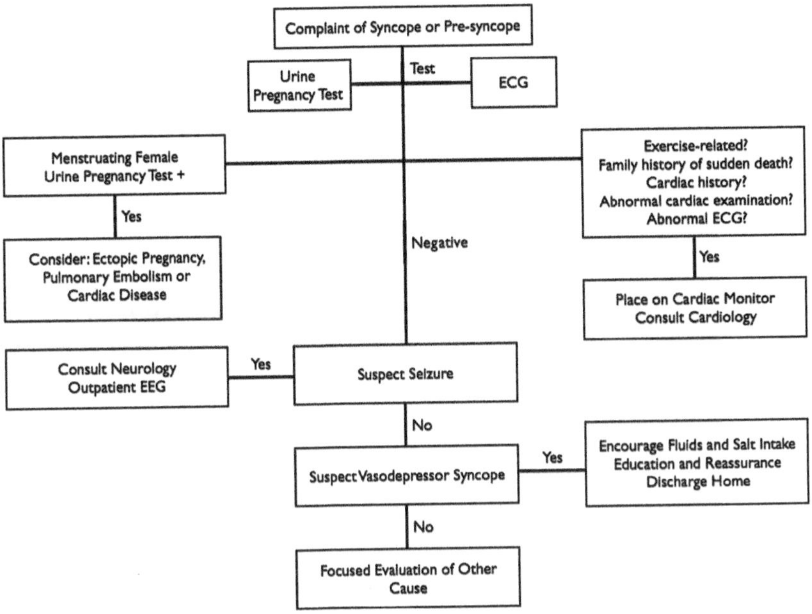

Fig. 1. Emergency department approach to pediatric syncope.

Witnesses, parents, relatives, friends, teachers, and coaches are often needed but may not always be present in the ED. Moreover, the nuances of the history (eg, did the tonic-clonic movement begin before or after loss of consciousness) may not be apparent to the lay-person and further confound the presentation. Despite these obstacles, the history and physical examination prove sufficient to define the cause of syncope in up to 77% of pediatric cases.[13,14]

WHAT ARE THE CRITICAL ELEMENTS OF THE PEDIATRIC SYNCOPE HISTORY?

The key elements or "red flags" the EP must elicit are a history of exercise-induced syncope, pre-syncope or chest pain, and/or a family history of sudden death, including dysrhythmia, drowning, sudden infant death syndrome (SIDS), or pacemaker placement. These historical elements and/or a history of congenital heart disease should prompt immediate cardiovascular monitoring, a cardiology consultation, and further testing.[15,16]

Healthy patients may experience vasodepressor syncope after vigorous exertion due to venous pooling, high ambient temperature, dehydration, and hyperventilation.[8] This condition must be differentiated from "mid-stride" syncope, which may indicate cardiac pathology.[17]

Patients with known cardiac pathology should be evaluated for interval change.[17] Patients who have previously undergone surgical repair or palliation of congenital heart disease may have acquired or residual structural lesions, myocardial dysfunction, and supraventricular or ventricular dysrhythmias.[16]

A detailed history should include the time of day, time of last meal, activities leading up to the event, and associated symptoms such as palpitations or racing heart beat, chest pain, headache, shortness of breath, nausea, diaphoresis, amnesia, visual changes, and auditory changes. The duration of symptoms, the patient's position when symptoms began, and the patient's appearance during and immediately following the episode are also important.[1]

In addition to the pertinent medical history, a family history should expose familial syncope, congenital heart disease, seizures, metabolic disease, and deafness.[1,16] A medication history including herbal, over-the-counter or illicit drug use, and access to other medications or toxins should be gathered.[1] Risk of pregnancy should be assessed by gathering a menstrual history.[13] Practitioners should also note the patient's syncope burden and the timing and frequency of episodes in patients with repeat syncope.[17]

WHAT ARE THE CRITICAL ELEMENTS OF THE PHYSICAL EXAMINATION?

Each patient should undergo a complete physical examination in the ED. Most examinations are normal, but physical findings can help identify cardiac and neurologic causes of syncope.[8,18]

Prehospital, triage, and orthostatic vital signs should be reviewed.

Cardiac auscultation should be performed in the supine and standing position to determine the presence of dynamic obstruction. Abnormalities of cardiac rhythm should also be sought.[17] The neurologic examination should focus on fundoscopy, cranial nerves, Romberg sign, gait, deep tendon reflexes, and cerebellar function.[8]

Physical features associated with cardiac disease (eg, abnormal facies, Marfan habitus, deafness, ataxia) or neurologic disease (eg, ash-leaf spots, cafe-au-lait spots, cleft palate) should be sought.[13]

WHAT DIAGNOSTIC STUDIES ARE NEEDED?

An electrocardiogram (ECG) should be obtained for *all* pediatric syncope patients. The ECG is low yield but is inexpensive, noninvasive, and highly sensitive. In combination with a detailed history and physical examination, the ECG has demonstrated a sensitivity of 96% for cardiac syncope.[19] Some forms of structural heart disease and primary electrical disorders may not otherwise be apparent.[17] Attention should be paid to the rhythm and the potential presence of a delta wave or a prolonged QT interval. Furthermore, the ECG may identify conduction disorders and cases of Brugada syndrome (**Table 2**).

Table 2
Selected electrocardiographic findings in pediatric syncope

Cause	ECG Findings
Wolff-Parkinson-White	Short PR interval, wide QRS complex, and a delta wave or positive slurring in the upstroke of the QRS complex
Long-QT syndrome	QTc >0.45
Brugada syndrome	ST elevation in anterior precordial leads, V_1 and V_2. Type 1 coved
Hypertrophic cardiomyopathy	LAE and LVH, ST-segment abnormalities, T-wave inversions, Q waves and diminished or absent R waves in the lateral leads.

Abbreviations: LAE, left atrial enlargement; LVH, left ventricular hypertrophy.

Data from Strickberger SA, Benson DW, Biaggioni I, et al. AHA/ACCF Scientific Statement on the evaluation of syncope: from the American Heart Association Councils on Clinical Cardiology, Cardiovascular Nursing, Cardiovascular Disease in the Young, and Stroke, and the Quality of Care and Outcomes Research Interdisciplinary Working Group; and the American College of Cardiology Foundation: in collaboration with the Heart Rhythm Society: endorsed by the American Autonomic Society. Circulation 2006;113(2):316–27; and Sharieff G. The pediatric ECG. Emerg Med Clin North Am 2006;24(1):195–208.

Any ECG abnormalities identified by the EP should be reviewed by a cardiologist before admission or ancillary testing. Despite low rates of discordance between EP and cardiologist ECG interpretation, suspected diagnoses can often be excluded by the cardiologist. Use of web-based or faxed ECG sharing can avoid unnecessary admission and testing.[20,21]

Other ED testing should be limited and patient focused. A urine pregnancy test should be sent for all menstruating females. A history suggesting electrolyte disturbance, malnutrition, an eating disorder, or endocrine abnormality should prompt serum electrolytes, including magnesium, calcium, and phosphate levels. Physical examination findings may guide the physician to check a hemoglobin level, a urine or serum toxicologic screen, or thyroid function tests.

Bedside ultrasound evaluation of fluid status and gross cardiac function may aid the EP in identifying dehydration, dilated cardiomyopathy, and hypertrophic cardiomyopathy.[22–26] Further studies are needed to determine the role of this evolving technology.

Ancillary tests are of limited use except for patients with a specific indication prompted by the history, physical or ECG.[19–21,27,28] Echocardiogram, Holter monitor, and tilt-table testing should only be ordered in consultation with a cardiologist. Electroencephalography (EEG), neuroimaging studies (including computer tomography or magnetic resonance imaging) and neurologic consultation may be indicated with specific neurologic findings.[20,29]

CASE 1: VASODEPRESSOR SYNCOPE

Sally is an 11-year-old girl brought in by ambulance to the ED after "fainting" this morning during math class. She describes feeling "dizzy" and "wobbly" when she stood up from her desk to answer a question. Witnesses report Sally became pale then collapsed into her chair, unconscious for 15 seconds. There was no abnormal movement or trauma noted. She woke up spontaneously feeling "weak." Sally was late for the school bus this morning and missed breakfast. Her mother denies any prior episodes of syncope or a family history of sudden cardiac death. Emergency medical services (EMS) report normal vital signs during transport and a point-of-care glucose of 92 mg/dL. Vital signs and physical examination are normal. An ECG is performed and interpreted as normal. Sally is diagnosed with vasodepressor syncope. Precautions and reassurance are given and she is discharged home.

How Does Vasodepressor Syncope Present?

Vasodepressor syncope is also known as vasovagal syncope, neurocardiogenic syncope, neurally mediated syncope, reflex syncope, and common fainting. Patients classically experience 3 distinct phases during an event: prodrome, loss of consciousness, and recovery. A good prodrome history can determine the diagnosis. This phase can last seconds to minutes and is usually recalled by the patient.[1,17]

Premonitory symptoms include a warm, hot, or cold sensation, lightheadedness, dizziness, nausea or abdominal pain, yawning, shortness of breath, pallor, diaphoresis, hearing or visual change (decreased acuity, tunnel vision, or double vision), headache, and anticipated loss of consciousness.[1,17,30] Any patient with abrupt syncope in which there is little or no premonitory symptoms must undergo a more extensive evaluation because of increased risk of serious cardiac disease and the risk of future injury.[17]

Actual loss of consciousness usually lasts somewhere between 5 and 20 seconds, but rarely extends to minutes. During this time patients appear pale or ashen, with cold skin and/or profuse sweating, and occasionally have dilated pupils and, rarely, seizure-like activity. In general, this phase is not recalled by the patient; although some patients may describe feeling "disconnected," or able to hear bystander voices but unable to respond.[17] The recovery phase lasts 5 to 30 minutes. Fatigue, dizziness, weakness, headache, and nausea are common. Episodes tend to be short but may recur if patients are helped up too quickly from the recumbent position.[1]

What Provokes Vasodepressor Syncope?

Several factors can provoke a common pathway causing vasodepressor syncope. These triggers include prolonged upright posture during sitting, standing, and walking; cough; menses; and carotid sinus pressure sensitivity.[1] Episodes may also be initiated by emotional stress, such as fear, anxiety, pain, phlebotomy, or the sight of blood. Precipitants that may contribute to an event include: anemia, relative dehydration, hunger, recent or concurrent illness, physical exhaustion, cessation of prolonged exercise, noxious stimuli, and/or crowded, warm, and poorly ventilated confines.[31] Patients with situational syncope generally have stereotypical triggers for recurrence such as swallowing, micturition, defecation, instrumentation (eg, colonoscopy), post-exercise, sneezing, diving, and pain.[17]

How Well Do We Understand the Mechanism for Vasodepressor Syncope?

Vasodepressor syncope is thought to be a normal reflex triggered at unintended situations.[32] There are 3 observed forms of vasodepressor syncope: primary bradycardia, which often includes transient asystole with subsequent hypotension; primary vasodepressor response with hypotension and relative preservation of heart rate; and a mixed response with simultaneous hypotension and bradycardia.[1] The common mechanism for all 3 forms has long been believed to be the Bezold-Jarisch phenomenon. Forceful contractions on an underfilled left ventricle causes excessive stimulation of the ventricular mechanoreceptors or C fibers, which leads to paradoxic signals to central nervous system pathways. A sudden conversion from vasoconstriction to vasodilation and bradycardia then follows.[32]

The magnitude of hypotension recorded may be substantial, with systolic blood pressure decreasing by 40 to 82 mm Hg. The average decrease in heart rate is variable, with an average decrease of 40 beats/min, and cardiac asystole lasting 3 to 40 seconds in 4% to 6% of patients.[33]

Mounting evidence suggests this neurocardiogenic pathway is inadequate to fully explain vasodepressor syncope. Aberrant autonomic regulation, endogenous vasodilators, disordered baroreflex function, paradoxic cerebral autoregulation, and low serum ferritin may all play a role.[32,34]

What is the Treatment for Vasodepressor Syncope?

Therapy in the ED is supportive, focusing on education and reassurance. Patients and caregivers should be encouraged to maintain adequate hydration and enhance dietary salt intake. Patients should learn to recognize prodrome symptoms and promptly sit or lie supine for up to 10 minutes or until symptoms resolve. Potential triggers should be identified and avoided. Recurrence in adolescence is common.

Referral to cardiology and subsequent medical therapy may be required for those with recurrent syncope unresponsive to behavioral modification, abrupt syncope associated with significant injury, or chronic dizziness.

Are There Similar Forms of Syncope?

Orthostatic hypotension results from a failure of compensatory mechanisms to maintain cardiac output with any postural change. These mechanisms (vasoconstriction, muscular contractions of the lower extremities, and venous valve competency) are mediated by increased sympathometic activity and parasympathometic inhibition. Symptoms include: dizziness, lightheadedness, blurred or tunnel vision, weakness, and syncope. Episodes occur frequently in the morning, after meals, or during exercise. Dehydration, blood loss, pregnancy, prolonged bed rest, and medication use (calcium channel blockers, vasodilators, phenothiazines, and diuretics) may contribute. Orthostatic testing is diagnostic. Standing blood pressures should be delayed to observe for possible, subsequent hypotension and syncope.[16]

Postural orthostatic tachycardia syndrome (POTS) is diagnosed by observing posturally induced symptoms with robust tachycardia and without significant blood pressure decline.[32] In POTS, the heart rate increases by more than 30 beats/min with the development of vasopressor symptoms.[8] The incidence is unknown. Patients may or may not develop frank syncope, and often complain of orthostatic palpitations, profound fatigue and exercise intolerance, lightheadedness, and cognitive impairment.[35] Symptoms improve with sitting. These patients have generalized malaise and are often misdiagnosed with chronic fatigue syndrome or psychiatric illness.[36]

CASE 2: NEUROPSYCHIATRIC DISEASE

Bill is a 3-year-old boy brought in by his mother to the ED after an episode of "fainting" this afternoon. His mother states Bill went into the bathroom to "pee pee." Two minutes later she heard the toilet seat bang and found him on the floor unresponsive. She witnessed no abnormal movement but his eyes were deviated to the left. He woke up 2 minutes later but remained confused for another 15 minutes. She noted he had wet his pull-ups but showed no visible signs of trauma. Bill had a febrile seizure at age 2 but is otherwise healthy. Review of systems is negative. Vital signs and physical examination are normal. An ECG is performed and interpreted as normal. Bill is diagnosed with a seizure. His primary care provider is contacted. Outpatient EEG and a follow-up with a neurologist is scheduled. Seizure precautions are given and he is discharged home.

How Does One Differentiate Seizure from Pediatric Syncope?

A detailed history and physical examination are typically sufficient to distinguish seizure from syncope. Typical seizures have a premonitory aura, generalized tonic-clonic activity, and a postictal period of lethargy and confusion. Patents with seizures do not experience the prodrome symptoms of syncope. Seizure findings typically include supine rather than upright posture at onset, convulsions before rather than after loss of consciousness, frothing at the mouth, tongue biting, incontinence, and warm, flushed, or cyanotic skin rather than pallor and diaphoresis.[16]

Can Pediatric Syncope Cause Seizure-Like Movements?

Syncope can cause stiffening, myoclonic, and limited clonic movements, known as *convulsive syncope*, and is a common reason for the misdiagnosis of pediatric epilepsy.[37] Transient global hypoxia leads to cortical suppression and disinhibition of limbic and subcortical structures.[38] Movements are usually during the loss of consciousness phase, not before or at the onset of that phase; and are brief with multifocal or 1 to 2 clonic jerks rather than prolonged clonic-tonic movements.[32] There is no postictal period.

Can Migraine Cause Pediatric Syncope?

Migraine can cause syncope; specifically, vertebrobasilar vascular spasm. Symptoms are atypical and may include severe a occipital headache before and/or after loss of consciousness, unilateral vision change, ataxia, emesis, and vertigo. These episodes are longer in duration with stable hemodynamics.[1] Scintillating scotomatas may precede onset.[13]

Are There Psychiatric Mimics of Pediatric Syncope?

Hyperventilation and *conversion syncope* commonly occur in adolescents, usually in a highly emotional setting, and can result in a loss of consciousness. Both conditions are rare in children younger than 10 years.

Hyperventilation begins with an apprehensive feeling and deep sighing respirations. These subtle changes may not be obvious to the patient.[8] Dyspnea, air hunger, and chest tightness may progress to loss of consciousness. Other symptoms include light-headedness, abdominal discomfort, palpitations, dizziness, paresthesias, and visual disturbances.[16]

Conversion syncope or hysteria typically occurs in the presence of an audience and rarely produces injury. Episodes are not posture dependent and may last up to an hour.[8,13] In addition, there are no neurologic, autonomic, or cardiovascular changes. Patients often describe feeling calm and may remember the surrounding environment during the episode.[16]

CASE 3: CARDIAC DYSRHYTHMIA

Frank is a 10-year-old boy brought in by ambulance to the ED after "fainting" this afternoon during recess. He says he was putting on his jacket and then woke up on the ground with a bleeding chin. Witnesses report Frank collapsed to the ground and failed to protect his chin from striking the floor. He was unconscious for 30 seconds before awaking spontaneously. There was no abnormal movement noted. His father states he has "fainted" twice this year but has never injured himself or visited a physician. There is no family history of sudden cardiac death. EMS report a point-of-care glucose of 90 mg/dL and normal vital signs during transport. Vital signs are normal. Physical examination reveals a 3-cm simple laceration to the chin. An ECG is performed with a delta wave, short PR interval with wide QRS complex identified. Frank is diagnosed with Wolff-Parkinson-White (WPW) syndrome and placed on a cardiac monitor. The laceration is repaired and he is admitted to the pediatric cardiology service.

Is Cardiac Syncope Common in Pediatric Patients?

Cardiac syncope is a serious concern but an uncommon diagnosis. A focused history and physical examination, screening ECG, and cardiology consultation when indicated can detect the majority of cardiac syncope and ultimately be life-saving. Cardiac causes account for 85% of sudden death in children and adolescent athletes, and 17% of young athletes with sudden death have a history of syncope.[39] The ECG should be reviewed for any abnormality, with specific attention to the corrected QT interval (QTc), evidence of an abnormal or irregular rhythm, ischemia, axis deviation, and hypertrophy.

What is the Correct Way to Calculate the QTc?

Bazet's formula, QTc = (QT)/square root (R-R) is the correct way to calculate the QTc. The QT interval should be measured from the beginning of the QRS complex to the end of the T wave in leads II, V5, or V6. The measured R-R interval should immediately precede the measured QT. Automated calculation from ECG machines cannot be relied on. The measurement should be averaged from several successive beats.

QTc calculation can be difficult to analyze in patients with very slow or fast heart rates, and those with sinus irregularities.

What if the ECG Reveals QTc >0.450 Milliseconds?

Long-QT syndrome (LQTS) is the prolongation of ventricular repolarization secondary to impaired ion channels in the myocardium. There are multiple genetic mutations that lead to dysfunction of potassium, sodium, and/or calcium ion channels which, in turn, leads to an overabundance of cations within the myocardium. LQTS puts the heart at risk for ventricular dysrhythmias such as torsades de pointes and ventricular fibrillation (**Fig. 2**). These ventricular dysrhythmias can cause syncope. If self-correction does not occur, then sudden death may follow.

What Congenital Syndromes are Associated with LQTS?

Romano Ward and Jervell-Nielsen-Lange are 2 commonly described syndromes associated with LQTS. Romano Ward is inherited in an autosomal dominant fashion, whereas Jervell-Nielsen-Lange is autosomal recessive and associated with congenital deafness; a family history of deafness is an important feature to ask about in screening for this syndrome. Cardiology referral and/or screening with an ECG is recommended for all identified family members of LQTS patients.[40]

Can Medications Induce or Exacerbate LQTS?

Several medications have been known to prolong the QT interval, including tricyclic antidepressants, antipsychotics, antibiotics (eg, macrolides), organophosphates, antihistamines, and antifungals.[41] Not all patients on these medications will develop LQTS. However, those with multiple risk factors are at greater risk for drug-induced LQTS. These risk factors include genetic predisposition, electrolyte abnormalities, female gender, multiple medications causing drug interactions, and structural heart disease.[42]

What is Brugada Syndrome?

Brugada syndrome is a heritable disorder of the cardiac sodium channels that creates a susceptibility to polymorphic ventricular tachycardia. This recurrent dysrhythmia can degenerate to ventricular fibrillation and cardiac arrest. Self-termination usually results in syncope or pre-syncope. The ECG is often dynamic with an ST elevation in the anterior precordial leads, that is, V_1 and V_2 being pathognomonic (**Fig. 3**).[8,43,44]

Patients who present with syncope have a 2-year risk of sudden cardiac death of approximately 30% if untreated. Placement of an internal defibrillator leads to an excellent prognosis with zero mortality at 10 years.[44] Systematic familial study can identify asymptomatic affected family members who can benefit from early treatment to prevent complications.[45]

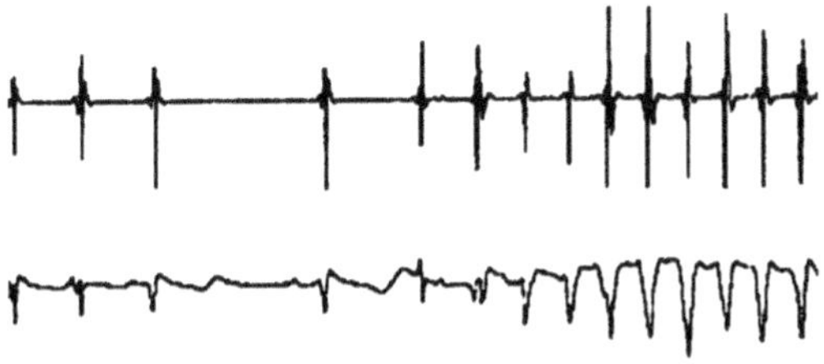

Fig. 2. Rhythm strip demonstrating long-QT syndrome and the degeneration to torsades de pointes. (*Courtesy of* Amandeep Singh, MD, Oakland, CA.)

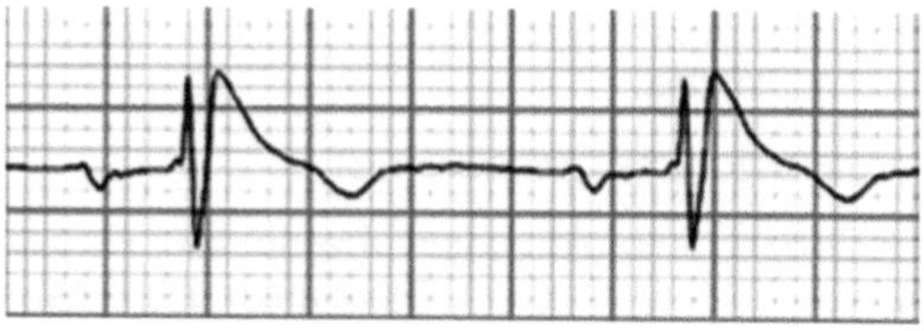

Fig. 3. Brugada syndrome. Coved ST elevation in anterior precordial leads, V_1 and V_2. (*Courtesy of* Nathan Irvin, MD, Oakland, CA.)

What Should One Consider if Heart Block is Found on the ECG?

First-degree heart block is usually an incidental finding in the setting of syncope, although it can be found in children with myocarditis, congenital heart disease, or cardiomyopathy.[41] Second- and third-degree heart block detected on ECG is of concern in the setting of syncope. Neonatal lupus syndrome can cause heart block secondary to the passage of anti-Ro or anti-La antibodies in infants and young children.[46] Maternal presence of these antibodies can occur with or without a history of maternal lupus. Congenital heart block may also be present in the setting of structural anomalies.

Acquired heart block can be caused by infectious myocarditis (most commonly Lyme disease), rheumatic heart disease, digoxin toxicity, and cardiac surgery. These cases require cardiology consultation for further testing and treatment. Symptomatic heart block may require pacing in the ED.

What is the Most Common Pediatric Dysrhythmia?

Supraventricular tachycardia (SVT) is the most common symptomatic pediatric dysrhythmia.[41,47] SVT is a narrow complex tachycardia with a heart rate of more than 220 beats/min for infants and young children and greater than 180 beats/min for older children and adolescents. SVT can be due to a junctional tachycardia, ectopic atrial tachycardia, or an accessory atrioventricular pathway that causes reentrant tachycardia, as described in WPW syndrome.

SVT creates a relative anoxia from compromised cardiac output that can lead to syncope. Narrow complex tachycardia, absent or polymorphic p waves, and lack of beat-to-beat variability are common ECG findings. When SVT has resolved (either spontaneously or with treatment in the ED), ECG findings may also suggest the presence of an accessory pathway. In WPW syndrome, a delta wave (due to accessory conduction through the Bundle of Kent), and other associated ECG findings can be seen (**Fig. 4**).

What Rare Dysrhythmias Cause or Mimic Pediatric Syncope?

Sick sinus or sinus node dysfunction can result in a variety of symptomatic arrhythmias and syncope. These arrhythmias can be caused by cardiac surgery (eg, Fontan procedure), infectious or postinfectious changes (eg, myocarditis, pericarditis), congenital heart disease (sinus venous atrial septal defect, Ebstein anomaly), antiarrhythmic drugs (eg, digitalis. propranolol), hypothyroidism, or can be idiopathic with an otherwise normal heart. Observed bradytachyarrhythmia is very concerning. Profound bradycardia following a period of tachycardia (overdrive suppression) can lead to syncope and even death.[8] Postoperative cardiac patients with a history of surgery involving the ventricles (eg, tetralogy of Fallot or a ventricular septal defect) are at risk for complete atrioventricular block or ventricular tachycardia.[10]

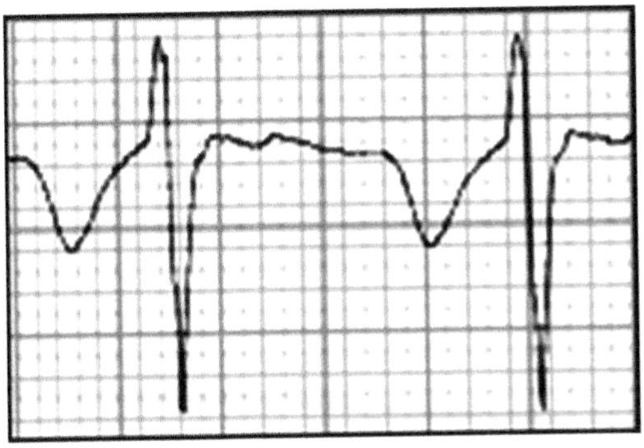

Fig. 4. Wolff-Parkinson-White syndrome. Lead V2 demonstrates a short PR interval, a wide QRS complex, and a delta wave or positive slurring in the upstroke of the QRS complex. (*Courtesy of* Aaron Harries, MD, Oakland, CA.)

Commotio cordis is a life-threatening dysrhythmia caused by a direct, nonpenetrating, often low-impact blow to the chest that may be confused with syncope. Two-thirds of cases occur during sporting events but reports include chest blows from physical abuse, fighting, snowballs, and hollow plastic toys.[48] Ventricular fibrillation is typical but heart block, ventricular tachycardia, bundle branch block, ST-T wave abnormalities, and asystole can also occur.[49] Patients are often amnestic to the event and have a contusion on the chest at the point of impact. Short-term observation and a cardiology release to return to athletics are required.[50]

CASE 4: STRUCTURAL CARDIAC DISEASE

Steve is a 14-year-old boy brought in by ambulance to the ED after "fainting" this evening while helping his dad with yard work. He says he was running to the garage and then woke up on the ground. His father reports Steve collapsed and was unconscious for 1 minute before awaking spontaneously. He had 3 to 4 clonic jerks during the event. Steve denies prior events but does endorse periodic chest discomfort when participating in recent neighborhood soccer games. There is no family history of sudden cardiac death. Review of systems is otherwise negative. EMS report a point-of-care glucose of 80 mg/dL and normal vital signs en route. Vital signs and physical examination are normal. ECG reveals left ventricular hypertrophy. An ECHO is performed that shows hypertrophic cardiomyopathy. He is placed on a cardiac monitor and admitted to the pediatric cardiology service.

What Congenital Cardiac Structural Anomalies are Important to Consider in Pediatric Syncope?

Important cardiac structural anomalies that can present as syncope include hypertrophic cardiomyopathy (HCM), valvular disease such as aortic stenosis, and coronary anomalies causing ischemic heart disease. Chest pain, dizziness, and shortness of breath (particularly in the setting of exercise) are important historical elements to elicit. On physical examination, a systolic murmur may be apparent in HCM and aortic stenosis. Cardiac auscultation should also be performed with various maneuvers to increase and decrease blood flow to the heart. In HCM, the systolic murmur will increase when venous return is decreased to the heart (eg, during Valsalva or in standing position). The murmur will decrease with increased flow to the heart (eg, sitting, or bringing legs to chest). The opposite is true for the murmur of aortic stenosis.

HCM results from a diverse group of mutations and phenotypes that ultimately leads to abnormal hypertrophy of cardiac tissue.[51] The estimated incidence is 1 in 500 individuals. Although obstruction can be the cause of syncope or sudden death in HCM, dysrhythmias from thickened muscle are more common. Left ventricular hypertrophy, axis deviation, and ST- or T-wave abnormalities may be identified on ECG (see **Table 2**).

Can Pediatric Patients Have Ischemic Heart Disease?

Myocardial ischemia or infarction is rare in children but must be considered. Syncope, chest pain (usually with exertion), shortness of breath, fatigue, and in infants, difficulty or sweating with feeds are all important historical features.

Anomalous left coronary artery from the pulmonary artery is a congenital cardiac anomaly in which the left coronary artery is attached to the pulmonary artery instead of the aorta. This anomaly results in deoxygenated blood being delivered to the myocardium, and potential ischemia and infarction. ECG findings of ST elevation, T or Q wave anomalies are consistent with infarction. Syncope and sudden death commonly present in infancy but may occur later in life.[52]

Moreover, Kawasaki disease and the development of coronary artery aneurysms can also lead to ischemia. Patients with a known history of aneurysms or those with previously undiagnosed Kawasaki disease are also at risk for ischemic heart disease. The EP should always be mindful of ECG interpretation, as it can clearly delineate ischemic disease.

CASE 5: ADDITIONAL CAUSES OF PEDIATRIC SYNCOPE

Jill is a 14-month-old girl brought in by her grandmother to the ED after "fainting" this evening. Her grandmother states Jill became "very upset" when it was time to go to bed and then collapsed into her crib. She was unconscious for 10 seconds before awaking spontaneously. She turned blue briefly but had no abnormal movements. Her mother arrives and confirms this has happened one other time while being dropped off at daycare. There is no family history of sudden cardiac death. Review of systems is negative. The vital signs and physical examination are normal. An ECG is performed and interpreted as normal. Jill is diagnosed with a breath-holding spell. Precautions are given and she is discharged home.

What is a Breath-Holding Spell?

Breath-holding spells occur when children typically aged 6 to 18 months are startled by an intense emotional trigger: pain, fright, or anger. The child holds their breath and becomes limp or falls to the ground within seconds. The entire event usually lasts less than a minute and ends with gasping breaths. Cyanosis is common but pallor may be observed due to the vasodepressor mechanism.[53] Convulsive syncope can occur.[54]

Breath-holding spells are reported in 2% to 5% of children. Therapy is rarely required.[55] Approximately 10% to 20% of children with a diagnosis of breath-holding spells develop more typical vasodepressor syncope in later life.[56]

Does Coughing Cause Pediatric Syncope?

Tussive syncope is associated with bronchospasm from an acute infection, asthma, pertussis, or cystic fibrosis.[13] Episodes are triggered by reduced cardiac output due to high intrathoracic pressures from the severe paroxysms of coughing. The transmission of high intrathoracic pressures to the subarachnoid space reducing cerebral blood flow may also contribute.[16]

Does Hypoglycemia Cause Pediatric Syncope?

Hypoglycemia does not cause isolated syncope, as symptoms have a gradual onset without spontaneous resolution.[57] Patients describe feeling weak, hungry, sweaty, agitated, and confused, and eventually develop altered mental status. Hypoglycemia is rare in children and adolescents except in the setting of fasting, insulin-dependent diabetes or suspected toxic ingestion. Measuring a serum glucose in all pediatric syncope patients is low yield and unnecessary.[20,58]

Does Pregnancy Matter in Pediatric Syncope?

All menstruating females should have a urine pregnancy test performed. Syncope and near-syncope are common with normal pregnancy, especially in the third trimester, but can be associated with ectopic pregnancy, pulmonary embolism, and pregnancy-related cardiac disease. These high-risk diagnoses must be ruled out.[59,60]

Can Carbon Monoxide Poisoning Present as Pediatric Syncope?

In the acute phase following carbon monoxide (CO) exposure, headache, nausea, and dizziness are common. As exposure increases, patients develop more pronounced and severe symptoms, including syncope. The brain and heart are the most oxygen-dependent organs and are also the most sensitive to the toxic effects of CO. A significant number of CO poisoning cases may go undetected as the signs and symptoms are diverse and easily confused with other illnesses.[61]

SUMMARY

Pediatric syncope is a common presentation in the ED, with a large differential diagnosis (see **Table 1**). Most causes are benign but an evaluation must exclude rare life-threatening disorders. The keys to identifying high-risk patients include a detailed history, a focused but thorough physical examination, and a screening ECG on all patients. Key features on history and physical examination for identifying high-risk patients include exercise-related symptoms, a family history of sudden death, a history of cardiac disease, an abnormal cardiac examination, or an abnormal ECG. Ancillary testing should be limited to corroborate concerning findings from the history and physical examination; routine blood work and diagnostic imaging are not indicated. Education and reassurance are important because recurrence is common.

REFERENCES

1. Lewis DA, Dhala A. Syncope in the pediatric patient. The cardiologist's perspective. Pediatr Clin North Am 1999;46(2):205–19.
2. McHarg ML, Shinnar S, Rascoff H, et al. Syncope in childhood. Pediatr Cardiol 1997;18(5):367–71.
3. Njemanze PC. Cerebral circulation dysfunction and hemodynamic abnormalities in syncope during upright tilt test. Can J Cardiol 1993;9(3):238–42.
4. Day SC, Cook EF, Funkenstein H, et al. Evaluation and outcome of emergency room patients with transient loss of consciousness. Am J Med 1982;73(1):15–23.
5. Ruckman RN. Cardiac causes of syncope. Pediatr Rev 1987;9(4):101–8.
6. Ganzeboom KS, Colman N, Reitsma JB, et al. Prevalence and triggers of syncope in medical students. Am J Cardiol 2003;91(8):1006–8, A8.
7. Driscoll DJ, Jacobsen SJ, Porter CJ, et al. Syncope in children and adolescents. J Am Coll Cardiol 1997;29(5):1039–45.

8. Park MK. Pediatric cardiology for practitioners [electronic resource]. Philadelphia: Mosby/Elsevier; 2008.
9. Massin MM, Bourguignont A, Coremans C, et al. Syncope in pediatric patients presenting to an emergency department. J Pediatr 2004;145(2):223–8.
10. Strickberger SA, Benson DW, Biaggioni I, et al. AHA/ACCF Scientific Statement on the evaluation of syncope: from the American Heart Association Councils on Clinical Cardiology, Cardiovascular Nursing, Cardiovascular Disease in the Young, and Stroke, and the Quality of Care and Outcomes Research Interdisciplinary Working Group; and the American College of Cardiology Foundation: in collaboration with the Heart Rhythm Society: endorsed by the American Autonomic Society. Circulation 2006;113(2):316–27.
11. Huff JS, Decker WW, Quinn JV, et al. Clinical policy: critical issues in the evaluation and management of adult patients presenting to the emergency department with syncope. Ann Emerg Med 2007;49(4):431–44.
12. Liberthson RR. Sudden death from cardiac causes in children and young adults. N Engl J Med 1996;334(16):1039–44.
13. Prodinger RJ, Reisdorff EJ. Syncope in children. Emerg Med Clin North Am 1998; 16(3):617–26, ix.
14. Kapoor WN, Karpf M, Wieand S, et al. A prospective evaluation and follow-up of patients with syncope. N Engl J Med 1983;309(4):197–204.
15. Chronister TE. Pediatric neurologist as consultant in evaluation of syncope in infants and children: when to refer. Prog Pediatr Cardiol 2001;13(2):133–8.
16. Tanel RE, Walsh EP. Syncope in the pediatric patient. Cardiol Clin 1997;15(2): 277–94.
17. Johnsrude CL. Current approach to pediatric syncope. Pediatr Cardiol 2000; 21(6):522–31.
18. Massin MM, Malekzadeh-Milani S, Benatar A. Cardiac syncope in pediatric patients. Clin Cardiol 2007;30(2):81–5.
19. Ritter S, Tani LY, Etheridge SP, et al. What is the yield of screening echocardiography in pediatric syncope? Pediatrics 2000;105(5):E58.
20. Goble MM, Benitez C, Baumgardner M, et al. ED management of pediatric syncope: searching for a rationale. Am J Emerg Med 2008;26(1):66–70.
21. Hue V, Noizet-Yvernaux O, Vaksmann G, et al. ED management of pediatric syncope. Am J Emerg Med 2008;26(9):1059–60.
22. Kosiak W, Swieton D, Piskunowicz M. Sonographic inferior vena cava/aorta diameter index, a new approach to the body fluid status assessment in children and young adults in emergency ultrasound—preliminary study. Am J Emerg Med 2008;26(3):320–5.
23. Chen L, Kim Y, Santucci KA. Use of ultrasound measurement of the inferior vena cava diameter as an objective tool in the assessment of children with clinical dehydration. Acad Emerg Med 2007;14(10):841–5.
24. Randazzo MR, Snoey ER, Levitt MA, et al. Accuracy of emergency physician assessment of left ventricular ejection fraction and central venous pressure using echocardiography. Acad Emerg Med 2003;10(9):973–7.
25. Ciccone TJ, Grossman SA. Cardiac ultrasound. Emerg Med Clin North Am 2004; 22(3):621–40.
26. Stewart GM, Nguyen HB, Kim TY, et al. Inter-rater reliability for noninvasive measurement of cardiac function in children. Pediatr Emerg Care 2008;24(7): 433–7.
27. Gordon TA, Moodie DS, Passalacqua M, et al. A retrospective analysis of the cost-effective workup of syncope in children. Cleve Clin J Med 1987;54(5):391–4.

28. Lerman-Sagie T, Lerman P, Mukamel M, et al. A prospective evaluation of pediatric patients with syncope. Clin Pediatr (Phila) 1994;33(2):67–70.
29. Matoth I, Taustein I, Kay BS, et al. Overuse of EEG in the evaluation of common neurologic conditions. Pediatr Neurol 2002;27(5):378–83.
30. Engel GL. Psychologic stress, vasodepressor (vasovagal) syncope, and sudden death. Ann Intern Med 1978;89(3):403–12.
31. Pratt JL, Fleisher GR. Syncope in children and adolescents. Pediatr Emerg Care 1989;5(2):80–2.
32. Weimer LH, Zadeh P. Neurological aspects of syncope and orthostatic intolerance. Med Clin North Am 2009;93(2):427–49, ix.
33. Berkowitz JB, et al. Tilt table evaluation for control pediatric patients: comparison with symptomatic patients. Clin Cardiol 1995;18(9):521–5.
34. Jarjour IT, Jarjour LK. Low iron storage in children and adolescents with neurally mediated syncope. J Pediatr 2008;153(1):40–4.
35. Grubb BP, Kosinski DJ, Boehm K, et al. The postural orthostatic tachycardia syndrome: a neurocardiogenic variant identified during head-up tilt table testing. Pacing Clin Electrophysiol 1997;20(9 Pt 1):2205–12.
36. Rowe PC. Orthostatic intolerance and chronic fatigue syndrome: new light on an old problem. J Pediatr 2002;140(4):387–9.
37. Zaidi A, Clough P, Cooper P, et al. Misdiagnosis of epilepsy: many seizure-like attacks have a cardiovascular cause. J Am Coll Cardiol 2000;36(1):181–4.
38. Lempert T, Bauer M, Schmidt D. Syncope: a videometric analysis of 56 episodes of transient cerebral hypoxia. Ann Neurol 1994;36(2):233–7.
39. Maron BJ, Shirani J, Poliac LC, et al. Sudden death in young competitive athletes. Clinical, demographic, and pathological profiles. JAMA 1996;276(3):199–204.
40. Petko C, Bradley DJ, Tristani-Firouzi M, et al. Congenital long QT syndrome in children identified by family screening. Am J Cardiol 2008;101(12):1756–8.
41. Doniger SJ, Sharieff GQ. Pediatric dysrhythmias. Pediatr Clin North Am 2006;53(1):85–105, vi.
42. Simko J, Csilek A, Karaszi J, et al. Proarrhythmic potential of antimicrobial agents. Infection 2008;36(3):194–206.
43. Dovgalyuk J, Holstege C, Mattu A, et al. The electrocardiogram in the patient with syncope. Am J Emerg Med 2007;25(6):688–701.
44. Brugada J, Brugada R, Antzelevitch C, et al. Long-term follow-up of individuals with the electrocardiographic pattern of right bundle-branch block and ST-segment elevation in precordial leads V1 to V3. Circulation 2002;105(1):73–8.
45. Gimeno JR, Lacunza J, Garcia-Alberola A, et al. Penetrance and risk profile in inherited cardiac diseases studied in a dedicated screening clinic. Am J Cardiol 2009;104(3):406–10.
46. Friedman DM, Rupel A, Buyon JP. Epidemiology, etiology, detection, and treatment of autoantibody-associated congenital heart block in neonatal lupus. Curr Rheumatol Rep 2007;9(2):101–8.
47. Samson RA, Atkins DL. Tachyarrhythmias and defibrillation. Pediatr Clin North Am 2008;55(4):887–907, x.
48. Maron BJ, Gohman TE, Kyle SB, et al. Clinical profile and spectrum of commotio cordis. JAMA 2002;287(9):1142–6.
49. Link MS, Wang PJ, Pandian NG, et al. An experimental model of sudden death due to low-energy chest-wall impact (commotio cordis). N Engl J Med 1998;338(25):1805–11.
50. Zangwill SD, Strasburger JF. Commotio cordis. Pediatr Clin North Am 2004;51(5):1347–54.

51. Washington R. Syncope and sudden death in the athlete. Clin Pediatr Emerg Med 2007;8(1):54–8.
52. Pena E, Nguyen ET, Merchant N, et al. ALCAPA syndrome: not just a pediatric disease. Radiographics 2009;29(2):553–65.
53. Lombroso CT, Lerman P. Breathholding spells (cyanotic and pallid infantile syncope). Pediatrics 1967;39(4):563–81.
54. DiMario FJ Jr. Breath-holding spells in childhood. Am J Dis Child 1992;146(1): 125–31.
55. Kelly AM, Porter CJ, McGoon MD, et al. Breath-holding spells associated with significant bradycardia: successful treatment with permanent pacemaker implantation. Pediatrics 2001;108(3):698–702.
56. Livingston S. Breathholding spells in children. Differentiation from epileptic attacks. JAMA 1970;212(13):2231–5.
57. Service FJ. Hypoglycemic disorders. N Engl J Med 1995;332(17):1144–52.
58. Steinberg LA, Knilans TK. Syncope in children: diagnostic tests have a high cost and low yield. J Pediatr 2005;146(3):355–8.
59. Gabbe SG, Niebyl JR, Simpson JL. Obstetrics: normal and problem pregnancies. 5th edition. Philadelphia: Churchill Livingstone/Elsevier; 2007.
60. Marx JA, Hockberger RS, Walls RM, et al. Rosen's emergency medicine: concepts and clinical practice, vol. 3. 6th edition. Philadelphia: Mosby/Elsevier; 2006.
61. Kao LW, Nanagas KA. Carbon monoxide poisoning. Emerg Med Clin North Am 2004;22(4):985–1018.

Seizures as a Cause of Altered Mental Status

David E. Slattery, MD[a,*],
Charles V. Pollack Jr, MA, MD[b]

KEYWORDS

• Seizure • Altered mental status • Status epilepticus

The differential diagnosis of altered mental status (AMS) in the emergency department (ED) is broad, and emergency physicians (EPs) must process the possibilities in an efficient and rapid manner. At the forefront of the ED evaluation is the prompt identification and treatment of the easily reversible causes of AMS: hypoxia, hypoglycemia, and opiate overdose. Ictal and postictal presentations are also often in the AMS differential, and, as with all patients in the ED, rapid assessment and intervention on impaired airway, breathing, and circulation issues take precedence in the seizing patient. After readily reversible causes are excluded and the immediate life threats are stabilized in these patients, the next priority is abating the seizure activity. This article reviews the breadth of disease states, metabolic abnormalities, ingestions, and physiologic derangements that may be of concern when a patient presents to the ED with AMS and seizure.

DEFINITION AND CLASSIFICATION OF SEIZURES

It is estimated that 6% of the population of the United States will experience at least 1 nonfebrile seizure during their lifetime. The annual incidence is 84 per 100,000 persons.[1] This number accounts for approximately 1% of all ED visits.[2] Roughly half of these patients will develop epilepsy. Seizures can be classified (**Fig. 1**) as generalized or partial. Generalized seizures result in a loss of consciousness because the abnormal electrical process involves both cerebral hemispheres. Partial seizures are differentiated into simple, affecting 1 area of the brain without impairment of cognition (perception, attention, emotion, memory, or executive function), or complex, affecting

Funding: None.
[a] Department of Emergency Medicine, University of Nevada School of Medicine, 901 Rancho Lane, Suite #135, Las Vegas, NV 89106, USA
[b] Department of Emergency Medicine, Pennsylvania Hospital, University of Pennsylvania, 800 Spruce Street, Philadelphia, PA 19107, USA
* Corresponding author.
E-mail address: dslatts@mac.com

Emerg Med Clin N Am 28 (2010) 517–534
doi:10.1016/j.emc.2010.03.011

emed.theclinics.com

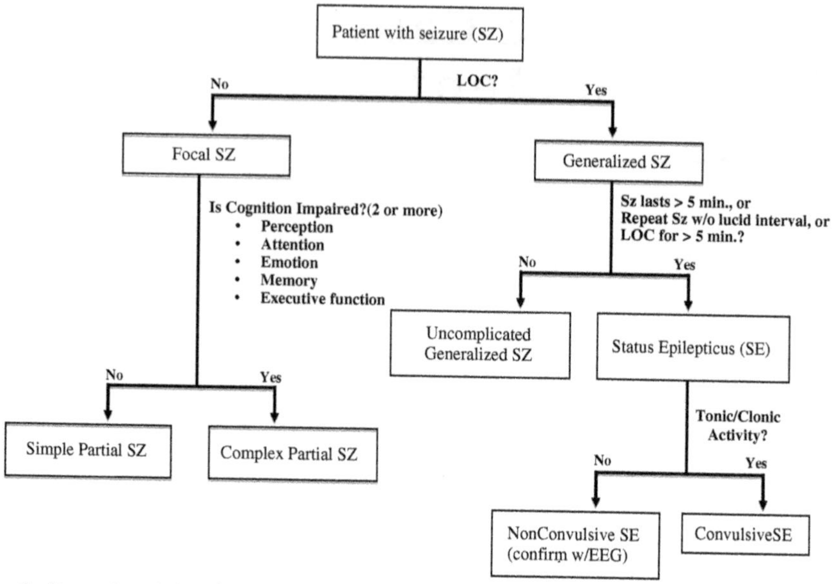

Fig. 1. Operational classification of seizures in the ED.

at least 2 or more areas of cognition.[3] However, simple focal seizures can progress and become generalized.[4]

There are several complicated seizure classification systems, but, for emergency medicine purposes, a clinically relevant framework is preferable (see **Fig. 1**). Specifically, it is helpful to determine whether the ictal event involves impairment of consciousness, whether it is a provoked event, and whether the event is simple or complicated. Seizures are classified as being uncomplicated if they last less than 5 minutes, if they do not recur without a lucid interval, and if they are not associated with a prolonged postictal state or focal deficit. Although the traditional neurology literature defines status epilepticus (SE) as a seizure lasting more than 30 minutes, the term impending SE is more appropriate in an ED setting and represents an ictal event that does not abate within 5 minutes, or repeats without a lucid interval.[5–8] SE is a true medical emergency, and prompt recognition and intervention are directly correlated with improvement in morbidity and mortality.[7] Generalized convulsive seizures (convulsive status epilepticus [CSE]) represent a unique challenge and portend a worse outcome for seizure patients. Mortality ranges from 19% to 27% with CSE. Elderly patients (age >65 years), those with anoxic seizures, and those with CSE lasting more than 1 hour have the highest mortality.[7] This clinical entity is easily identified and, hence, can be more aggressively treated. Animal data suggest that γ-aminobutyric acid (GABA) receptors, which inhibit cortical neurons, undergo a conformational change after a certain amount of time that makes them less responsive to benzodiazepine treatment.[9,10] In addition, GABA receptor sensitization, trafficking (movement from the synaptic membrane into endozomes), decreases in synaptic inhibitory receptor concentrations, along with concurrent increases in excitatory receptors (ie, *N*-methyl-D-aspartate [NMDA] receptors) all contribute to pharmacoresistance.[5] Hence, a heightened urgency to stop active seizing with more aggressive and rapid use of antiseizure medications is the emerging paradigm.[5,7]

CSE management begins with airway support and breathing while protecting the cervical spine, identifying and treating hypoglycemia and hypoxia, and initiation of antiseizure medications (**Table 1**). Benzodiazepenes are the preferred initial treatment because of their prompt action and broad effect on stimulated neurons, which is largely independent of the specific stimulus. In the ED, lorazepam is generally preferred (0.1 mg/kg intravenously [IV]), because of its rapid onset but longer duration of action than other benzodiazepines. Other options include midazolam 0.1 to 0.2 mg/kg IV, intramuscularly (IM), or intranasally, or diazepam 5–10 mg IV (pediatric dose 0.25–0.50 mg/kg IV up to a maximum of 5 mg).[5,7,11] If the seizure does not abate after repeated benzodiazepine doses, then anticonvulsant therapy should be initiated. Initial choice depends on the suspected cause. In most non–toxin-related seizures, the patient should be given 18 to 20 mg/kg of IV phenytoin, not exceeding 50 mg/min, or fosphenytoin 18 to 20 phenytoin equivalents (PE) at 100 to 150 mg/min.[7,11] If seizures persist, or in the case of a suspected toxin-induced seizure, patients should be given phenobarbiatal 20 mg/kg IV at 100 mg/min. If ictal activity continues, patients should be intubated, and other pharmacologic options should be considered:

Table 1
Drugs used in the abortive treatment of status epilepticus in the ED

Generic Name	Brand Name	Adult Dose	Comments
Diazepam	Valium	5–10 mg IV every 10 min, up to 30 mg per 8-h period	May be given per rectum in pediatrics (0.3–0.5 mg/kg)
Lorazepam	Ativan	0.1 mg/kg IV (usually 4 mg in adults); may repeat in 10 min, then 0.01–0.1 mg/kg/h infusion	Preferred benzodiazepine owing to its longer duration of action
Midazolam	Versed	0.1–0.2 mg/kg IV bolus, then 0.02–0.1 mg/kg/h IV	Midazolam for seizure is an unlabeled use. May be given intranasally (0.2 mg/kg)
Phenytoin	Dilantin	20 mg/kg IV at <50 mg/min	Cardiac and blood pressure monitoring during infusion; large-bore IV line
Fosphenytoin	Cerebyx	20 PE/kg IV at 150 mg PE/min	Cardiac monitoring. Less risk of infusion site reaction; may be IM
Phenobarbital	Luminal	20 mg/kg IV, then 5–10 mg/kg every 20 min, up to 2 g	May be given as IM loading dose
Valproate	Depakote	Loading dose 15–45 mg/kg administered at <6 mg/kg/min Maintenance dose: IV infusion: 1–4 mg/kg/hour	Titrate dose as needed based upon patient response and evaluation of drug-drug interactions.
Propofol	Diprivan	1–2 mg/kg IV bolus, then 0.3–0.6 mg/kg/h infusion	Intubation required; monitor hemodynamics
Pentobarbital	Nembutal	10–20 mg/kg IV load over 1–2 h, then 0.5–1 mg/kg/h infusion	Intubation required; monitor hemodynamics
Isoflurane	Forane, Terrell	Via general endotracheal anesthesia	Monitor with EEG

Abbreviations: EEG, electroencephalogram; IM, intramuscularly; IV, intravenously; PE, phenytoin equivalents.

Data from Owenstein DH. Treatment options for status epilepticus. Curr Opin Pharmacol 2005;5:334; Engel J Jr, Pedley TA, editors. Epilepsy: a comprehensive textbook. 2nd edition. Philadelphia: Lippincott Williams & Wilkins; 2008.

midazoloam 0.2 mg/kg bolus followed by a drip at 0.02 to 0.1 mg/kg/h; propofol 1 to 2 mg/kg bolus followed by a maintenance dose of 0.3 to 0.6 mg/kg/h; pentobarbital 10 mg/kg loading dose followed by 0.5 to 1 mg/kg/h; thiopental 100 to 250 mg bolus over 20 seconds, then 50 mg boluses every 3 minutes until seizure control, followed by infusion at 3 to 5 mg/kg/h.[7,11]

Nonconvulsive status epilepticus (NCSE) represents an under-recognized and more clinically challenging type of generalized status seizure.[12] This is an important diagnosis to consider for any patient with AMS, especially those patients with seizure disorders, histories of recent seizures, or patients who are comatose with no readily identifiable structural, metabolic, or traumatic causes.[13–15] NCSE is estimated to account for up to 20% of all cases of SE.[16] However, in one study, 8% to 10% of all unconscious patient admissions to an intensive care unit had NCSE.[17] The true prevalence of NCSE in ED patients with no apparent cause of AMS is unknown.[16] NCSE results in a wide spectrum of clinical presentations and therefore should be prominent on the list of differential considerations for AMS in the ED.[12] Clues to the diagnosis include prolonged (>1 hour) postictal state in patients with a recent convulsive seizure; behavioral abnormalities such as agitation or bizarre behavior; and subtle myoclonus, chewing, blinking, staring, nystagmus, somnolence, or coma. In some instances, confusion, personality change, or nystagmus may be the only presenting signs.

It is estimated that approximately 14 % of patients with CSE evolve into NCSE after their tonic-clonic event ceases.[12] Husain and colleagues[15] prospectively identified signs and symptoms predictive of NCSE in patients for whom an urgent electroencephalogram (EEG) was requested during a 6 month period. All patients were evaluated by neurology residents before the EEG. Patients were dichotomized into those with and those without NCSE. Remote risk factors for seizures, ocular movement abnormalities, and a low Glasgow coma scale (GCS) score were the only 3 variables that reached a statistically significant difference. Ocular movement abnormalities had the greatest specificity (86%). There were no differences recent seizure risk factors, tonic-clonic activity, history of epilepsy, or subtle motor activity.

In the elderly, NCSE can be challenging to diagnose because clinical findings are often inappropriately attributed to other causes (cerebrovascular accident, transient ischemic attack).[16] Therefore, the diagnosis can be delayed for as many as 5 days. Although NCSE does not usually result in secondary complications of convulsive SE such as hyperthermia, rhabdomyolysis, hyperkalemia, and cardiovascular collapse, it nonetheless represents a neurologic emergency that must be identified and treated rapidly; delay in management (as in CSE) can lead to an increasingly refractory state.

Prompt management of NCSE may be hindered by the requirement of an EEG for confirmation of diagnosis.[12,15,18] Although some institutions have incorporated abbreviated EEGs in the ED evaluation of patients with AMS,[19] most hospitals do not have this capability on a 24/7 basis. The reliance on obtaining a cumbersome test such as an EEG on a comatose, intubated ED patient poses a significant logistical barrier to rapid diagnosis in the ED. Advanced imaging technology such as dynamic brain perfusion computed tomography (PCT) may provide a more clinically relevant mode of rapidly securing this subtle diagnosis. Hauf and colleagues[20] showed that PCT-acquired perfusion maps of patients with NCSE have a significantly higher regional cerebral blood flow compared with the similarly matched patients who are comatose and without NCSE. They found a 78% sensitivity of PCT for diagnosing NCSE. However, until this approach is prospectively validated and widely available there is no substitute for astute clinical suspicion and empirical therapy in the challenging patient with AMS. Treatment mirrors that of convulsive SE with initial benzodiazepines followed by traditional antiepileptic drug (AED) regimens. The long-term neurologic outcomes of patients with NCSE are not known[14] because many of these patients have concomitant, equally critical conditions such as hypoxic brain injury, shock, and metabolic derangements. Published mortality proportions are as varied as the clinical spectrum, with percentages as low as 6% and as high as 44%.[20] Despite the paucity of robust, long-term neurologic outcome data, expert consensus opinion is that NCSE must be treated in an expeditious fashion.[7,13,14]

PROVOKED SEIZURES

There are a variety of conditions and exposures associated with seizure activity. Provoked seizures can be caused by extrinsic or intrinsic factors (**Box 1**). Provoked seizures, by definition, do not recur once the inciting event or condition is removed. Because treatment is aimed at concurrently abating the seizure and removing the inciting cause, it is helpful to approach patients with provoked seizure based on cause. Inciting factors such as metabolic derangements, drugs, toxins, withdrawal syndromes, infectious and inflammatory causes, and structural lesions represent most provoked seizures. This article provides a brief overview of each of the major causes, and when appropriate, cause-specific ED intervention beyond standardized ED seizure management.

PSEUDOSEIZURES

Psychogenic seizures, or pseudoseizures, are functional events that may be associated with AMS, abnormal movements, and autonomic changes. They are not the result of abnormal central nervous system (CNS) electrical activity. Psychogenic seizures may be primarily motor and mimic convulsive generalized seizures, including refractory SE, or they may be nonconvulsive and resemble absence or complex partial seizures.

The ED evaluation of these patients is difficult, because seizures and pseudoseizures can coexist. All but obviously functional abnormalities should be treated as for true ictus pending formal neurologic evaluation. Many patients with pseudoseizures are not deliberately attempting to mislead the examining physician. Confirmation of the diagnosis may require simultaneous video and EEG recording, and long-term treatment may include intensive psychotherapy.

METABOLIC CAUSES

At the most fundamental level of evaluating a patient with AMS in the ED is an assessment for 2 easily identifiable and reversible metabolic insults: hypoglycemia and hypoxemia. Oxygen and glucose are essential substrates for proper brain function and, when absent, can result in diminished mental status and seizures.[21] Hypoxemia can be caused by numerous disease states, most of which are readily reversed with supplemental oxygen, with active assisted breathing or by positive pressure ventilation. Hypoxemic seizures can result from systemic disease (pulmonary, systemic, or cardiac-induced hypoxemia) and cardiac arrhythmias including bradyarrhythmias (heart block, sick sinus syndrome) and tachydysrhythmias (nonsustained ventricular tachycardia and torsade de pointes).

With universal availability of bedside glucometers, hypoglycemia and hyperglycemia can be assessed in less than a minute in the out-of-hospital and ED environments. Although hypoglycemia is the more important and time-sensitive glucose abnormality, extreme hyperglycemia can also result in AMS and seizures. Hyperosmolar

Box 1
Causes of provoked seizures

- Drugs of Abuse
  - Alcohol
  - Stimulants
    - Amphetamine/methamphetamine
    - Cocaine
  - Lysergic acid diethylamide (LSD)
  - Phencyclidine (PCP)
  - Ecstasy
  - Herbal products
    - Guarana
    - Ma huang
- Iatrogenic (medications)
  - Antibiotics
    - Penicillins
    - Rifampin
    - Isonazid
  - Antiarrhythmic agents
    - Local anesthetics
      - Lidocaine
      - Procainamide
      - Bupivicaine
    - Cardiac medications
      - Propafenone (Rythmol)
  - Pain medications
    - Aspirin
    - Tramadol (Ultram)
    - Demerol
    - Propoxyphene
  - Antidepressants
    - Cyclic antidepressants
    - Bupropion
  - Antipsychotics
    - Cozapine
    - Haloperidol
- Metabolic Disorders
  - Hypoglycemia/hyperglycemia
  - Hypoxia
  - Hyponatremia/hypernatremia
  - Hypocalcemia[a]
  - Hypomagnesemia[a]
- Infectious/Inflammatory
  - Meningitis
    - Bacterial
    - Viral
    - Fungal
  - Cerebral abscess
  - Cerebritis
    - Lyme disease
    - Neurosyphillis
    - Lupus
  - Encephalitis
    - Herpes viruses
    - Cytomegalovirus
    - West Nile Virus
  - Non–central nervous system (CNS) infections
    - Salmonella
    - Rotovirus
- Lesions
  - Tumors
  - Intracranial hemorrhage
  - Ischemic stroke
- Systemic Causes
  - Eclampsia
  - Extreme fever
  - Thyrotoxicosis
- Miscellaneous
  - Trauma
  - Posterior reversible encephalopathy syndrome

[a] Seizure may be hypoxic and from prolonged QT syndrome with nonsustained torsade de pointes. Please refer to the text.

hyperglycemic states (HHS) can result in AMS and seizures secondary to profound dehydration.[22] After initial airway, breathing, and circulation stabilization, treatment focuses on volume replacement, insulin therapy, potassium replacement, and identification and treatment of inciting factors such as infection and myocardial infarction.[22]

Several electrolyte abnormalities can cause AMS and seizures.[22,23] Seizures are most commonly seen with abnormalities in sodium, calcium, magnesium, and phosphorous balance. Hyponatremia, defined as serum sodium concentrations less than 135 mEq/L, is caused by a broad variety of conditions that are also discussed in an article by Jennifer J. Casaletto elsewhere in this issue. In general, the causes are in 4 general categories: the syndrome of inappropriate antidiuretic hormone (SIADH) secretion, renal salt wasting, medication associated, and water intoxication.[24] The rapidity of the decrease in concentration, in addition to the absolute level, determines the clinical presentation, with the former being the more influential factor. As with all electrolytes and osmotically active particles, rapid changes result in more profound effects. In the case of sodium, a decline of greater than 0.5mEq/L/h is believed to result in serious effects.[23] Cerebral osmolar homeostasis can be maintained for slow changes in sodium by excretion of other ions and osmotically active particles. When the rate of decline exceeds the homeostasic capabilities of brain tissue, intracellular water shifts and results in cerebral edema.[23] Patients may start to become symptomatic at sodium concentrations less than 129 mEq/L; however, most symptomatic patients have levels less than 120 mEq/L.[23,24] Symptoms can include confusion, nausea, vomiting, lethargy, hypothermia, and, in the most severe cases, seizures, coma, brain herniation, and death.

Treatment depends on the clinical symptoms and degree of hyponatremia. It is important not to correct sodium too rapidly, especially for the most common presentation, which is chronic hyponatremia. Overaggressive correction of chronic and acute hyponatremia can result in development of the osmotic demyelination syndrome (ODS). ODS is believed to be caused by extreme osmotic stress in the areas of the brain that are least resistant to these changes; the central pons, basal ganglia, and cerebellum. Clinically, this syndrome has a spectrum of presentation ranging from AMS to focal abnormalities as extreme as quadraparesis or pseudobulbar palsy, coma, or death. Avoidance of ODS depends on tightly controlling the rate of sodium correction to less than 8 mEq/L/24 h.

In situations in which the sodium must be corrected emergently (ie, hyponatremia-related seizures), treatment should be initiated using 3% saline infusion. Kacprowicz and Lloyd[23] describe a simple formula for emergency sodium correction, 1 mL/kg body weight of 3% saline per hour, which will result in an increase of 1 mEq/L Na per hour. Kacprowicz and Lloyd[23]also advocate treatment until 1 of 3 end points are reached: resolution of symptoms, serum sodium reaches 120 mEq/L, or the daily limit of 8 mEq/L is reached. It is essential to monitor the serum sodium hourly during infusion to avoid overshooting the target sodium level.

Hypernatremia, defined as a serum sodium greater than 150 mEq/L, can be a cause of AMS, coma, and seizures. As serum sodium levels increase to more than 158 mEq/L, neurologic symptoms progress from irritability and restlessness to ataxia and hyperreflexia, and, ultimately, seizures and coma.[24] Emergency treatment of hypernatremia-related seizures is volume resuscitation with normal saline until adequate tissue perfusion occurs. One of the best indicators of adequate perfusion is urine output of at least 0.5 mL/kg/h. It is important not to exceed 10 to 15 mEq/L/d reduction, especially in cases of chronic hypernatremia.

Calcium abnormalities can also lead to AMS and seizures. Hypocalcemia, defined as an ionized serum calcium level less than 2.0 mEq/L, can cause many neurologic signs, including impaired memory, confusion, tetany, and seizures. It will also result in a prolonged QT interval, which may incite the development of torsade de pointes. This polymorphic ventricular tachycardia may lead to a hypoxemic seizure and represents an important seizure mimic to consider. In patients with suspected hypocalcemia-induced seizures, in addition to standard ED antiseizure care, administration of 10 mL of 10% calcium chloride solution can be given IV over 10 to 20 minutes.

Hypercalcemia, defined as serum ionized calcium levels in excess of 2.7 mEq/L, is usually due to hyperparathyroidism or malignancy. It can also cause AMS and seizures. Although definitive normalization of serum calcium levels involve numerous medications, for emergency hypercalcemia-related seizures and mental status changes, the highest priority is to replenish volume status, correct associated electrolyte abnormalities (hypokalemia and hypomagnesemia can be seen in up to one-third of patients with significant hypercalcemia), and increase the renal elimination of calcium. Normal saline rehydration, followed by low-dose furosemide, addresses the most time-sensitive issues. The remainder of hypercalcemia regimens (pamidronate, zoledronate, calcitonin, glucocorticoids) can be delayed until after stabilization is achieved. In patients with acute or chronic renal failure, emergency hemodialysis should be considered.[23] Although cardiac manifestations usually predominate in the clinical picture of patients with hypomagnesemia, low magnesium and phosphate levels can present with AMS, coma, and seizures.

DRUGS/TOXINS

In addition to metabolic derangements leading to seizures, EPs must also consider over-the-counter and prescription medications, drugs of abuse, toxins, and herbal preparations as potential causes for patients who present with AMS and concomitant seizure activity. A comprehensive review of all potential seizure-causing agents is beyond the scope of this article, but the interested reader will find excellent reviews by Wills and Erickson[25] and Kunisaki and Augenstein[26] useful. **Box 2** shows 2 helpful mnemonics of the more commonly encountered causes of toxin-induced seizures.[25] Those toxins that should provoke important or unique ED seizure management are discussed in the next section.

Several neurochemical pathways (**Table 2**) are associated with toxin-induced seizures. Although all of the mechanisms are important, a few ED-relevant mechanisms deserve special consideration. First, GABA serves as a primary inhibitory neurotransmitter of the brain. There are 2 classes of GABA receptors, $GABA_A$ and $GABA_B$. The former receptor is primarily responsible for inhibitory effects most relevant to seizure-related problems. When agonists bind to the $GABA_A$ receptor, chloride ions enter the cell causing the cell membrane to be hyperpolarized (ie, creates a more negative resting potential across the cell membrane), which in turn inhibits depolarization. Benzodiazepines (the cornerstone of seizure therapy), most sedative hypnotics, barbiturates, and alcohol exert their inhibitory effects by binding allosterically (ie, binding to a site other than its active site) to the $GABA_A$ receptor, making it more sensitive to the effects of GABA.[27] Next, glutamate, an excitatory amino acid neurotransmitter, binds to its receptors, resulting in influx of sodium or calcium ions that, in turn, leads to depolarization.[25] NMDA receptors bind glutamate and play an important role in withdrawal seizures, as discussed later. Phencyclidine (PCP) and ketamine are NMDA antagonists, and their use in healthy patients induces AMS characterized by dissociation, disorganization, hallucinations, and delusions. Sodium channel blockade, autonomic overstimulation by norepinephrine (NE), and cholinergic overstimulation may also play a role in certain ingestion and withdrawal syndromes.[25]

Box 2
Mnemonics for drug- and toxin-associated seizures

Otis Campbell

- **O**rganophosphates
- **T**ricyclic antidepressants (TCAs)
- **I**soniazid (INH), insulin
- **S**ympathomimetics
- **C**ocaine, camphor
- **A**mphetamines, anticholinergics
- **M**ethylxanthines (theophylline, caffeine)
- **P**CP
- **B**enzodiazepine withdrawal, botanicals (water hemlock)
- **E**thanol withdrawal
- **L**ithium, lidocaine
- **L**ead, lindane

With la Cops

- **W**ithdrawal from alcohol, benzodiazepines, or barbiturates
- **I**NH
- **T**heophylline and TCA
- **H**ypoglycemia, hypoxia
- **L**ead, local anesthetics, and lithium
- **A**nticholinergics, aminophylline, alpostadil, amphetamines, analgesics (meperidine, propoxyphene)
- **C**holinergics, camphor, carbon monoxide, cimetidine
- **O**granophosphates,
- **P**henothiazines, penicillins, PCP
- **S**ympathomimetics, salicylates, and strychnine

Data from Wills B, Erickson T. Chemically induced seizures. Clin Lab Med 2006;26:185–209.

ALCOHOL WITHDRAWAL SEIZURES

With chronic alcohol and GABA agonist use, GABA receptor concentrations and numerous other neurotransmitter receptor alterations occur in the brain. In acute alcohol withdrawal, multiple receptor and neurotransmitter alterations culminate in a generalized hyperexcitable state that may lead to seizures.[28] Alcohol withdrawal seizures usually occur within 6 to 48 hours after the last alcoholic drink,[29] and these are treated with supportive care and benzodiazepines titrated to control withdrawal symptoms. Large doses of benzodiazepines may be required. Folate, thiamine, and magnesium administration remain important adjuncts to consider when treating these patients. Unless complicated by SE, routine alcohol withdrawal seizures do not require acute or chronic subsequent anticonvulsant therapy.[8] See also the article by Pitzele and Tolia elsewhere in this issue for further exploration of this topic.

Table 2
Mechanisms of drug/toxin–induced seizures

Receptor Mechanism	Effect	Examples
GABA	Inhibitory	Alcohol and benzodiazepine withdrawal
NMDA receptor	Excitatory	Glutamate, glycine
Sodium channel blockade	Therapeutic levels: seizure protective Overdose: leads to seizure	Lidocaine Bupivicaine Carbamazepine Tricyclic antidepressants Propoxephene
Norepeinephrine	Excitatory	Alcohol withdrawal Sympathomimetics
Acetylcholine	Excitatory in acetylcholine overstimulation	Carbamates Organophosphates Nerve agents
Adenosine receptors	Agonists: inhibit glutamate release and cause an anticonvulsant effect Antagonism: increased seizures	Theophylline Caffeine
Histamine	Anticonvulsant effects	Antihistamines (toxic levels)

Stimulant Drugs of Abuse

There are numerous stimulant drugs that, in overdose, can cause seizures and AMS. They are categorized as direct acting, which bind to and directly stimulate α and β receptors, or indirect, which cause a presynaptic release of catecholamines and transmitters (NE, dopamine, and serotonin) to exert their effects. Cocaine, methamphetamine, and amphetamines represent indirect-acting sympathomimetic drugs of abuse. There are also numerous herbal preparations that produce similar effects.[30] These include ma huang, which contains ephedrine alkaloids similar in structure to amphetamine but are direct-acting sympathomimetics. Ephedra alkaloids are structurally similar to, weaker in potency than, and used as a precursor in the manufacturing of methamphetamine.[30] Khat, *Catha edulis*, is a plant in East Africa that is widely used as a stimulant. Its active component, cathinone, acts as an indirect sympathomimetic by stimulating presynaptic release of dopamine and other neurotransmitters. Dependence, toxicity, and withdrawal symptoms are similar to those of other sympathomimetics.

In excess concentrations, the methylxanthines, caffeine and theophylline, can also cause seizures and AMS. They exert their effect via an indirect mechanism (release of NE), by adenosine antagonism, and through phosphodiesterase inhibition.[30,31] In addition to the usual commercial preparations of caffeine, there are herbal preparations that are more potent. Guarana, *Paullina cupana*, is a shrub that has a large amount of caffeine and other xanthine alkaloids. Guarana seeds are ground into a powder and used to brew a variety of beverages. Mate is a stimulant made from the South American plant *Ilex paraguariensis*, and its leaves contain caffeine as well as theobromine and theophylline. As with other causes of caffeine toxicity, these patients have many of the classic symptoms of the sympathomimetic syndrome and may manifest cardiac arrhythmias, AMS, and seizures.

Stimulant drugs of abuse can result in a classic sympathomimetic toxidrome that includes agitation, tachycardia, hypertension, hyperthermia, diaphoresis, and mydriasis. It can further progress to rhabdomyolysis, seizures, and coma.[25,29,30] Cocaine and amphetamines cause an increase in the release of NE and serotonin. Seizures are believed to be secondary to the serotonergic effects. Treatment involves hydration, sedation with benzodiazepines, and aggressive hyperthermia control. For suspected cocaine toxicity, β-blockers are contraindicated because they would leave the α-agonist activity of cocaine unopposed. If SE develops, phenobarbital is the preferred anticonvulsant.[25]

There are numerous medications that lead to seizures as idiosyncratic reactions or from CNS toxicity when their concentrations are increased. Antibiotics, analgesics, psychiatric medications, local anesthetics, cellular toxins, and medications with anticholinergic and cholinergic profiles are discussed later in this article.

Antibiotics

Penicillin has been associated with seizures when given intramuscularly and intravenously in high doses.[32] This ictal activity is believed to result from a penicillin-induced allosteric change in the GABA receptor, resulting in decreased inhibition. Treatment is with GABA agonist agents such as benzodiazepines and barbiturates.

Isoniazid (INH) is an antituberculosis medication that is structurally similar to nicotinic acid, nicotinamide adenine dinucleotide (NAD), and pyridoxine (vitamin B_6). INH alters the metabolism of pyridoxine and creates a functional deficiency of this important cofactor. Specifically, pyridoxine is used by glutamic acid decarboxylase to synthesize GABA from glutamic acid. In toxicity, INH-induced seizures are believed to be a result of this GABA depletion. In addition, INH inhibits oxidative phosphorylation and causes a profound metabolic acidosis in toxic doses.[25,33] Toxicity can develop following 20 mg/kg ingestions, and seizures are almost universally present after ingestions of more than 35 mg/kg. The classic clinical triad for INH toxicity is intractable seizures, profound anion gap metabolic acidosis, and coma. Toxicity is treated supportively with airway management, activated charcoal, benzodiazepines, and fluids, in addition to the antidote, pyridoxine.[25] The dose is a gram-for-gram replacement with pyridoxine if the INH dose is known. The initial dose in cases with an unknown INH dose is 5 g for adults and 70 mg/kg for children (not to exceed 5 g). Pyridoxine is given at a rate of 1 g over 2 to 3 minutes. If seizures do not abate, an additional 5 g should be administered.[33] In addition to aborting the seizures, pyridoxine will also improve the metabolic acidosis and reverse the comatose state.[33,34] In terms of logistics, it is important to know the availability of pyridoxine at your institution. Many hospital pharmacies do not have sufficient stocks to treat a seriously poisoned patient. Borrowing from other community hospitals, state stockpiles, and crushing the pill form of pyridoxine to deliver the dose via gastric tube are all potential solutions.

Analgesics

Propoxyphene, meperidine, and tramadol are all opioids that can cause seizures. Ten percent of patients will develop seizures after overdosing on propoxyphene. The exact mechanism is unknown, the EP must remember that propoxyphene has sodium channel blockade effects, which in overdose can manifest as tricyclic antidepressant (TCA)–like toxicity. Analogous to TCA overdose (discussed later), QRS widening and cardiotoxicity should be expected; however, propoxyphene overdoses with these cardiac manifestations do respond to sodium bicarbonate.[35] Treatment of seizures involves standard approaches such as benzodiazepines, with phenobarbital if needed.[36] Propoxyphene formulations are combined with aspirin or acetaminophen, so it is important to maintain a high clinical suspicion for these cotoxins when evaluating patients. Meperidine is metabolized to normeperidine, which, in toxic doses, can cause seizures through excitatory neurotoxicity. These seizures do not abate with naloxone, but are usually responsive to standard antiseizure management. Tramadol, a synthetic analgesic with opioid and nonopioid properties, differs from propoxyphene and meperidine because of its ability to cause seizures at therapeutic doses. These seizures may occur in the first 24 hours of initiation of therapy, although the exact mechanism is unknown.[36]

Salicylates (eg, acetylsalicylic acid [ASA]) represent the most important nonopiate analgesic that, in toxic doses, can result in AMS and seizures. Following a toxic ingestion, ASA causes stimulation of the respiratory center in the brainstem and uncoupling of oxidative phosphorylation, resulting in a profound metabolic acidosis. In addition, ASA toxicity can cause hypoglycemia by increasing glucose consumption, inhibition of gluconeogenesis, and enhancing insulin secretion. CNS excitation predominates during the initial phase of salicylate toxicity. Seizures can be seen as a result of cerebral edema, hypoxia, or low CNS glucose.[37] Treatment of seizures related to salicylate toxicity is aimed at rapid management of hypoglycemia, early airway management, alkalinization of the urine to facilitate ion trapping and to decrease CNS salicylate concentrations, and standard antiseizure management with benzodiazepines, and, if needed, phenobarbitol or phenytoin.

Psychiatric Medications

Cyclic antidepressant (CA) medications lead to seizures due to their numerous pharmacologic effects. TCAs, in particular, possess anticholinergic, NE reuptake inhibition, sodium channel blockade, antihistamine, and antidopaminergic effects, all of which can contribute to AMS and seizures associated with overdose. Moreover, CA medications can have serious cardiac and CNS toxicity. AMS, seizures, and coma can be seen in CA overdose. Seizures are usually generalized and occur within 1 to 2 hours after ingestion.[38] Although most CA-related seizures are self-limited, when prolonged they can be associated with an increased risk of ventricular dysrhythmias and hypotension. Sodium loading and serum alkalinization with sodium bicarbonate is the mainstay treatment of CA-related cardiotoxicity.[38,39] If seizure treatment is necessary, CA-related seizures generally respond to benzodiazepines. Phenobarbital or propofol can be used if initial benzodiazepines are ineffective.[38] Phenytoin should be avoided because it may worsen the cardiotoxic effects of CA overdose.[25,38] Buproprion is classified as an atypical antidepressant; it inhibits the reuptake of dopamine, NE, and serotonin by an unclear mechanism. Seizures can occur in overdose, probably caused by the metabolite hydroxybuproprion. Seizures are treated with benzodiazepines and phenobarbital.[25,40]

Many of the atypical and typical antipsychotic medications can result in generalized seizures in overdose. In general, these seizures are usually self-limited and respond favorably to benzodiazepines and phenobarbital. As with all medications that are proconvulsant and cardiotoxic, rapid termination of the seizure is critical because, as the seizure persists, a more profound metabolic acidosis develops, further potentiating cardiac toxicity from these agents.[38]

Lithium deserves special mention as a psychiatric medication that can lead to AMS and seizures in toxic doses. Lithium is a monovalent cation that is used to treat bipolar disorder. Although its exact mechanism of action is unknown, the strongest theory suggests that lithium causes depletion of inositol, a sugar involved in a variety of cellular signaling mechanisms. Lithium can increase serotonin release and receptor sensitivity and stabilizes intracellular c-AMP.[41] Neurotoxicity manifests as tremors, AMS, and seizures. Treatment of lithium-related seizures involves treating the underlying cause with IV fluids, hemodialysis, and standard seizure management with benzodiazepines.[25,41,42]

Local Anesthetics

Another commonly used class of medications that can cause seizures and AMS are the local anesthetics. Medications that produce sodium channel blockade can result in seizure activity. Lidocaine and related anesthetics exert their effects through such sodium channel blockade, readily cross the blood-brain barrier, and can cause seizures when inadvertently injected intravascularly or when administered in toxic doses. It is not clear whether the proconvulsant action occurs by blocking of normal inhibitory processes (GABA inhibition)[43] or by some other unknown mechanism.[25] Anatomically, they block inhibitory neurons in the amygdala, resulting in a decrease in the seizure threshold.[43,44] CNS toxicity is directly related to the potency of the anesthetic (bupivicaine>tetracaine>lidocaine) and the rate of administration. For lidocaine, CNS symptoms begin to appear at serum concentrations between 5 and 9 μg/mL, and seizures occur at 10 μg/mL.[44] Signs and symptoms of CNS and cardiac toxicity appear in a predictable sequence during gradual increases in serum lidocaine levels. Initially, numbness of the tongue, lightheadedness, and visual and auditory symptoms predominate; then muscle twitching, AMS, loss of consciousness, seizures, coma, respiratory arrest, and cardiac arrest occur.[43,44] It is therefore critical for EPs to maintain a high vigilance for these progressive symptoms during injection of local anesthetics because they signal systemic toxicity, and, with the exception of direct vertebral or carotid injection, these minor symptoms usually herald seizures and cardiac toxicity.[43,44] Most anesthetic-related seizures are self-limited; however, when they are sustained, treatment with benzodiazepines or thiopental (induction dose 3–5 mg/kg IV) has been advocated. Propofol, because of its delivery in a lipid emulsion, has been advocated by some investigators for management of CNS and cardiac toxicity, but this remains controversial and there is insufficient evidence to recommend its routine use in this setting.[25,43,45]

Cellular Toxins

Any cellular toxin can cause seizures secondary to cellular hypoxia. Because of their unique ED treatments, carbon monoxide (CO) and iron toxicities are discussed here. CO toxicity can manifest with decreased mental status and seizures.[25,46] These seizures are believed to be a direct result of cellular and tissue hypoxia from toxic carboxyhemoglobin levels. Treatment of CO-related seizures involves early airway management with 100% oxygen, benzodiazepines, and hyperbaric oxygen treatment, if available.[46,47] Iron toxicity disrupts mitochondrial oxidative phosphorylation and results in a series of metabolic and physiologic effects including a profound metabolic acidosis, hypovolemia, and shock.[47] Iron toxicity is classically categorized into 5 stages. Patients with a serious iron overdose can develop seizures during the third phase (12–24 hours after a major ingestion) of the iron toxicity syndrome. These stages are not distinct, and treatment should be based on the patient's clinical presentation rather than their perceived stage of toxicity. Treatment of iron overdose includes aggressive fluid resuscitation, whole bowel irrigation, administration of deferoxamine, correction of coagulopathy, and routine seizure control with benzodiazepines.[25,47,48]

Medications Affecting Nicotinic and Muscarinic Receptors

Anticholinergic agents, including antihistamines such as diphenhydramine, can result in AMS and seizures at toxic doses. Seizures should be treated with repeated doses of benzodiazepines and, in refractory cases, phenobarbital or propofol.[49] Although physostigmine may have additional benefits in managing delerium in anticholinergic poisoning,[50] there is insufficient evidence to recommend routine use in patients exhibiting seizures, and consultation with a toxicologist is recommended.

Toxicity from organophosphates (OGP) such as dichlorodiphenyltrichloroethane (DDT) and hexachlorocyclohexane (lindane) can result in seizures, presumably from GABA receptor antagonism. Treatment should be aimed at skin decontamination, early airway management, and standard seizure regimens with benzodiazepines and barbiturates.[25,51] With severe OGP toxicity, muscarinic symptoms are controlled with IV atropine 1 mg (pediatric dose 0.01 mg/kg) IV every 5 minutes until secretions are dry and pralidoxime (2-PAM) to displace the OGP from the cholinesterases. The 2-PAM dose is 1 to 2 g (pediatric dose 25 mg/kg given at 10–20mg/kg/h; up to 1 g) in normal saline given over 10 minutes.[51]

SYSTEMIC CAUSES OF PROVOKED SEIZURES

Infectious Causes

Various systemic and CNS infections can be associated with AMS and seizures. Systemic infections, such as gastroenteritis caused by Shigella and rotavirus, are associated with seizures.[52] These seizures are usually self-limited and do not require long-term anticonvulsant therapy. Shigellosis can be associated with encephalopathy, hypoglycemia, and sepsis, all of which may contribute to an ictal episode. Priorities include recognition and treatment of hypoglycemia, appropriate broad spectrum antibiotics, and aggressive sepsis resuscitation.[53,54] CNS pathologies include infections and inflammation of the meninges (meningitis), the brain tissue (encephalitis), the spinal cord (myelitis), and cerebral or epidural abscesses.[55] Initial treatment is targeted at treating bacterial causes using appropriate broad spectrum antibiotics followed by antiviral agents until exact organisms and antibiotic sensitivities are known. Seizures usually respond to standard benzodiazepine and antiseizure regimens.[55]

Structural Lesions

Seizures in cancer patients can occur with primary or metastatic brain tumors, metabolic derangements, or as a result of radiation or chemotherapy. Patients with CNS tumors may present with AMS, signs or symptoms of increased intracranial pressure, NCSE, or seizures.[56,57] New-onset seizure is the presenting symptom in 20% to 40% of patients with CNS tumors. Depending on the tumor type, 30% to 60% of CNS tumor patients will manifest a seizure at some point in their clinical course, as will 13% of all cancer patients.[56] In general, seizures caused by structural lesions are most often simple partial or complex partial seizures. CSE is rare, usually due to metabolic derangements, and, when occurring in the setting of a CNS tumor, carries a high mortality. Chemotherapeutic agents and hemorrhage into CNS tumors can also cause seizures in cancer patients. Posterior reversible encephalopathy (PRS), previously known as reversible posterior leukoencephalopathy syndrome, is associated with some chemotherapy agents and numerous nonmalignant conditions such as lupus, chronic renal failure (dialysis disequilibrium syndrome), high-dose steroid use, hypertensive encephalopathy, and eclampsia.[56,58,59] It is classically described as a clinical pentad consisting of headache, AMS, generalized seizures, visual symptoms, and computerized tomography (CT)/magnetic resonance imaging (MRI) findings of posterior cerebral white matter vasogenic edema. Altered mental status can span the entire spectrum from confusion to generalized seizures and coma.[56,58] Treatment is aimed at lowering blood pressure and achieving routine seizure control with benzodiazepines.[58] Encephalitis, meningitis, and leptomeningeal metastatic (LM) disease can all result in seizures and AMS. LM disease occurs in 8% of all cancer patients. Although any metastatic cancer can spread to the meninges, those cancers that most commonly lead to LM disease are leukemia, breast cancer, non–small cell carcinoma, and melanoma.[56] Similar to multiple sclerosis presentations, LM disease classically presents with poorly localized and diffuse neurologic symptoms. Cerebral spinal fluid (CSF) findings are important for the EP to consider because approximately 50% of patients have increased opening CSF pressure, 70% have a pleocytosis, and 80% have an increased CSF protein.[56] Definitive diagnosis is based on cytology, and the prognosis is generally poor.

Eclampsia is a pregnancy-associated complication that causes AMS and seizures in 0.1% of deliveries in the United States, and can occur ante partum (91% of cases occur after 28 weeks of gestation), in the peripartal period, or up to 4 weeks post partum.[60] Abortive treatment of eclamptic seizures is with magnesium sulfate, which is superior to diazepam or phenytoin in limiting maternal mortality and preventing further seizures.[61] Because hypermagnesemia may cause respiratory arrest, it is essential to monitor patients for hyporeflexia, which precedes respiratory compromise. Simultaneous reduction in blood pressure is also recommended.[62]

SUMMARY

The differential diagnosis and empirical management of AMS often overlap with that for seizures. AMS may accompany seizures or simply be the manifestation of a postictal state. Ictal activity or concern for NCSE in a patient with AMS should prompt immediate consideration for anticonvulsant therapy (typically with benzodiazepines) and a search for a reversible cause (hypoxemia, hypoglycemia, toxic exposure). Traditional definitions of SE are impractical, and EPs should use a more appropriate operational definition of SE that prompts early aggressive treatment after 5 minutes of sustained seizure activity. Successful cessation of SE is dependent on time, in part because of the rapid development of receptor pharmacoresistance. Emergency physicians should maintain a high level of suspicion for NCSE for those patients who are comatose with no readily identifiable structural, metabolic, or traumatic cause. For many toxin-related seizures unresponsive to benzodiazepines, phenobarbital is the preferred first-line AED. As with all medications that are proconvulsant and cardiotoxic, rapid termination of the seizure is critical because prolonged seizures potentiate cardiac toxicity from these agents. Other special cases such as pregnancy-related seizures or seizures from CO poisoning, with accompanying AMS, necessitate an overall approach to management tailored to the specific situation.

REFERENCES

1. Engel JJ, Starkman S. Overview of seizures. Emerg Med Clin North Am 1994;12(4):895–923.
2. Huff J, Morris D, Kothari R, et al. Emergency department management of patients with seizures: a multicenter study. Acad Emerg Med 2001;8(6):622–8.
3. Duviver EH, Pollack CV. Seizures. In: Marx JA, editor. Rosen's emergency medicine: concepts and clinical practice. 7th edition. Philadelphia: Mosby Elsevier; 2010. p. 1346–55.
4. Goldstein JN, Greer DM. Rapid focused neurological assessment in the emergency department and ICU. Emerg Med Clin North Am 2009;27(1):1–16, vii.
5. Chen J, Wasterlain C. Status epilepticus: pathophysiology and management in adults. Lancet Neurol 2006;5(3):246–56.
6. Lowenstein D, Bleck T, Macdonald R. It's time to revise the definition of status epilepticus. Epilepsia 1999;40(1):120–2.

7. Millikan D, Rice B, Silbergleit R. Emergency treatment of status epilepticus: current thinking. Emerg Med Clin North Am 2009;27(1):101–13, ix.
8. Catlett C. Seizures and status epilepticus in adults. In: Tintinalli JE, editor. Emergency medicine: a comprehensive study guide. 6th edition. New York (NY): McGraw-Hill; 2004. p. 1409–17.
9. Goodkin H, Kapur J. Responsiveness of status epilepticus to treatment with diazepan decreases rapidly as seizure duration increases. Epilepsy Curr 2003;3(1):11–2.
10. Kapur J, Macdonald R. Rapid seizure-induced reduction of benzodiazepine and Zn^{2+} sensitivity of hippocampal dentate granule cell GABAA receptors. J Neurosci 1997;17(19):7532–40.
11. Knake S, Hamer H, Rosenow F. Status epilepticus: a critical review. Epilepsy Behav 2009;15(1):10–4.
12. Bearden S, Eisenschenk S, Uthman B. Diagnosis of nonconvulsive status epilepticus (NCSE) in adults with altered mental status: clinico-electroencephalographic considerations. Am J Electroneurodiagnostic Technol 2008;48(1):11–37.
13. Drislane FW, Lopez MR, Blum AS, et al. Detection and treatment of refractory status epilepticus in the intensive care unit. J Clin Neurophysiol 2008;25(4):181–6.
14. Drislane FW. Evidence against permanent neurologic damage from nonconvulsive status epilepticus. J Clin Neurophysiol 1999;16(4):323–31 [discussion: 353].
15. Husain AM, Horn GJ, Jacobson MP. Non-convulsive status epilepticus: usefulness of clinical features in selecting patients for urgent EEG. J Neurol Neurosurg Psychiatry 2003;74(2):189–91.
16. Beyenburg S, Elger CE, Reuber M. Acute confusion or altered mental state: consider nonconvulsive status epilepticus. Gerontology 2007;53(6):388–96.
17. Towne A, Waterhouse E, Boggs J, et al. Prevalence of nonconvulsive status epilepticus in comatose patients. Neurology 2000;54(2):340–5.
18. Praline J, Grujic J, Corcia P, et al. Emergent EEG in clinical practice. Clin Neurophysiol 2007;118(10):2149–55.
19. Bautista RE, Godwin S, Caro D. Incorporating abbreviated EEGs in the initial workup of patients who present to the emergency room with mental status changes of unknown etiology. J Clin Neurophysiol 2007;24(1):16–21.
20. Hauf M, Slotboom J, Nirkko A, et al. Cortical regional hyperperfusion in nonconvulsive status epilepticus measured by dynamic brain perfusion CT. AJNR Am J Neuroradiol 2009;30(4):693–8.
21. Bazakis AM, Kunzler C. Altered mental status due to metabolic or endocrine disorders. Emerg Med Clin North Am 2005;23(3):901–8, x–xi.
22. Graffeo C. Hyperosmolar hyperglycemic state. In: Tintinalli J, editor. Emergency medicine: a comprehensive study guide. 6th edition. New York (NY): McGraw-Hill; 2004. p. 1307–11.
23. Kacprowicz R, Lloyd J. Electrolyte complications of malignancy. Emerg Med Clin North Am 2009;27(2):257–69.
24. Londner M. Fluid and electrolyte problems. In: Tintinalli J, editor. Emergency medicine: a comprehensive study guide. 6th edition. New York (NY): McGraw-Hill; 2004. p. 167–79.
25. Wills B, Erickson T. Chemically induced seizures. Clin Lab Med 2006;26:185–209.
26. Kunisaki T, Augenstein W. Drug- and toxin-induced seizures. Emerg Med Clin North Am 1994;12(4):1027–56.
27. Morrow E, Roffman J, Wolf D, et al. Psychiatric neuroscience: incorporating pathophysiology into clinical case formulation. In: Stern TA, Rosenbaum JF, Fava M, et al, editors. Stern: Massachusetts General Hospital comprehensive clinical psychiatry. 1st edition. Philadelphia (PA): Mosby; 2008. p. 562.

28. Hughes J. Alcohol withdrawal seizures. Epilepsy Behav 2009;15(2):92–7.
29. Tetrault J, O'Connor P. Substance abuse and withdrawal in the critical care setting. Crit Care Clin 2008;24(4):767–88, viii.
30. Richardson WH, Slone CM, Michels JE. Herbal drugs of abuse: an emerging problem [abstract ix]. Emerg Med Clin North Am 2007;25(2):435–57.
31. Perrone J. Cocaine, amphetamines, caffeine, and nicotine. In: Tintinalli J, editor. Emergency medicine: a comprehensive study guide. 6th edition. New York (NY): McGraw-Hill; 2004. p. 1075–9.
32. Jalbert E. Seizures after penicillin administration. Am J Dis Child 1985;139(11): 1075.
33. Ew B. Antituberculosis medications. In: Flomenbaum NE, Goldfrank LR, Hoffman RS, et al, editors. Goldfrank's toxicologic emergencies. 8th edition. New York (NY): McGraw-Hill; 2006. p. 861–71.
34. Brent J, Vo N, Kulig K, et al. Reversal of prolonged isoniazid-induced coma by pyridoxine. Arch Intern Med 1990;150(8):1751–3.
35. Stork C, Redd J, Fine K, et al. Propoxyphene-induced wide QRS complex dysrhythmia responsive to sodium bicarbonate–a case report. J Toxicol Clin Toxicol 1995;33(2):179–83.
36. Nelson L. Opioids. In: Flomenbaum NE, Goldfrank LR, Hoffman RS, et al, editors. Goldfrank's toxicologic emergencies. 8th edition. New York (NY): McGraw-Hill; 2006. p. 591–613.
37. Henry K, Harris C. Deadly ingestions. Pediatr Clin North Am 2006;53(2):293–315.
38. Liebelt E. Cyclic antidepressants. In: Flomenbaum NE, Goldfrank LR, Hoffman RS, et al, editors. Goldfrank's toxicologic emergencies. 8th edition. New York (NY): McGraw-Hill; 2006. p. 1083–97.
39. Michael J, Sztajnkrycer M. Deadly pediatric poisons: nine common agents that kill at low doses. Emerg Med Clin North Am 2004;22(4):1019–50.
40. Stork C. Serotonin reuptake inhibitors and atypical antidepressants. In: Flomenbaum NE, Goldfrank LR, Hoffman RS, et al, editors. Goldfrank's toxicologic emergencies. 8th edition. New York (NY): McGraw-Hill; 2006. p. 1070–82.
41. Greller HA. Lithium. In: Flomenbaum NE, Goldfrank LR, Hoffman RS, et al, editors. Goldfrank's toxicologic emergencies. 8th edition. New York (NY): McGraw-Hill; 2006. p. 1052–61.
42. Mokhlesi B, Leikin J, Murray P, et al. Adult toxicology in critical care: part II: specific poisonings. Chest 2003;123(3):897–922.
43. Dorf E, Kuntz AF, Kelsey J, et al. Lidocaine-induced altered mental status and seizure after hematoma block. J Emerg Med 2006;31(3):251–3.
44. Schwartz DR, Kaufman B. Local anesthetics. In: Flomenbaum NE, Goldfrank LR, Hoffman RS, et al, editors. Goldfrank's toxicologic emergencies. 8th edition. New York (NY): McGraw-Hill; 2006. p. 1004–15.
45. Harden C, Huff J, Schwartz T, et al. Reassessment: neuroimaging in the emergency patient presenting with seizure (an evidence-based review): report of the Therapeutics and Technology Assessment Subcommittee of the American Academy of Neurology. Neurology 2007;69(18):1772–80.
46. Kao L, Nañagas K. Carbon monoxide poisoning. Med Clin North Am 2005;89(6): 1161–94.
47. Perrone J. Iron. In: Flomenbaum NE, Goldfrank LR, Hoffman RS, et al, editors. Goldfrank's toxicologic emergencies. 8th edition. New York (NY): McGraw-Hill; 2006. p. 629–37.
48. Holstege C, Dobmeier S, Bechtel L. Critical care toxicology. Emerg Med Clin North Am 2008;26(3):715–39, viii–ix.

49. Tomassoni AJ. Antihistamines and decongestants. In: Flomenbaum NE, Goldfrank LR, Hoffman RS, et al, editors. Goldfrank's toxicologic emergencies. 8th edition. New York (NY): McGraw-Hill; 2006. p. 785–93.
50. Burns M, Linden C, Graudins A, et al. A comparison of physostigmine and benzodiazepines for the treatment of anticholinergic poisoning. Ann Emerg Med 2000; 35(4):374–81.
51. Robe WC, Meggs WJ. Insecticides, herbicides, rodenticides. In: Flomenbaum NE, Goldfrank LR, Hoffman RS, et al, editors. Goldfrank's toxicologic emergencies. 8th edition. New York (NY): McGraw-Hill; 2006. p. 1134–43.
52. Ben-Ami T, Sinai L, Granot E. Afebrile seizures and rotavirus gastroenteritis: an infrequently recognized association. Clin Pediatr (Phila) 2007;46(2):178–80.
53. Bennish M. Potentially lethal complications of shigellosis. Rev Infect Dis 1991; 13(Suppl 4):S319–24.
54. Salam M, Bennish M. Antimicrobial therapy for shigellosis. Rev Infect Dis 1991; 13(Suppl 4):S332–41.
55. Somand D, Meurer W. Central nervous system infections. Emerg Med Clin North Am 2009;27(1):89–100, ix.
56. Damek DM. Cerebral edema, altered mental status, seizures, acute stroke, leptomeningeal metastases, and paraneoplastic syndrome. Emerg Med Clin North Am 2009;27(2):209–29.
57. Antunes NL, De Angelis LM. Neurologic consultations in children with systemic cancer. Pediatr Neurol 1999;20(2):121–4.
58. Leroux G, Sellam J, Costedoat-Chalumeau N, et al. Posterior reversible encephalopathy syndrome during systemic lupus erythematosus: four new cases and review of the literature. Lupus 2008;17(2):139–47.
59. Servillo G, Bifulco F, De Robertis E, et al. Posterior reversible encephalopathy syndrome in intensive care medicine. Intensive Care Med 2007;33(2):230–6.
60. Zhang J, Meikle S, Trumble A. Severe maternal morbidity associated with hypertensive disorders in pregnancy in the United States. Hypertens Pregnancy 2003; 22(2):203–12.
61. Duley L, Henderson-Smart D. Magnesium sulphate versus diazepam for eclampsia. Cochrane Database Syst Rev 2003;4:CD000127.
62. Sibai B. Diagnosis, prevention, and management of eclampsia. Obstet Gynecol 2005;105(2):402–10.

Central Nervous System Infections as a Cause of an Altered Mental Status? What is the Pathogen Growing in Your Central Nervous System?

Sharon E. Mace, MD[a,b,c,d,e,*]

KEYWORDS

- Central nervous system • Pathogens
- Altered mental status • Infections

EPIDEMIOLOGY OF CENTRAL NERVOUS SYSTEM DISEASES

Despite antibiotics and vaccines for immunoprophylaxis, bacterial meningitis is still a common disease worldwide, with high morbidity and mortality. Meningitis can occur at any age and in previously healthy immunocompetent individuals, although some patients have a greater risk of meningitis, including the immunocompromised patient and individuals at the extremes of age (eg, the geriatric patient [age >60 years] and the pediatric patient [age <5 years]). Immunocompromised patients with an increased risk of meningitis include asplenic patients (eg, status after splenectomy or sickle cell disease), those with cirrhosis and other liver disorders, alcoholics, diabetics, anyone with immunologic disease (such as immunoglobulin deficiency, complement deficiency), individuals on immunosuppressive drugs, those with an underlying malignancy, and patients who are positive for the human immunodeficiency virus (HIV) or

[a] Department of Emergency Medicine, Cleveland Clinic Lerner College of Medicine of Case Western Reserve University, 9500 Euclid Avenue, Cleveland, OH 44195, USA
[b] Emergency Medicine Residency Program, MetroHealth Medical Center/Cleveland Clinic, 9500 Euclid Avenue, Cleveland, OH 44195, USA
[c] Pediatric Education/Quality Improvement, Cleveland Clinic, 9500 Euclid Avenue, Cleveland, OH 44195, USA
[d] Observation Unit, Cleveland Clinic, 9500 Euclid Avenue, Cleveland, OH 44195, USA
[e] Rapid Response Team, Cleveland Clinic, 9500 Euclid Avenue, Cleveland, OH 44195, USA
* Emergency Services Institute, Cleveland Clinic, E19, 9500 Euclid Avenue, Cleveland, OH 44195.
E-mail address: maces@ccf.org

Emerg Med Clin N Am 28 (2010) 535–570
doi:10.1016/j.emc.2010.03.002

who have AIDS. Encephalitis and brain abscess are less common than meningitis, although it is likely that the incidence of encephalitis is underestimated because patients with mild cases may not seek medical attention or be overlooked. Furthermore, it can be difficult to identify a specific cause in many cases of encephalitis.

DEFINITIONS

The various infections of the central nervous system (CNS) are defined based on anatomy (**Box 1, Fig. 1**). Meningitis, also known as arachnoiditis or leptomeningitis, is an inflammation of the membranes surrounding the brain and spinal cord. Thus, meningitis is an inflammation of the 2 CNS membranes (the pia mater and the arachnoid) and the interposed cerebrospinal fluid (CSF). Encephalitis is an inflammation of the brain itself, whereas myelitis is an inflammation of the spinal cord. A CNS abscess refers to a focal intracerebral collection of pus surrounded by a well-vascularized capsule (see **Fig. 1**). In reality, an infection may be more diffuse, involving more than one discrete anatomic area, which may also make it more difficult to diagnose and treat the underlying CNS infection. For example, meningoencephalitis refers to a CNS inflammation of the membranes of the brain and the brain itself, whereas encephalomyelitis denotes inflammation involving the brain and spinal cord.

PATHOPHYSIOLOGY OF CNS INFECTIONS

For any pathogen to successfully cause an infection in the CNS, the invading organism must be able to avoid the defenses of the host and to navigate through several steps. These phases include (1) colonize or enter the body, (2) travel to and gain access to the CNS, (3) multiply or replicate usually within the CNS, and (4) incite an inflammatory response (**Box 2, Fig. 2**).

First, the pathogen has to have a local portal of entry. With meningitis, most pathogens are transmitted by the respiratory route from person to person.[1] The most common bacteria that cause meningitis are *Streptococcus pneumoniae* and *Neisseria meningitides*. Both of these bacteria initially attach to the host's nasopharyngeal mucosal epithelium and colonize in the upper respiratory tract. For viruses, the initial site of entry varies.

After attaching to and colonizing the host, the pathogen must travel to and enter the CNS. There are 3 routes to the CNS: hematogenous, direct extension, or neuronal. Hematogenous spread is the most common method for pathogens, whether bacterial or viral. Bacteria may also gain entry to the CNS by direct extension from a contiguous focus, such as sinusitis, otitis media, mastoiditis, or when the integrity of the skull and meninges are breached, whether from trauma, neurosurgical procedures, or congenital malformation. The rabies virus and herpes simplex virus (HSV) gain access to the CNS from the periphery by neuronal spread: rabies via a peripheral wound to the dorsal root ganglion to the brain and HSV by the cranial nerves (either trigeminal or olfactory) to the brain.

Primary viremia or bacteremia allows the respective pathogen to seed distant locations in the body. The organism circulates in the vascular system attached either to or within host cells or as an unattached free pathogen.

The specific bacterial or viral pathogen must not only survive but also multiply in the host's tissue to obtain a critical mass or sufficient quantity to invade the CNS. With hematogenous spread, the virus often replicates at the local site of entry in addition to a primary viremia.[2] Later in the disease process, a secondary viremia or bacteremia sends high titers of the pathogen throughout the bloodstream, which seeds organs throughout the body. After attaching to the cell of the host, the virus must enter the cell then undergo replication. The host cell must be permissive to provide conditions sufficient for or an adequate environment for viral replication to occur. There are multiple steps in the viral multiplication cycle. Attachment to the host cell, then penetration into the host cell, assembly of the virions, and finally their release from the host cell by the process of budding.[2] Bacteria must also undergo multiplication to be a successful pathogen (although unlike viruses, they multiply outside the host cell).

The blood-brain barrier under normal conditions provides a physiologic boundary between CNS neuronal cells and changes outside the CNS. The endothelial cells and tight junctions act as a physical barrier to most pathogens. Whether bacterial or viral, any blood-borne pathogen must cross the blood-brain barrier from the bloodstream to cause CNS disease. Pathogens can transverse the blood-brain barrier via several mechanisms: (1) transport across the cell by endocytosis (transcellular passage) (eg, meningococci or *Streptococcus* pneumococci), (2) transport between the cells (paracellular passage) can occur after endothelial injury or following disruption of the intracellular endothelial connections, and (3) within WBCs during diapedesis. During certain disease states, the endothelial cells become damaged and the blood-brain barrier becomes porous, allowing pathogens to transverse the blood-CSF barrier (see **Fig. 2**).

Once the pathogen breaches the blood-brain barrier and enters the CNS, whether by hematogenous or nonhematogenous spread, it sets off an inflammatory reaction. Many of the manifestations and complications of CNS infections are attributed to the body's immune response to the invading organism instead of any direct pathogen-induced tissue injury.

Components of the pathogen, such as the cell wall of bacteria, trigger an inflammatory cascade. Many brain cells, including resident macrophages, endothelial cells, ependymal cells, glial cells, and astrocytes, all secrete proinflammatory molecules (specifically cytokines and chemokines) in response to a pathogen. Some of the physiologic effects of cytokines include breakdown of the blood-brain barrier, increased cerebral metabolism/oxygen consumption/cerebral blood flow, and trigger neutrophilic inflammation. Chemokines are specific types of cytokines that induce chemotactic migration in leukocytes. Some of the cytokines released with bacterial meningitis include tumor necrosis factor (TNF), and various interleukins (ILs) (eg, IL-1β, IL-6, IL-8, IL-10). These cytokines, in turn, will stimulate the release of various inflammatory mediators, ranging from NO, ROS, MMPs, to other interleukins, prostaglandins, chemokines, and platelet-activating factor.

The pathophysiologic events that result from these inflammatory processes include disruption of the blood-brain barrier, vasculitis of the arteries, thromboses of inflamed veins, cerebral ischemia from local and global changes in cerebral blood flow, loss of autoregulation of the cerebral blood flow, and even brain cell death. Early increases in cerebral blood flow in meningitis are followed by a decrease in cerebral blood flow and then a loss of autoregulation. Moreover, increased intracranial pressure (ICP) can then lead to herniation of the brain and death.

Host Defenses in the CNS

Once in the CNS, invading organisms can multiply or replicate rapidly. Reasons for this include: normal CSF contains only small amounts of immunoglobulins and complement proteins, and a limited number of WBCs; complement and immunoglobulins are needed for opsonization of bacteria, an essential first step in the phagocytosis of bacteria by neutrophils; in addition, solid tissue substrate provides a better environment for phagocytosis than fluid substrates like CSF; impaired phagocytosis enables bacteria to multiply rapidly and is one reason for poor host defenses in the CSF.

Box 1
Differential diagnosis of infections of the CNS

- Meningitis
  - Bacterial
  - Aseptic: infections with a negative Gram stain and culture or noninfectious causes
    - Infections
      - Viral
      - Bacteria with negative Gram stain and culture: bacteria with negative Gram stain with usual stain and technique and not culturable with usual media
        - Organisms not able to grow on routine culture media: *Mycobacteria*, *Treponema* (syphilis), *Mycoplasma* (tuberculosis), *Chlamydia*, *Borrelia burgdorferi* (Lyme disease)
      - Nonviral
        - Fungal
        - Meningeal inflammation secondary to adjacent pyogenic infections
        - Eosinophilic meningitis (parasitic CNS infections)
    - Noninfectious cause
      - Neoplasms (meningeal carcinomatosis or leptomeningeal carcinomatosis)
      - Systemic diseases that affect the CNS: systemic lupus erythematosis, sarcoidosis, others
      - Drugs
- Encephalitis
  - Infections
    - Viral
    - Nonviral
      - Bacteria: bacteria with negative Gram stain and culture
      - *Rickettsia*
      - Fungi
      - Protozoa
      - Helminths
- Brain abscess
  - Bacterial
  - Nonbacterial
    - Fungi
    - Protozoa
    - Parasites
- Parameningeal infections
  - Brain abscess
  - Subdural empyema
  - Epidural abscess

- Acute disseminated encephalomyelitis (ADEM)
- CNS disease
  - Hemorrhage
  - Strokes
  - Venous thrombosis
  - Aneurysms
  - Migraines/Other headaches
- Hematologic disorders
  - Hyperviscosity syndromes
    - Polycythemia
    - Leukocytosis/leukostasis
    - Platelet disorders
      - Thrombocytosis
    - Coagulopathy
- Encephalopathies
  - Metabolic
  - Hypoxia
  - Ischemia
  - Intoxications
  - Organ dysfunction
  - Systemic infection
- Delirium/dementia
- Seizures
  - Nonconvulsive status epilepticus
- Legionnaire disease
- Posttransplant lymphoproliferative disorder
- Prion diseases
- Other disorders
  - Epstein-Barr virus
  - Legionnaire disease
  - Posterior fossa syndrome

Proteases made by various bacteria, notably *Haemophilus influenza*, *N meningitides*, and *S pneumoniae*, inactivate the host's immunoglobulin A by cleaving the antibody. This destruction enables the pathogen to attach to and colonize the nasopharyngeal mucosa.

Once a virus gains access to the CNS, it must enter the cell to replicate and then be released by the host cell. The presence of viral proteins in the host cell membrane triggers an immunologic response. The host immune response may then focus on and destroy the infected CNS cells. This process minimizes spread of the virus but causes apoptosis and may worsen CNS damage. Thus, neuronal cell death may result from the body's attempt to fight the invading pathogen.

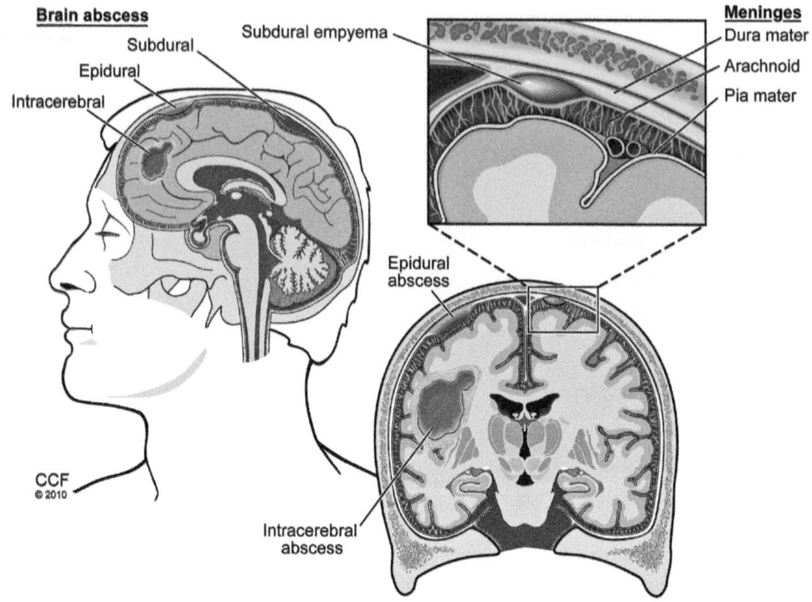

Fig. 1. CNS infections: meningitis, encephalitis, brain abscess, myelitis. (*Courtesy of* Sharon E. Mace, MD, Emergency Services Institute, Cleveland Clinic and Dave Schumick, Cleveland Clinic Center for Art and Medical Photography.)

With postinfectious encephalitis, there is no evidence of virus or viral antigens in the CNS and no direct viral damage. However, the body's immune response is erroneously directed against the brain itself.

There are several properties of successful pathogens that allow them to invade the CNS. The first step is attachment to the host's mucosal epithelium followed by colonization of the host. Upper respiratory tract viruses destroy ciliated cells in the nasopharynx, which impairs the host's ability to eliminate pathogens. The fimbriae or pili of *N meningitides* allow it to adhere to the nasopharyngeal mucosa, whereas several proteins on the cell surface of *S pneumoniae* enable it to attach to the nasopharyngeal mucosa.

Pneumolysin, a compound secreted by *S pneumoniae*, is a virulence factor that has several harmful effects: it induces apoptosis in brain cells, has proinflammatory effects (ranging from the release of NO in neutrophils to activation of the complement pathway), and limits the respiratory burst in polymorphonuclear leukocytes, chemotaxis, and bactericidal activity. The phagocytosis of bacteria by the body's neutrophils followed by complement-mediated killing of the invading bacteria are critical mechanisms in the body's ability to defend against invading pathogens. These 2 steps are inhibited by the polysaccharide capsule of certain bacteria such as *S pneumoniae*, *H influenzae*, and *N meningitidis*.

Certain bacteria including *S pneumoniae* can attach to the cerebral capillary endothelial cells with subsequent passage through or between these cells to enter the CSF. *S pneumoniae* bacteria also produce hyaluronidase, an enzyme (the spreading enzyme) that degrades hyaluronic acid, which is a constituent of the extracellular matrix. Components in the polysaccharide capsule of meningitides limit activation of the alternative complement pathway. The fimbria that are part of *Escherichia coli* and *N meningitides* allow these pathogens to adhere to the glycoproteins on brain

Box 2
Pathophysiology of CNS infections

- Bypass or attach to and enter host's cells (avoid the body's barriers to pathogens)
  - Travel and enter CNS
  - Replicate or multiply in the host
  - Initiate inflammatory cascade
    - Release of cytokines, chemokines
    - Activation of inflammatory mediators (eg, nitric oxide [NO], reactive oxygen species [ROS], matrix metalloproteinases [MMPs])
    - Recruitment of white blood cells (WBCs) to the site of infection
    - Cytotoxic events
- Damage to CNS
  - By direct invasion
  - By inflammatory cascade
- Inflammatory mediators:
  - Direct neurotoxicity
  - Increase vascular permeability
  - Increase cerebral blood flow
- Physiologic events
  - Cerebral edema
    - Vasogenic edema: loss of blood-brain barrier
    - Cytotoxic edema: from cellular swelling and destruction
    - Obstruction to CSF outflow at arachnoid villi
  - Cerebral hypoperfusion from local vascular inflammation and/or thrombosis
  - Loss of autoregulation

endothelial cells. Several pathogens, including *E coli*, *H influenzae*, and pneumococci, can all have a cytopathic effect on cerebral microvascular endothelial cells.

Host Defenses Against CNS Pathogens

WBCs form the first line of defense against invading organisms (eg, neutrophils against bacteria, lymphocytes against viruses). Although the CNS has few WBCs, during an infection when the blood-brain barrier is breached, WBCs can then readily enter. Some of the pericytes and glial support cells in the CNS can transform to monocyte-macrophage antigen-presenting cells.

Antibodies secreted by host cells enhance the opsonization of bacteria followed by phagocytoses of bacterial by polymorphonuclear leukocytes and macrophages. Activation of the complement system is another host defense against encapsulated pathogens.

CLINICAL PRESENTATION OF CNS INFECTIONS

The clinical presentation of a patient with a CNS infection can be extremely variable and may include headaches, fever, a stiff neck, and focal neurologic deficits, or an

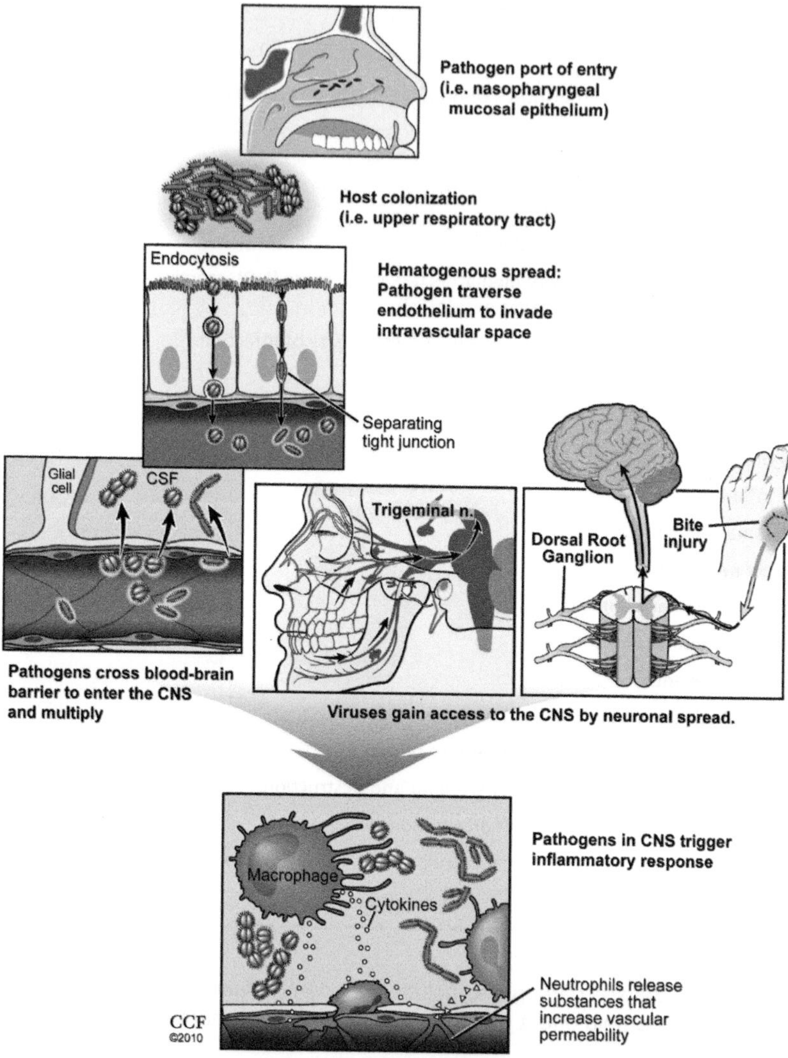

Fig. 2. Pathophysiology. (*Courtesy of* Sharon E. Mace, MD, Emergency Services Institute, Cleveland Clinic and Dave Schumick, Cleveland Clinic Center for Art and Medical Photography.)

altered mental status that includes lethargy, confusion, obtunded, unresponsive, or coma.[3] When classic signs and symptoms are present as with the meningitis triad of fever, neck stiffness, and altered mental status, the diagnosis is more straightforward. Such classic signs and symptoms are often not present, which makes the diagnosis difficult.

The classic triad of fever, neck stiffness, and altered mental status occurred in less than half (44%) of adult patients with meningitis.[3] However, 95% of patients had at least 2 of the 4 meningitis symptoms of fever, headache, neck stiffness, and altered mental status.[3] In another older study of adults with meningitis, the classic triad of meningitis was present in two-thirds of the patients.[4] The most common element of the triad (in 95%) was fever, a nonspecific finding.[4] Other reports, also in adults, had similar findings. In adult patients with meningitis one study noted only 51% had the classic triad,[5] whereas another reported 66% had fever, stiff neck, and headache.[6] According to a report that pooled 11 studies, the classic triad was present in less than half of the patients (46%).[7] In one of these more recent adult meningitis studies fever was noted in only about three-fourths (77%) of the patients.[3]

Further confounding the diagnosis of meningitis is the fact that many patients, especially those at the extremes of age (eg, geriatric and pediatric patients, especially infants) may lack the classic signs and symptoms of meningitis.[8–10] Such patients may only have a fever, be afebrile, or even be hypothermic. Moreover, the immunocompromised individual may also be afebrile or hypothermic. Similarly, the patient who has been on antibiotics and has partially treated meningitis may not present with a fever.

Confusion or any abnormal mental status suggests the possibility of meningitis or encephalitis, especially if a fever is present.[8–11] Confusion or an abnormal mental status may be the only finding in meningitis in elderly people[12] and the only presenting symptom with a patient of any age with encephalitis.[13]

Seizures as the initial complaint have been reported in one-third of pediatric patients with bacterial meningitis and in 5% to 28% of adults with meningitis.[4,6,14] Seizures may also be the presenting symptom in patients with encephalitis.[13]

Nuchal rigidity is a hallmark of meningitis yet is found merely 30% of the time.[15] The Kernig and Brudzinski signs are classic findings in meningitis, yet they are present in only about half of adults with meningitis.[16] If purpura or petechiae are present, meningococcal meningitis should be in the differential, although these skin findings may be present with other bacterial causes of meningitis.[17]

CLINICAL PRESENTATION OF ENCEPHALITIS VERSUS MENINGITIS

The clinical signs and symptoms in patients with encephalitis can be similar to patients with meningitis, and there is much overlap.[9,18] Furthermore, meningitis and encephalitis (meningencephalitis) can occur in the same patient.[11,19] Headache, photophobia, vomiting, lethargy, altered mental status, fever, seizures, neck stiffness, and focal neurologic findings may occur with either meningitis or encephalitis.[9,11,13] However, altered mental status, seizures, focal neurologic deficits, and especially new psychiatric symptoms and/or cognitive deficits are more common with encephalitis.[11] The dyad of an altered mental status and focal neurologic findings is more predictive for encephalitis than meningitis.[11,13] Furthermore, certain viruses have a predilection for a specific part of the CNS. Typically, the HSV causes the onset of new psychiatric symptoms as a result of frontal lobe involvement but may also cause temporal lobe seizures,[20] whereas the West Nile virus may attack the anterior horn cells, causing a Guillain-Barré-like paralysis.[21]

A clinical presentation similar to encephalitis with focal neurologic signs might occur with meningitis if complications (eg, vascular occlusion causing stroke or cerebral edema) are present.[9]

SPECIFIC PATIENT POPULATIONS

Pediatric Patients

Pediatric patients present additional difficulties in the diagnosis of CNS infections because typical clinical signs and symptoms are often absent, and findings tend to be nonspecific and subtle.[10] Although nuchal rigidity has been reported in 60% to 70% of pediatric meningitis patients, this finding is likely to be absent in infants, especially in neonates. Infants with meningitis may be afebrile or present only with a fever or even be hypothermic. Nonspecific presentations are common in infants with meningitis and range from irritability, lethargy, rash, or poor feeding to apnea, seizures, or a bulging fontanelle.[10] Infants and young children are also unable to verbalize their complaints such as headache, neck pain, or photophobia.[9]

Geriatric Patients

Elderly patients can also present a diagnostic dilemma. The patient with a stroke or Alzheimer disease may be unable to express a chief complaint such as headache. Fever may also be absent in the geriatric patient or they may be hypothermic.[12] If fever is present in elderly patients with meningitis, it is commonly attributed to other infections, including urinary tract infections, viral illness, respiratory infections (pneumonia or bronchitis), bacteremia, and sepsis.[12] These various infections can coexist with meningitis, and meningitis may result from the seeding of the bloodstream that occurs with some of these infections.

Nuchal rigidity and meningeal signs are often unreliable in the older patient.[12] False-positive signs (eg, positive Kernig or Brudzinski sign and/or neck stiffness) can occur in healthy geriatric individuals, likely from cervical musculoskeletal disease causing restrictive neck mobility.[22] Conversely, nuchal rigidity and meningeal signs are less likely to be present in the elderly patient with meningitis than in the nongeriatric adult with meningitis.[23–25] The elderly patient with meningitis may present with altered mental status, seizures, neurologic deficit, or hydrocephalus.[23–25]

Because of the unreliable clinical signs and symptoms and the nonspecific often subtle clinical presentation, the diagnosis of meningitis in patients at the extremes of age is frequently delayed or even missed, resulting in increased morbidity and mortality.[23–25]

DIFFERENTIAL DIAGNOSIS OF CNS INFECTIONS

Making the diagnoses of a CNS infection is further confounded because many other disorders or disease processes may mimic a CNS infection (see **Box 1**).[19]

Meningitis has been classified into bacterial and aseptic meningitis. Bacterial or pyogenic meningitis is caused by a bacterial infection that usually causes a polymorphonuclear response in the CSF. Aseptic meningitis is defined as meningeal inflammation without evidence of pyogenic bacterial infection on Gram stain or culture of the CSF. Aseptic meningitis is further subdivided into infectious (generally nonbacterial) causes and noninfectious causes of meningeal inflammation. Infectious causes of aseptic meningitis characteristically have a mononuclear pleocytosis and are usually caused by viruses or rarely fungi, a partially treated bacterial meningitis, or a bacteria that is unable to grow on the usual culture media; such as *B burgdorferi* (Lyme disease), *Treponema* (syphilis), or *Mycobacterium* (tuberculosis), *Rickettsia*, or ehrlichoses (see **Box 1**).

Eosinophilic meningitis is a meningitis with a significant percentage of eosinophils in the CSF (defined as >10 eosinophils in the CSF or ≥10% of CSF leukocytes are eosinophils) and is usually caused by a parasitic infection of the meninges. Eosinophilic meningitis is found primarily in the Pacific Islands and Southeast Asia and is caused by a nematode infection of the CSF, specifically a rodent lungworm with terrestrial freshwater shrimp, fish, snails, or slugs serving as intermediate hosts for the parasites.[26]

Noninfectious causes of aseptic meningitis include tumors or malignancy (neoplastic meningitis or leptomeningeal carcinomatosis), systemic diseases that cause meningeal inflammation (for example, neurosarcoidosis or sarcoid meningitis, and lupus cerebritis), and drugs or toxins.[19,27] Drug-induced aseptic meningitis can be a result of the instillation of contrast materials (during diagnostic procedures) or the ingestion of medications. Medications implicated in drug-induced aseptic meningitis include nonsteroidal antiinflammatory drugs, trimethoprin-sulfamethioxazole, azathioprine, timonacic, and OKT3.[19]

The differential diagnosis of CNS infections also includes parameningeal infections: brain abscesses, subdural empyema, and epidural abscess (see **Fig. 1**).

Malignancies that can cause meningeal carcinomatosis may be primary or metastatic to the CNS. Tumors that have been reported as a cause of leptomeningeal carcinomatosis include primary CNS lymphomas and metastatic tumors from leukemias (acute myelogenous, acute lymphocytic), lymphomas (Hodgkin, non-Hodgkin), breast, lung (bronchogenic carcinoma), melanoma, renal cell carcinoma, and germ cell tumors.[19]

Patients with high red blood cell (RBC) counts or polycythemia, and patients with disorders of the WBCs who have high peripheral WBC counts with leukostasis, can also develop CNS symptoms as a result of hyperviscosity that mimic a CNS infection.[19]

The posterior fossa syndrome occurs in patients after craniotomy.[19] They present similarly to patients presenting with bacterial meningitis but with a negative CSF Gram stain and culture. Posterior fossa syndrome is a type of aseptic meningitis caused by RBCs in the CSF resulting from the craniotomy procedure. In general, symptoms are directly proportional to the number of RBCs in the CSF. The patient's symptoms resolve as the RBCs in the CSF are cleared by the body's normal physiologic mechanisms.

Other noninfectious CNS disorders, including strokes (whether embolic or thrombotic), CNS venous thrombosis, and vascular aneurysms, can also present similarly to a CNS infection.[19]

When the combination of fever and altered mental status occurs, the possibility of a CNS infection must be considered. However, a wide differential diagnosis comprises infections within the CNS and outside the CNS and even noninfectious processes that can mimic a CNS infection. Furthermore, patients with an infection outside the CNS may have a coexistent fever and altered mental status. The classic picture of this is the confused elderly patient with a urinary tract infection.

Fever by itself may cause an abnormal mental status. Conversely, not every patient with a CNS infection presents with altered mental status and a fever.

ADEM, also known as postinfectious encephalitis, is believed to be caused by an autoimmune response to a preceding antigenic challenge.[19] The precipitating antigenic stimulus may be a preceding infection or possibly an immunization. The neurologic symptoms generally begin within 1 week after the rash appears during an exanthematous illness or within 1 to 14 days after an immunization. Some of the numerous viral infections associated with ADEM are influenza, enteroviruses, hepatitis A, herpes simplex, Epstein-Barr virus, measles, mumps, rubella, varicella zoster, and cytomegalovirus.[13] Although a cause and effect relationship has not been established, several immunizations have been temporally associated with ADEM. These immunizations include the vaccines against influenza, rabies, measles, smallpox, and yellow fever. Patients presenting with ADEM usually do not have a fever, have a variable mental status from confusion or stupor to coma, and have multifocal neurologic signs involving the brain, spinal cord, and optic nerves. CSF findings with ADEM are similar to viral encephalitis (eg, normal glucose, increased protein level, and lymphocytic pleocytosis). Currently, high-dose intravenous corticosteroids (eg, methylprednisolone, 1 g intravenously every day for at least 3 to 5 days) are recommended, so it is important to make a timely and accurate diagnosis and initiate therapy.

DIAGNOSTIC EVALUATION: MENINGITIS

CSF

CSF is essential in the definitive diagnosis and treatment of meningitis (**Table 1**). However, treatment of bacterial meningitis should not be inordinately delayed to obtain CSF. If obtaining CSF will result in an unacceptable delay in antibiotic administration, empirical antibiotic therapy should be administered first with lumbar puncture (LP) to follow as soon as possible.[10,11]

In most patients with acute bacterial meningitis, an LP can be safely performed without antecedent neuroimaging. In patients with a CNS mass lesion, such as a brain abscess, tumor, or CNS bleed, or increased ICP from any cause, neuroimaging may be indicated before the LP.[9,28] Patients at risk of possible CNS mass lesion or increased ICP in whom neuroimaging before LP might be warranted include those age more than 60 years, immunocompromised patients, those with a history of CNS disease, recent seizure (<1 week), abnormal level of consciousness or abnormal sensorium and cognition, papilledema, focal neurologic deficit(s), head trauma, history of CNS mass lesion, focal CNS infection, or stroke.[28] When bacterial meningitis is a possibility, studies on CSF should include Gram stain and culture, cell count with differential, glucose and protein (see **Table 1**). Depending on the clinical scenario, other diagnostic tests may also be warranted (**Box 3**).[18]

General Diagnostic Studies

Additional laboratory studies include blood glucose, electrolytes, serum urea nitrogen (BUN), creatinine, and blood cultures. With bacterial meningitis, the WBC count is usually increased, with a leftward shift. The exceptions may be patients at the extremes of age (infants, elderly patients) and immunosuppressed patients, who may have a normal or depressed WBC count.[12,23,24,29] Serum glucose is needed for comparison with the CSF glucose (normal CSF/blood glucose ratio >0.40) and to rule out hypoglycemia in septic patients. Kidney function tests (BUN, creatinine) are useful when calculating medication dosages and can help assess renal function and perfusion. There may be abnormalities of the electrolytes, including hyponatremia, from many causes, including the syndrome of inappropriate antidiuretic hormone (SIADH) and dehydration. Because blood cultures may be positive when CSF cultures are negative, they are usually indicated in patients with bacterial meningitis.[18] The urinanalysis gives data about renal function and hydration status, and may detect a urinary tract infection, which could be a nidus for bacteremia, meningitis, and sepsis. Chest radiograph yields information on comorbidities, including congestive heart failure or tumors and any concurrent pneumonia, which may lead to hematogenous seeding of the meninges. Other studies may include an electrocardiogram or echocardiogram to assess for dysrhythmias and cardiac function, an EEG if seizures have occurred, or computed tomography (CT) of the head if complications are present.

DIAGNOSTIC EVALUATION: ENCEPHALITIS

Neuroimaging

Neuroimaging, either magnetic resonance imaging (MRI) or CT, must be performed in patients with encephalitis.[30] In the emergency department (ED), if MRI is not immediately available, then CT can be the initial study and MRI performed later. MRI is more

Table 1
CSF diagnostic studies with CNS infections

	Gram Stain	Culture	WBC Count	Differential	Glucose (mg/dl)	Glucose CSF Blood Ratio	Protein	Other
Normal (adult)	–	–	<5	0% polys	>40	>0.4	<50	
Bacterial meningitis	+	+	↑ ↑ (>1000)	↑ ↑ (>80% polys)	↓ (<40)	↓ (<0.4)	↑ ↑ (>200)	
Viral meningitis	–	–	↑ (<1000)	↑ (1%–50% polys)	N	N	↑ (<200)	Viral studies
Fungal meningitis	–	–	Mild ↑ (<500)	↑ (1%–50% polys)	↓ (<40)	↓ (<0.4)	Mild ↑ (<200)	+ fungal culture
Eosinophilic meningitis (helminths)	–	–	Mild ↑	↑ eos >10%	↓ (<40)	↓ (<0.4)	↑ (<200)	↑ eos
Encephalitis	–	–	Mild ↑	↑ lymph or N typical ≈ 20 (20%–100% lymphs)	N	N	N or mild ↑	
Herpes encephalitis	–	–	Mild ↑	↑ lymphs	N	N	↑ (>40)	↑ RBC
Acute disseminated encephalomyelitis	–	–	Mild ↑	↑ lymphs typical <100 (5–200)	N	N	>40 (mild ↑ ↑) typical <100 (20–500)	
Neoplastic	–	–	Mild ↑ (<500)	↑ (1%–50% polys)	↓ (<40)	↓ (<0.4)	↑ (>200)	+ cytology

Usual range is given.
Abbreviations: eos, eosinophils; lymphs, lymphocytes; N, normal; polys, polymorphonuclear leukocytes.

Box 3
Encephalitis: history, physical examinations, diagnostic testing and causes

Relevant history[a]

- Age of patient
- Immunization status
- Temporal progression of illness and symptoms
- Immunologic status
- If child, history of maternal infections during pregnancy (TORCH: toxoplasmosis, other [listeria], rubella, cytomegalovirus, herpes simplex 2)
- Travel history
- Exposure to vectors (ticks/mosquitos), animal reservoirs
- Location: endemic area
- Any recent outbreaks, local epidemics, case clusters

Relevant physical examination[a]

- Neurologic
  - Include cranial nerves, spinal nerves, peripheral nerves,
- Mucous membranes
- Skin: rashes, petechiae, purpura
- Lymphoid tissue
- Signs of increased ICP cerebral edema
- Cardiopulmonary
- Abdominal

Diagnostic testing for encephalitis

- Neuroimaging[b]
- CSF[c]
  - Gram stain
  - Culture
  - Cell count with differential
  - Glucose
  - Protein
- Other:
  - Electroencephalogram (EEG)
  - General Diagnostic Studies[d]
  - Complete blood count/differential
  - Glucose
  - Renal function tests
  - Liver function tests
  - Coagulation studies
- Cultures
  - Blood: bacterial, fungal

Other: nasopharyngeal, sputum, skin scraping, stool

Chest roentgenogram

Electrocardiogram

Causes of encephalitis

Viruses (most common cause)

Bacteria (unable to be grown on usual culture media)

Mycobacteria

Rickettsia/ehrlichioses

Spirochtes: neurosyphilis, Lyme disease

Fungi

Protozoa

Helminths

[a] Additional history and physical examination in addition to usual history and physical examination.
[b] CT scan may be performed initially and MRI can be performed after admission, although MRI is more sensitive than CT scan.
[c] With encephalitis, CSF analysis is usually indicated but (unlike meningitis) is generally performed after a CT scan or MRI.
[d] General diagnostic studies suggested depending on clinical situation.

sensitive and specific than CT, but may not be so readily available and may be contraindicated in some patients with pacemakers or other implants (see **Box 3**).

Some types of encephalitis have characteristic neuroimaging patterns that may suggest a specific pathogen.[30] For example, bilateral temporal lobe involvement is nearly pathognomonic for herpes simplex encephalitis, whereas encephalitis caused by the flaviruses and eastern equine encephalitis characteristically affect the thalamus, basal ganglia, and not on midbrain, showing mixed intensity on hypodense lesions. The usual pattern on MRI with enterovirus 71 encephalitis shows hyperintense lesions in the midbrain, pons, and medulla.

MRI is also helpful in the differential diagnoses of encephalitis by documenting the typical lesions of ADEM (showing multiple areas of enhancing signal abnormalities in the subcortical white matter), nonenhancing white lesions with progressive multifocal leukoencephalopathy, or subcortical white matter lesions of multiple sclerosis.[30]

Positron emission tomography scanning is not routinely recommended for patients with encephalitis because it has not been helpful in delineating encephalitis from other CNS disorders or disease.[30]

Electroencephalography

The EEG may show cerebral involvement in early encephalitis because it does indicate cerebral dysfunction but is usually nonspecific. The exception is herpes simplex encephalitis, in which there is a temporal focus with characteristic epileptiform discharges.[30] The EEG may also be valuable in the differential diagnosis of the patient with an altered mental status ranging from confusion or obtundation to coma because it can detect nonconvulsive status epilecticus.

CSF Analysis

In all patients with encephalitis, as with meningitis, CSF analysis is critical, and LP to obtain CSF should be performed unless there are contraindications (see **Table 1**).[19,30,31] Typical CSF findings with viral encephalitis show normal glucose level, a mild to moderate increased protein level, and mild mononuclear pleocytosis. A decreased CSF glucose level is unusual in viral encephalitis and raises the suspicion for a bacterial (*Listeria* or *Mycobacterium*), fungal, cryptococcal, or protozoan (for example, *Naegleria*) pathogen.

A polymorphonuclear cell predominance may occur early in the course of viral encephalitis and may persist in patients with West Nile virus. An increase in RBC in the CSF is characteristic of herpes encephalitis. CSF eosinophilia suggests a helminth as the pathogen, although a lesser CSF eosinophilia can occur with *Treponema*, *Rickettsia*, *M pneumoniae*, coccidiomycosis, and *Toxoplasma*.[26] Because the automated cell count performed by machine can confuse eosinophils and neutrophils, and eosinophils are easily deformed or destroyed during the processing of specimens, consider using a special stain (Wright or Giemsa) for detecting eosinophils and requesting the laboratory or pathologist to perform a manual differential. CSF should be sent for Gram stain and culture, especially if bacterial or fungal meningitis is suspected. In up to 10% of patients with viral encephalitis, the CSF findings might be completely normal.[30]

Viral cultures are generally not helpful because the yield is extremely low[30] (5.7% in one study[32]) and are not routinely recommended. For nonviral (eg, bacterial or fungal) causes of encephalitis, CSF cultures are recommended even though some bacteria, specifically *Rickettsia*, *Ehrlichia*, *Bartonella*, *Mycoplasma*, and *Treponema pallidum*, cannot be reliably isolated in routine cultures.[9,30]

Antibody Testing

Depending on the specific clinical situation, other CSF studies may be useful. Because immunoglobulin M (IgM) antibodies do not readily diffuse across the blood-brain barrier the finding of IgM antibodies by enzyme-linked immunosorbent assay (ELISA) assay is diagnostic of CNS disease.[30] However, the absence of such virus-specific IgM antibodies on CSF does not rule out a particular pathogen as a cause of neuroinvasive disease. IgM antibodies by ELISA testing are available for several pathogens including varicella zoster and the flaviruses. The flaviviruses include West Nile virus, Japanese encephalitis virus, St Louis encephalitis virus, Murray Valley encephalitis virus, Powassan virus, and tick-borne encephalitis virus.

Nucleic Acid Amplification Tests

Polymerase chain reaction (PCR) assays are based on the amplification of microbial nucleic acids. PCR assays for herpes simplex are useful in diagnosing herpes encephalitis and have a high sensitivity and specificity (95% to 99%), although false-positive and false-negative tests can occur.[30]

Brain Biopsy

Brain biopsy is rarely performed to diagnose encephalitis except in a few instances, for example, in patients with encephalitis of unknown cause who are deteriorating despite treatment.[30]

General Diagnostic Studies

Serum (acute and convalescent) titers for West Nile virus should be sent for serology when West Nile virus is a consideration.[30] Other diagnostic studies outside the CNS may provide valuable clues to suggest a cause for the encephalitis and should be performed in most cases, based on the clinical scenario (see **Box 3**).[30]

CNS ABSCESSES

The clinical presentation of patients with an intracranial abscess usually differs from patients with meningitis or encephalitis.[33–35] Generally, these patients seem nontoxic and have a subacute onset of illness. Less than half of the patients have a fever, and a stiff neck is rare. Unlike other CNS infections, focal deficits are frequently present and papilledema is not uncommon. Neuroimaging, usually a CT scan with contrast, is essential to diagnose a brain abscess. The typical finding on CT scan or MRI is a hypodense lesion with a contrast-enhancing ring. A brain abscess is the only CNS infection in which an LP is never recommended and may even be contraindicated.[33] This advice is not only because an LP does not help in the diagnosis but also because increased ICP is often present as a result of the mass effect, which increases the likelihood of herniation. The management of a brain abscess requires appropriate antibiotics and neurosurgical consultation. Empirical antibiotics should include coverage for anaerobic pathogens, such as a third-generation cephalosporin and metronidazole, plus vancomycin if there is a history of penetrating trauma or a recent neurosurgical procedure. Mortality from a brain abscess has recently decreased from about 50% to 20%, mostly as a result of earlier diagnosis from readily available CT scanning.[34,35] Brain abscess is still associated with high morbidity, including seizures (up to 80%), persistent altered mental status, and focal motor deficits.

CNS abscesses occur either by direct spread from a contiguous site or by hematogenous seeding (**Fig. 3**). Spread from a contiguous site generally causes a solitary brain abscess, whereas hematogenous spread typically causes multiple CNS abscesses. Hematogenous spread usually leads to multiple abscesses located in the distribution of the middle cerebral artery. Some of the primary infections that can lead to a brain abscess(es) from hematogenous seeding are chronic pulmonary infections (often a lung abscess or empyema), skin infections, intra-abdominal (including pelvic) infections, endocarditis, and cyanotic congenital heart disease. Moreover, primary infections that can lead to a brain abscess include dental infections (usually spreads to the frontal lobe), ethmoid or frontal sinusitis (usually spreads to the frontal lobe), and subacute or chronic otitis media or mastoiditis (usually spreads to the inferior temporal lobe and cerebellum). Penetrating head trauma, facial trauma, or postneurosurgical procedures can also serve as foci for a brain abscesses. Cryptic brain abscesses in which no obvious source can be identified occur in 20% to 30% of all brain abscesses.[33]

CAUSATIVE ORGANISMS IN CNS INFECTIONS

Meningitis

The pathogens that cause meningitis generally enter the CNS via hematogenous seeding of the meninges and occasionally by direct extension from a contiguous focus. The median age and pathogens responsible for causing meningitis have changed since the introduction of newer vaccines. Before the introduction of the *H influenza* type b (Hib) vaccine, the median age of patients with meningitis was 15 months (in 1986), which reflects the increased incidence of and risk for meningitis in infants and young children compared with adults (except for elderly patients).[36] After widespread use of Hib, the median age was cited as 25 years (in 1995).[37]

Before the introduction of the Hib vaccine, approximately half of all bacterial meningitis cases were caused by *H influenza* (45%), with the causative organism being *S*

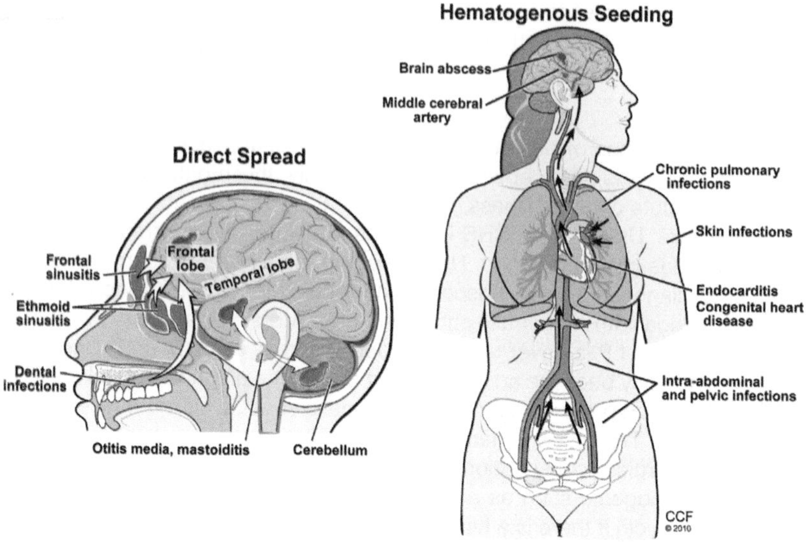

Fig. 3. Brain abscess: contiguous and hematogenous spread. (*Courtesy of* Sharon E. Mace, MD, Emergency Services Institute, Cleveland Clinic and Dave Schumick, Cleveland Clinic Center for Art and Medical Photography.)

pneumoniae in 18% and *N meningitides* in 14%.[36] Since the introduction of Hib in 1995, the most common pathogens responsible for bacterial meningitis are *S pneumoniae* (47%), *N meningitides* (25%), group β streptococci (12%), and *Listeria monocytogenes* (8%).[37]

The Hib vaccine introduced in the early 1990s in the United States altered the incidence of meningeal pathogens. It seems likely that the introduction of the *S pneumoniae* vaccine (approved in 2000 by the US Food and Drug Administration) will again alter the relative incidence of pathogens causing meningitis.

Meningitis: Causative Organisms Based on Clinical Scenario

In postoperative neurosurgery patients, those with penetrating head trauma, and patients with CSF shunts, staphylococci are the most common pathogens of meningitis. Neonatal (age ≤30 days) meningitis is often caused by group B-β hemolytic streptocci, gram-negative enteric bacteria, and *L monocytogenes*. The geriatric patient in a nursing home may have a methicillin-resistant *Staphylococcus aureus* or a vancomycin-resistant enterococcus. *L monocytogenes* should be considered as a possible pathogen in patients in the extremes of age (eg, the neonate and the geriatric patient), the patient with HIV and others with impaired immunity. Consider *S pneumoniae*, various streptococci, and *H influenza* in individuals with a basilar skull fracture or a CSF leak. Patients with a CSF shunt (such as ventriculoperitoneal shunt) are especially prone to infections with coagulase-negative *Staph aureus*, *Staph aureus*, and aerobic gram-negative bacilli (such as *Pseudomonas aeruginosa* and *Propionbacterium acnes*) (**Table 2**).[18]

Encephalitis: Causative Organisms Based on Clinical Scenario

Many pathogens can cause encephalitis including viruses (the most common cause), fungi, bacteria unable to be cultured on the usual culture media, mycobacteria, *Rickettsia* and ehrlichioses, spirochetes, protozoa, and helminthes (see **Box 3**; **Table 2**). However, the most frequent cause is the arboviruses, followed closely by HSV. The common arboviruses encountered in the United States are West Nile virus, St Louis encephalitis, western equine encephalitis, and eastern equine encephalitis. Recently in the United States, West Nile virus has been the most common epidemic encephalitis. Pathogens responsible for encephalitis may enter the CNS via hematogenous spread, from a contiguous foci, or by neuronal spread (**Fig. 4**).

Transmission: Zoonoses

Encephalitis is often caused by a zoonosis, a disease transmitted by animals (**Fig. 5**).[38] Insect vectors with animal reservoirs often serve as a means of entry for a virus to bypass the body's protective epithelial layer.[38] For example, with the arthropod-borne encephalitides including the arboviruses, the virus is infected into the host's bloodstream via the bite of a mosquito (West Nile virus, St Louis, eastern equine, and western equine encephalitis) or a tick (tick-borne encephalitis), whereas the rabies virus is transmitted via the bite of (or secretions from) an infected animal (whether a rabid bat, raccoon, skunk, fox, dog, or cat) (see **Tables 2** and **3**).[27]

The bite of a tick is essential for such viral encephalitides as Lyme disease, Rocky Mountain spotted fever, or Colorado tick fever.[38] Exposure to the secretions of infected mice, rats, or hamsters that are carrying the rodent-borne areanavirus can lead to the human acquired zoonosis lymphocytic choriomeningitis virus (LCMV). Exposure to pet birds can lead to psittacosis caused by *Chlamydia psittacosis*. Inhalation of infected particles into the respiratory tract is a site of entry for LCMV and psittacosis. Bartonellosis is spread by the bite of an arthropod that disrupts the skin's protective layer. The animal reservoirs for bartonellosis include dogs, cattle, cats, and body lice. The gastrointestinal tract is the entry site for brucellosis from ingestion of unpasteurized dairy products and Q fever caused by the *Coxiella burnetii* organism. Amoebic meningoencephalitis caused by *Acanthamoeba* or *Naegleria fowleri* can enter the body when an individual swims in a lake or pond or nonchlorinated water (see **Tables 2** and **3**).

Brain Access: Causative Organisms Based on Clinical Scenario

There is a wide range of pathogens that can cause a brain abscess.[33–35] Common organisms are anaerobic pathogens (often by direct spread from mouth flora and otorhinolaryngeal infections but also via hematogenous spread from intra-abdominal/pelvic infections) and aerobic gram-positive cocci (often following trauma or status after neurosurgical procedure). Common anaerobes include anaerobic streptococci, *Bacteroides* spp, *Prevotella melaninogenica*, *Propionibacterium*, *Fusobacterium*, and *Actinomyces*. The aerobic gram-positive cocci that are frequent pathogens are *Streptococcus viridans*, *Streptococcus milleri*, and *Staph aureus*. *Staph aureus* is common in brain abscesses after a neurosurgical procedure or head trauma but aerobic gram-negative rods (*Klebsiella*, *Pseudomonas*, *E coli*, *Proteus*) may also be found. When the primary source is a dental infection, aerobic gram-negative rods may also be present (see **Box 3**).

Immunocompromised hosts can have a vast array of pathogens from the usual organisms to other more unusual pathogens including *Toxoplasma*, *Listeria*, *Nocardia*, *Aspergillosus*, *Cryptococcus*, *Coccidioides*, and other fungal pathogens. Consider parasites (such as cysticercosis from *Taenia*, *Entoamoeba histolytica*, *Schistosoma*, and *Paragonismus*) in immigrants or travelers from an underdeveloped part of the world with a brain abscess(es) (see **Table 2**).

Table 2
Pathogens based on clinical scenario: meningitis, encephalitis, and brain abscess

Clinical Setting/Risk Factor	
Meningitis	Pathogen
Neonate (≤30 days)	Group β streptococcus Gram-negatives: *E coli*, *Klebsiella* Listeria
Infants and very young children (1–23 months)	*S pneumoniae* N meningtidis Group β streptococcus H influenzae *E coli*
Children (2–18 years)	S pneumoniae *N meningitidis*
Adult (nongeriatric) 18–50 years	S pneumoniae *N meningitidis*
Adult (elder) >50 years	S pneumoniae *N meningitidis* *L monocytogenes* Consider other pathogens
HIV/other immunocompromised patients	S pneumoniae Gram-negative bacilli *L monocytogenes*
CSF shunt	Coagulase-negative staphylococci *Staph aureus* Aerobic gram-negative bacilli
Basilar skull fracture or CSF leak	S pneumoniae Streptococci *H influenzae*
Penetrating head trauma or S/P neurosurgical procedure	*Staph aureus* Coagulase-negative staphylococci Aerobic gram-negative bacilli
Encephalitis	Pathogen
Neonates	TORCH
Infants/children	Eastern equine encephalitis Japanese encephalitis Murray Valley encephalitis Influenza La Crosse virus
Geriatric	West Nile virus, eastern equine encephalitis, St Louis encephalitis, Listeria, Creutzfeldt-Jakob disease
Insect vector: mosquitoes	West Nile virus, eastern equine encephalitis, western equine encephalitis, St. Louis encephalitis, Murray Valley encephalitis, La Crosse virus, plasmodium
Insect vector: ticks	*B burgdorferi* (Lyme disease), *Rickettsia rickettsii*, *Ehrlichia*, tick-borne encephalitis
Insect vector: sand flies	Bartonella
Insect vector: tsetse flies	Trypanosomiasis
Exposure to rabies: bats, raccoons, dogs, cats, or skunks, or their saliva	Rabies

(*continued on next page*)

Table 2
(continued)

Clinical Setting/Risk Factor	
Animal reservoir: horses	Eastern equine encephalitis, western equine encephalitis, *Bartonella*, tick-borne encephalitis, Japanese encephalitis
Animal reservoir: deer	*B burgdorferi* (Lyme disease)
Animal reservoir: rodents	Tick-borne encephalitis, *Bartonella*
Animal reservoir: birds	West Nile virus, Eastern equine encephalitis, western equine encephalitis, St Louis encephalitis, Japanese encephalitis, *Cryptococcus* (bird droppings)
Gastrointestinal tract: unpasteurized milk	*Listeria*, *C burnetti*, tick-borne encephalitis
Raw or partially cooked meat	Toxoplasma gondii
Recreation outdoors: camping/hunting	Any mosquito or tick vector disease
Swimming in warm unchlorinated body of water	Amoebic meningoencephalitis (*Naegleria*)
Brain abscess	Pathogen
Dental infection, otorhinolaryngeal infection, intra-abdominal or pelvic infection	Anaerobic: *Bacteroides*, *Prevotella melaninogenica*, *Propionibacterium*, *Fusobacterium*, *Actinomyces*
Status post penetrating head trauma or neurosurgical procedures	*Staph aureus*
Dental infection	Gram-negative bacilli
Immigrants	Parasites: *Taenia*, *Entoamoeba*, *Schistosoma*, *Paragonimus*
Immunocompromised	*Toxoplasma*, *Listeria*, *Nocardia*, *Aspergillosis*, *Cryptococcus*, *Coccidiodes*, other fungal

MANAGEMENT OF CNS INFECTIONS

Empirical Treatment of CNS Infections

Meningitis

For suspected bacterial meningitis, begin antibiotic therapy in all patients with adjunctive dexamethasone in specific patients (**Table 4**).[9–11,18,39–41] If the specific pathogen is unknown, empirical therapy can be given. A typical empirical antibiotic regimen includes a cephalosporin (third- or fourth-generation such as cefotaxime or ceftriaxone) plus vancomycin.[39,40] If listeria is a possibility, ampicillin is administered as a third antibiotic. Elderly patients, newborns and patients with impaired immunity such as HIV are those in whom *Listeria* is a possible pathogen. Alternative drugs include a carbepenem (eg, meropenum) for the cephalosporins, trimpethoprim-sulfamethoxazole for ampicillin (trimethoprim-sulfamethoxazole is not recommended in newborns), or chloramphenicol plus vancomycin for the cephalosporins. Rifampin is generally not given alone because resistance develops quickly. Therefore, it should be used in combination with other antibiotics. Rifampin is also often added to the antimicrobial regimen when dexamethosone is given because it is theorized that dexamethasone may lead to a higher therapeutic failure rate by decreasing the CSF level of antibiotics such as vancomycin.[10,18] Adjunctive dexamethasone is given immediately before or concurrently with antibiotics in certain patients with meningitis (see **Table 4**).[39–41]

Encephalitis

Begin treatment with acyclovir in all patients with encephalitis pending results of diagnostic studies because acyclovir can improve the outcome in patients with herpes encephalitis.[9,13,30,41] In addition to acyclovir, corticosteroids have also been recommended by some experts to treat herpes simplex encephalitis.[42] Begin treatment with doxycycline in patients with encephalitis with suspected rickettsial or ehrlichial infections during the appropriate season.[30] In addition, corticosteroids have been recommended by some experts in the treatment of specific types of encephalitis.[9,41]

Brain abscess

Brain abscesses usually require drainage in addition to appropriate microbial therapy, so early neurosurgical consultation is recommended.[33]

CONTROVERSIES WITH CNS INFECTIONS

Controversy: Neuroimaging Before LP

The risk of brain herniation following LP has long been a source of controversy.[9,11] There have been anecdotal case reports noting a temporal association between an LP and brain herniation.[9] However, recent studies have challenged this association. No significant adverse events were reported in several large series of patients with increased ICP and even papilledema in whom an LP was performed.[43–45] A series of 200 patients with increased ICP secondary to brain tumors reported no complications following LP.[43] Other studies had similar results: no complications from an LP in patients with increased ICP and/or papilledema.[44,45] Patients with meningitis may herniate without undergoing LP[46,47] and patients with normal CT scans may herniate.[48] Furthermore, in patients with pseudotumor cerebri who have increased ICP, an LP is diagnostic and therapeutic.[9]

A CT scan not only assists in identifying patients at risk for brain herniation but also may diagnose disorders that would eliminate the need for LP, and/or diagnose diseases (such as cerebral abscess or brain tumor) that would be missed if only LP was done.

Decision rules for CT before LP have been suggested.[28,49,50] As per these clinical guidelines, a head CT before LP should be performed in patients with recent seizures ($\leq$1 week), an immunocompromised state, history of CNS disease, altered mental status, abnormal gaze or facial palsy, abnormal language or inability to answer 2 questions or follow 2 commands, visual field abnormalities, and arm or leg drift.[28] Some experts have criticized this nonvalidated decision rule, noting that in a small group of 96 patients without these findings, an abnormal CT scan occurred in 9% (1 of 11) patients.[9] Moreover, a decision rule may be unable to diagnose all patients with an intracranial lesion for several reasons.[9] A parameningeal infection (such as a brain abscess) may have WBCs in the CSF and could be mistakenly diagnosed as meningitis if neuroimaging was not performed. Frequently, patients (especially patients in the ED) with HIV or AIDS may not be cognizant of their HIV infection, yet they are at risk for CNS disease including CNS lymphoma and toxoplasmosis, both of which can be diagnosed with neuroimaging.[9]

Two caveats should be noted when discussing neuroimaging and LPs. First, pediatric patients may be at a greater lifetime risk from CT scans than adults and may be at a lesser risk for such disorders as HIV/AIDS when it may be necessary to obtain a CT

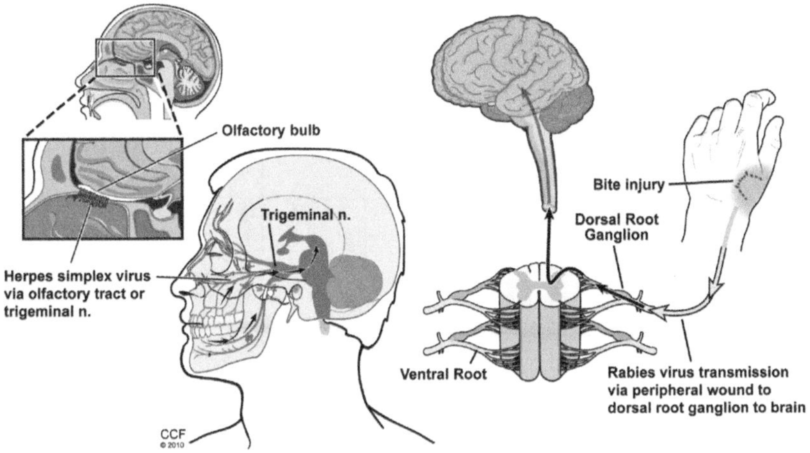

Fig. 4. Encephalitis: hematogenous, contiguous, and neuronal spread. (*Courtesy of* Sharon E. Mace, MD, Emergency Services Institute, Cleveland Clinic and Dave Schumick, Cleveland Clinic Center for Art and Medical Photography.)

scan. Secondly, patients with encephalitis almost always need neuroimaging; a CT scan is often the initial study because it is easier and faster to obtain a CT than an MRI.[30] The MRI with contrast, however, is better at delineating and diagnosing the underlying encephalitis.[30]

A CT scan does not need to be performed before every LP especially if the diagnosis of meningitis is straightforward and there are no focal findings or signs of increased ICP.

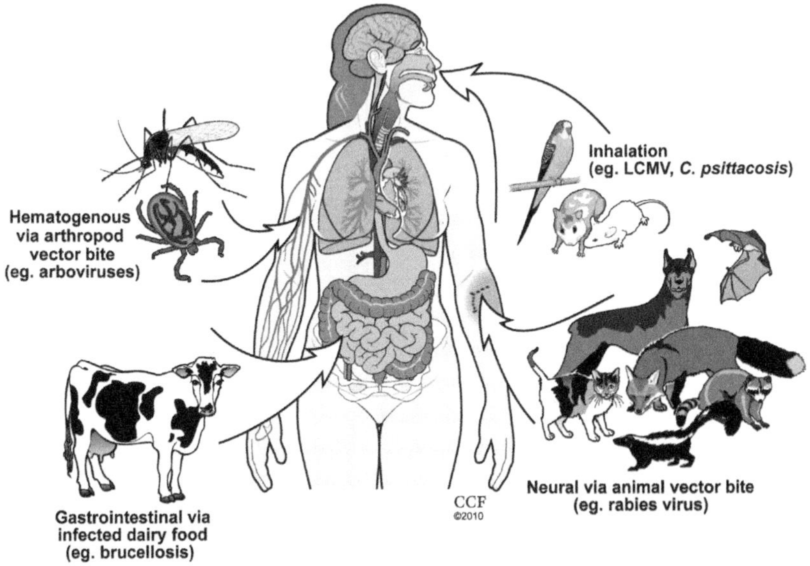

Fig. 5. Encephalitis: transmission. (*Courtesy of* Sharon E. Mace, MD, Emergency Services Institute, Cleveland Clinic and Dave Schumick, Cleveland Clinic Center for Art and Medical Photography.)

Table 3
Transmission of encephalitis

	Disease	Pathogen	Spread or Vector	Reservoir or Host	Seasonal Other Factors	Geographic Distribution	Exposure, Age Predilection	Diagnosis	Comments	Clinical	Treatment
Viruses											
HSV	HSV 1 (except neonates: HSV 2)	Herpes viridae	Via trigeminal nerve or olfactory tract to CNS	With primary, recurrent, or latent HSV infection	Any season	United States Worldwide Most common cause fatal sporadic encephalitis	All ages, occurs after HSV infection	PCR-HSV in CSF, brain biopsy rarely performed except if patient deteriorating	Perform LP for CSF for PCR in any encephalitis patient	Fever, headache, seizures, focal neuro signs, impaired LOC	Acyclovir 10 mg/kg every 8 h empirical tx for any suspected HSV encephalitis
Arbovirus (arthropod-borne)	Eastern equine encephalitis	Toga viridae	Mosquitoes	Birds	Summer/fall (Aug–Sep)	Americas United States: Atlantic/Gulf coasts	Sporadic small outbreaks each summer	CSF IgM Ab, >4-fold ↑ serum Ab titers Isolate virus, viral Ag	Most severe arboviral encephalitis, mortality >30%	Fever, headache, nausea, vomiting	Supportive, complete recovery is uncommon
Arbovirus (arthropod-borne)	Western equine encephalitis	Toga viridae	Mosquitoes	Birds Rabbits	Summer/fall	Americas Recent ↓ incidence: equine vaccine, ↑ vector control, ↓ horse population	Infants/children at greatest risk Low mortality	CSF IgM Ab, >4-fold ↑ serum Ab titers Isolate virus, viral Ag	Large outbreaks in humans/horses in 1950s/1960s	Headache, vomiting, stiff neck, backache	Supportive
Arbovirus (arthropod-borne)	St Louis encephalitis	Flavi viridae	Mosquitoes	Birds	Summer/fall number 2 cause of epidemic viral encephalitis in United States	Americas United States: midwest, south	Elderly OH-Miss valley, eastern TX, FL	Serology (IgM-ELISA) CSF IgM Ab	↑ risk ↑ mortality in elderly and ↑ mortality eastern versus western United States	Fever, headache, malaise, myalgias respiratory sx,/urinary sx in some	Supportive

Arbovirus (arthropod-borne)	La Crosse encephalitis	*Bunyaviridae* (California encephalitis group)	Mosquitos	Rodents, chipmunks, squirrels, foxes	Summer/fall (Jul–Sep)	United States: central, eastern	School-age children	CSF IgM Ab, >4-fold ↑ serum Ab Isolate virus, viral Ag	Low mortality	Fever, headache, vomiting, disorientation, seizure, focal neuro signs	Supportive
Arbovirus (arthropod-borne)	West Nile encephalitis	Flavi vridiae	Mosquitoes	Birds	Summer/fall	Worldwide	Elderly	Serology, CSF for IgM Ab (ELISA)	Number one cause of epidemic viral encephalitis in United States	Fever, headache, myalgias, back pain, MP rash (some), flaccid paralysis	Supportive
Arbovirus (arthropod-borne)	Colorado tick fever	Reo viridae	Ticks Transmission: woodtick	Rodents, small mammals	Mar–Sep, peak Apr–Jun	Western United States and western Canada	Children Mountain areas 1200–3000 m (4000–10,000 feet) elevations	PCR tests + from day 1 of sx Serology + in 10–14 d	History of tick bite in 90%	Headache, fever, chills, myalgias, prostration, rash (15%)	Supportive
Neurotropic virus	Rabies	Rhabdo viridae	Rabid animals Rare Transmission via transplant of tissues	United States: main reservoirs: bats, raccoons, skunks, foxes	Any season Consult: CDC, and United States state health department if overseas exposure	Worldwide, developing countries: reservoir, dogs	All ages Virus travels from peripheral wound to dorsal root ganglion to brain	Clinical dx Must test several specimens eg, saliva, skin, serum, CSF	Highest case fatality rate of any disease Specimens: potentially infectious	Prodrome: flulike sx, pain, paresthesias, pruritus at entry site Neurologic: encephalitic or paralytic rabies	No survivors (1 exception) if not vaccinated before onset of sx Supportive, experimental Prevention: after exposure
Rickettsia (tick-borne)	Rocky Mountain spotted fever (RMSF)	*Rickettsia rickettsii*	Ticks	Dog tick (east, south central United States) Wood tick (west of Miss River)	Spring/early summer	United States: southeast, south central states especially NC, AR	Children Exposure to dogs Live near wooded areas	Clinical features in appropriate setting (endemic area) Spotless RMSF 10% of patients	No reliable dx test early Serology + Ab After 7–10 d, obtain at 14–21 d	Typical rash, fever, headache, malaise, arthralgias	Doxycycline (if pregnant chloram-phenicl)

(continued on next page)

Table 3
(continued)

	Disease	Pathogen	Spread or Vector	Reservoir or Host	Seasonal Other Factors	Geographic Distribution	Exposure, Age Predilection	Diagnosis	Comments	Clinical	Treatment
Spirochete (tick-borne)	Lyme disease (tick-borne)	*B burgdorferi*	Ticks	Deer	Spring/summer /fall	Worldwide United States: first reported Lyme, CT	All ages 3 stages: early localized, early disseminated, late	Clinical dx if EM rash present, never dx by serology alone, PCR test on CSF	Most common tick-borne disease in United States and Europe	Early local: rash (80%) nonspecific sx, headache, fatigue early disseminated multiple EM lesions, neuro sx, cardiac sx Late: arthritis, neuro sx	Doxycycline, amoxicillin, cefuroxime
Bacteria	Cat scratch disease	*Bartonella hensalae* (fastidious slow growing, gram-negative)	Cat bite, or cat scratch, or flea bite	Cats	Any season Consider in FUO	Worldwide In 1 study, third most common FUO in children	All ages Elderly: atypical sx Cat or flea contact	Clinical dx + hx of exposure, + serology, lymph node biopsy	Regional lymphad-enopathy, sometimes visceral organ/ neurologic/ ocular involvement	Local skin lymph node near entry site (85%) Dissemination (15%) neuro sx, liver, spleen, eyes, MSK	[a]Azithromycin alternatives: clarithromycin, rifampin, bactrim, cipro (adults)
Mycobacterium	TB	CNS TB	Primary infection or reactivation	Outcome depends on stage when tx initiated → need early tx	Abnormalities on CXR in 50%, negative skin test does not rule out TB, new blood test for TB	Worldwide Developed world: mostly adults with reactivation	Immuno-suppressed Newer rapid tests detect TB nucleic acids	Gold standard: AFB on CSF CSF: AFB stain/culture ↑ monos ↓ glucose, ↑ protein	Signs of active TB outside CNS are helpful but often absent or nonspecific	CNS TB: meningitis, intracranial tuberculoma, arachmoiditis	4-drug therapy, may be drug-resistant TB, consider glucortico-steroids
Chlamydophilia	Psittacosis (ornithosis)	Chlamydophilia	Birds as pets, vets, poultry workers	Contact with birds (pigeons in spring)	May be transmitted without direct contact	All ages Worldwide	Exposure to birds as pets or occupation or in nature	Culture is dangerous, highly infectious, not encouraged, so do serology	Clinical dx + hx of bird contact, All diagnostic tests have limitations	Fever, HA, myalgias, dry cough, CXR usually +	[a]Doxycycline, tetracycline (avoid children <8 y), Alternative: chloram-phenicol

Parasite	*Naegleria fowleri* (primary amebic meningo-encephalitis)	Ameba (can be cultured but not by routine methods)	Because of swimming/ water activities may be seen more often in summer	Ponds, man-made lakes, hot springs, thermally polluted streams, rivers, unchlorinated pools	Ameba not found in sea water, enters CNS via olfactory epithelium	Worldwide, especially in warm bodies of water	Previously healthy children/young adults, presents like bacterial meningitis	Clinical dx + hx of recent water/sports activities All diagnostic tests have limitations	CSF wet mount: trophozoite form on Wright or Giemsa stain (not seen on Gram stain)	Fever, headache, neck stiffness, nausea, vomiting, altered taste/smell	Amphotericin B plus rifampin Does not respond to routine antibiotics, fatal in >95%
Fungal	Cryptococus	Cryptococcal meningoen-cephalitis	Inhalation via respiratory tract then hematoge-nenous spread	Presentation differs HIV versus non-HIV: HIV > number of organisms ↓ inflammatory response	Cryptococcal meningoe-ncephalitis is the most common manifestation of cryptococcosis	Worldwide, consider in immuno-competent patients with subacute or chronic meningitis	Opportunistic infection in immuno-suppressed patients	CSF: + culture +Ag, India ink: encapsulated yeast forms ↑ OP, ↓ glu ↑ monos ↑ protein Serum: + Ag	Must perform LP to diagnose Perform blood cultures because they may be positive	Subacute onset, nonspecific signs/sx, fever, headache, CNS signs/sxs	Initial tx: amphotericin B + flucytosine

This is not an all-inclusive table but is intended to list some of the important causes of encephalitis that may be encountered in North America.

Abbreviations: Ab, antibody; AFB, acid fast bacilli; Ag, antigen; AR, Arkansas; CDC, Center for Disease Control; CT, Connecticutt; CXR, chest radiograph; dx, diagnosis; EM, erythema migrans; FL, Florida; FUO, fever of unknown origin; glu, glucose; HA, headache; hx, history; LOC, level of consciousness; Miss, Mississippi; monos, monocytes; MP, maculopapular; MSK, musculoskeletal; N, nausea; NC, North Carolina; neuro, neurologic; OH, Ohio; sx, symptoms; OP, opening pressure; TB, tuberculosis; tx, treatment; TX, Texas; V, vomiting.

[a] Drug of choice, other alternatives may be listed.

Table 4
Specific therapy for meningitis and encephalitis[a] when the pathogen is known

Meningitis: Pathogen	Recommended	Alternative
Empirical Therapy: Meningitis[a]		
Need coverage for *S pneumoniae* and *N meningitides* (most common causes of meningitis in children and adults)	Third-generation cephalosporin (cefotaxime or ceftriaxone) plus vancomycin (if *Staph* is a consideration)	Add ampicillin in elderly patients (>50 years) and in newborns (coverage for *Listeria*) Vancomycin for *Staph* coverage
In neonates also need coverage for *Listeria*	Ampicillin plus cefotaxime or ampicillin plus gentamicin	Ceftriaxone not recommended in neonates Trimethaprim-sulfamethoxazole for gentamicin
In elderly patients, also need coverage for *Listeria*	Ampicillin plus vancomycin plus third-generation cephalosporin	
Recent neurosurgery or anatomic defects or penetrating head trauma or recent CSF shunt	Third-generation cephalosporin plus vancomycin plus aminoglycoside (gentamicin)	Aminoglycioside for gram-negatives, Vancomycin for *Staph aureus*, coagulase-negative *Staph* (*Staph epdermidis*)
Meningitis: Specific Pathogen		
Enterobactericeae: *E coli*, others	Third-generation cephalosporin	Meropenem
H influenzae (β-lactam positive)	Third-generation cephalosporin	Chloranphenicol
L monocytogenes	Ampicillin or penicillin G	Meropenem, if pen allergic, bactrim (avoid in newborns)
N meningitides	Third-generation cephalosporin: cefotaxime or ceftriaxone	Chloramphenicol, meropenem, penicillin G (if sensitive)
Other *Streptoocci* (β hemolytic *Streptococci*)	Ampicillin or penicillin G	
Pseudomonas aeruginosa	Ceftazidime	Meropenem
Staphylococci	Vancomycin (if methicillin-resistant)	Nafcillin or oxacillin if methicillin sensitive, linezolid
S pneumoniae	Third-generation cephalosporin plus vancomycin	

Adjunctive Corticosteroids	
Infants/children Hib meningitis	Recommended[b]
Infants/children >6 weeks old Pneumococcal meningitis	Consider corticosteroids[b]
Adults Pneumococcal meningitis	Recommended[c]
Drug Dosages: Antibiotics	
Corticosteroids dose: 0.15 mg/kg per dose every 6 h for 2–4 d	Give first dose of corticosteroids just before (eg, 15–20 min) or concurrently with the first dose of antibiotics
Ampicillin: 100 mg/kg every 6 h (maximum 2 g per dose)	
Cefotaxime 50 mg/kg every 6 h	
Ceftriaxone 50 mg/kg every 12 h	
Chloramphenicol 50 mg/kg every 6 h (maximum 1 g every dose)	
Gentamicin pediatric 2.5 mg/kg every 8–12 h (maximum 1 g every dose, 4 g every day) adult 1–2 g every 8–12 h	
Meropenem 40 mg/kg every 8 h (maximum 2 g per dose)	
Nafcillin pediatric 25–50 mg/kg every 6 h (maximum 12 g daily), adult 1–2 g every 6 h	
Oxacillin (same dose as for nafcillin)	
Penicillin pediatric: 100,000 U/kg every 6 h, adult: 4 million units every 6 h (maximum 4 million units every dose)	
Quinolones: adults 400 mg every 8 h or 600 mg every 12 h (maximum 1200 mg every 6 h)	
Rifampin: pediatric 5–10 mg/kg given once or twice daily, adult 600 mg/d	

(continued on next page)

Table 4
(continued)

Trimethaprin-sulfamethoxazole 5 mg/kg every 12 h (based on trimethoprim component) (avoid in neonates)		
Tobramycin: pediatric 2.5 mg/kg every 8 h; adult 1–2 mg/kg every 8 h		
Vancomycin: pediatric 15 mg/kg every 8–12 h (maximum 1 g every dose, 4 g every day), adult 1 g every dose		
Encephalitis: Pathogen	Recommended[b]	Consider[b]
Viruses		
Herpes simplex	Acyclovir	
Varicella zoster	Acyclovir	
Cytomegalovirus	Ganciclovir plus foscarnet	
Epstein-Barr virus		Corticosteroids
Human herpes virus 6	Ganciclovir or foscarnet if immunocompromised	Consider gancyclovir or foscarnet if immunocompetent
Influenza		Oseltamivir
St Louis encephalitis		Interferon-α
Measles		Ribavirin
Subacute sclerosing panencephalitis		Intrathecal Ribavirin
Bacteria		
L monocytogenes	Ampicillin plus gentamicin (if penicillin allergy trimethoprim-sulfamethoxazole)	
Mycobacterium tuberculosis	4-drug antituberculous therapy, if meningitis adjunctive dexamethasone	

Mycoplasma pneumoniae	Macrolides: azithromycin, clarithromycin or erthromycin	Alternatives to macrolides include tetracycline and doxycycline. Fluroquinolones may be used in adults but are not recommended as first-line agents for children
Rickettsioses ehrlichioses		
Rickettsia rickettsii	Doxycycline (alternative chloramphenical if during pregnancy)	
Spirochetes		
B burgdorferi	Ceftriaxone or cefotaxime or penicillin G	
Treponema palladium	Penicillin G (ceftriaxone as alternative)	
Fungi		
Coccidoides	Fluconazole (alternatives itraconazole, voriconazole, amphotericin B)	
Cryptococcus neoformans	Amphotericin B plus flucytosine	
Histoplasma capsulatum	Amphotericin followed by itraconazole	
Protozoa		
Naegleria fowleri	Amphotericin plus rifampin	
Plasmodium flaciparum	Quinine, quinidine or artemether	
Toxoplasma gondii	Pyrimethamine plus either sulfadiazine or clindamycin	
Helminth		
Taenia solium	Albendazole and corticosteroids	

This is not an all-inclusive list but gives some of the pathogens encountered in North America. This is for immunocompetent patients. Other sources may be consulted for a more extensive list.

[a] A common currently suggested empirical regimen is given. Pathogens and their sensitivities to drugs and dosages may change so other sources should be consulted.

[b] Based on Red Book.[37,38]

[c] Based on clinical practice guidelines (2008) by the Infectious Disease Society of America.[16]

Controversy: Distinguishing Bacterial from Viral Meningitis Based on Laboratory Studies

There are distinct CSF findings that suggest bacterial meningitis. The identification of an organism on a Gram stain of CSF is helpful in deciding on a specific antibiotic therapy for a given pathogen. With bacterial meningitis, a positive Gram stain is reported in 50% to 90% of patients but declines to 7% to 41% if the patient has been on oral antibiotics.[9] Other CSF results that suggest bacterial meningitis include glucose level less than 40 mg/dL or CSF blood glucose ratio less than 0.40, protein level greater than 200 mg/dL, WBC count greater than 1000/μL, more than 80% polymorphonuclear neutrophils, or an opening pressure greater than 300 mm.[18] Viral meningitis tends to have CSF findings as follows: WBC count less than 300 cell/mm,[3] less than 20% polymorphonuclear neutrophils, normal protein level, and a normal glucose level on CSF.[18] A CSF lympocytic pleocytosis and increased CSF RBCs are characteristic of HSV encephalitis.[9]

The classic CSF findings may not always be present in a patient with bacterial meningitis.[9] In one study, 12% (83 of 696) of adult patients with bacterial meningitis had none of the CSF findings typical of bacterial meningitis.[3] Conversely, up to half (30%–50%) of patients with viral meningitis show predominance of CSF neutrophils, which is the classic finding for bacterial meningitis.[51–53]

PCR technology has become available and may be helpful in some cases.[30,54] For example, a rapid (<3 hour) qualitative test for enteroviral RNA in the CSF has recently become available that could be useful because enteroviruses are the most common cause of viral meningitis.[54] When encephalitis is in the differential, CSF should be tested for HSV-PCR even although this is not a rapid test. If the clinical situation warrants, serology for West Nile virus can be performed.[30]

Other studies including acute phase reactants such as C-reactive protein or procalcitonin levels have been suggested as a tool in distinguishing bacterial from viral meningitis. Because these studies have a high specificity but low sensitivity for bacterial meningitis, most experts do not recommend using these biomarkers or acute phase reactants to make decisions regarding a given patient.[9]

Because there is no one test or constellation of tests that has 100% accuracy in distinguishing bacterial from viral meningitis, decisions in any specific patient require clinical judgment, with test results being part of the data that are integrated into the overall clinical picture.

Controversy: Adjunctive Corticosteroids

The use of corticosteroids for the treatment of meningitis and encephalitis has been a subject of debate for many years.[9–11] Inflammation in the CNS can have devastating consequences (see pathophysiology section) and the hope is that antiinflammatory agents, specifically corticosteroids, can decrease the inflammation associated with CNS infection.

The administration of corticosteroids in animal models of meningitis caused a decrease in cerebral edema, in CSF pressure, and in CSF lactate levels.[55] Administration of antibiotics to patients with meningitis kills the pathogenic bacteria, thereby releasing components of the bacterial cell wall. These cell wall components promote the production and release by the body of proinflammatory cytokines into the subarachnoid space. Once the body's cells have been stimulated into making and releasing these proinflammatory cytokines, dexamethasone has no effect.[56,57] Timing is critical. For dexamethasone to have an effect, it must be given before the body's cells have started marking inflammatory cytokines.[56] For this reason the recommendation is that dexamethasone be given immediately before (eg, 15–20 minutes) or concurrently with antibiotic administration.

The evidence favors the use of corticosteroids at least in some patients.[16,41] Improved patient outcomes were documented in a large, prospective, randomized, placebo-controlled double-blind multicenter trial of adult bacterial meningitis when dexamethasone was given before or with the first antibiotic dose.[55] A Cochrane meta-analysis of adult patients with bacterial meningitis given dexamethasone also documented decreased morbidity and mortality.[41]

Pediatric studies have had some conflicting results with dexamethasone use in bacterial meningitis. Decreased morbidity (eg, lower incidence of long-term hearing loss) was noted with dexamethasone administration in 2 randomized, double-blind, placebo-controlled studies of childhood bacterial meningitis.[58] A meta-analysis of dexamethasone use in pediatric patients with bacterial meningitis[59] and several other pediatric studies[60,61] noted a benefit, specifically a decreased incidence of hearing loss.

Contrary to these reports, a study of neonatal (age ≤30 days) meningitis documented negative results with dexamathesone.[62] Two large trials, 1 in adults and 1 in pediatric patients with bacterial meningitis, did not find a benefit with dexamethasone.[63,64] These 2 studies were undertaken in sub-Saharan Africa, where there are high rates of HIV (from 28% to 90%). It may be that these unique patient populations with a large incidence of HIV-positive patients affected the study's results.[11]

The effect of the introduction of the various vaccines (HIV and streptococcal vaccines) on the epidemiology of meningitis on infants and children in the developed world remains to be determined.

Dexamethasone can be used in adult patients with proven or suspected pneumococcal meningitis, [18] in infants and children more than 6 weeks of age with Hib meningitis[39]; and dexamethasone may be considered in infants and children more than 6 weeks of age with pneumococcal meningitis.[40] If dexamethasone is to be given, it should be administered before or concurrently with the first dose of antibiotics.

SUMMARY

The clinical presentation of any of the CNS infections including meningitis, encephalitis, and brain abscess, may include an altered level of consciousness as well as a range of other symptoms from headache and fever to focal neurologic deficits. Early recognition and treatment of such infections is critical to improve patient outcome.

REFERENCES

1. Leib SL, Tauber MG. Pathogenesis and pathophysiology of bacterial infections. In: Scheld WM, Whitley RJ, Marra CM, editors. Infections of the central nervous system. 3rd edition. Philadelphia: Lippincott, Williams & Wilkins; 2004. p. 331–46.
2. Cassady KA, Whitley RJ. Pathogenesis and pathophysiology of viral infections of the central nervous system. In: Scheld WM, Whitley RJ, Marra CM, editors. Infections of the central nervous system. 3rd edition. Philadelphia: Lippincott, Williams & Wilkins; 2004. p. 57–74.
3. van de Beek D, De Gans J, Spanjaard L, et al. Clinical features and prognostic factors in adults with bacterial meningitis. N Engl J Med 2004;351(18):1849–59.
4. Durand ML, Calderwood SB, Weber DJ, et al. Acute bacterial meningitis in adults: a review of 493 episodes. N Engl J Med 1993;328:21–8.
5. Sigurdardottir B, Bjornsson OM, Jonsdottir KE, et al. Acute bacterial meningitis in adults. A 20-year overview. Arch Intern Med 1997;157(4):425–30.

6. Hussein AS, Shafran SD. Acute bacterial meningitis in adults. A 12 year view. Medicine (Baltimore) 2000;79(6):360–8.
7. Attia J, Hatala R, Cook DJ, et al. The rational clinical examination. Does this adult patient have acute meningitis? JAMA 1999;282(2):176–81.
8. Valmari P, Peltola H, Ruuskanen O, et al. Childhood bacterial meningitis: initial symptoms and signs related to age, and reasons for consulting a physician. Eur J Pediatr 1987;146(5):515–8.
9. Fitch MT, Abrahamian FM, Moran GJ, et al. Emergency department management of meningitis and encephalitis. Infect Dis Clin North Am 2008;22:33–52.
10. Mace SE. Acute bacterial meningitis. Emerg Med Clin North Am 2008;26(2): 281–317.
11. Somard D, Meuer W. Central nervous system infections. Emerg Med Clin North Am 2009;27:89–100.
12. Choi C. Bacterial meningitis. Clin Geriatr Med 1992;8(4):889–902.
13. Silvia MT, Licht DL. Pediatric central nervous system infections and inflammatory white matter disease. Pediatr Clin North Am 2005;52:1107–26.
14. Pfister HW, Feiden W, Einhaulp KM. Spectrum of complications during bacterial meningitis in adults. Results of a prospective clinical study. Arch Neurol 1993; 50(6):578–81.
15. Ziai WC. Advances in the management of central nervous system infections in the ICU. Crit Care Clin 2006;22(4):661–94.
16. Lavoie FW, Caucier JR. Central nervous system infections. In: Marx JA, Hockberger RS, Walls RM, et al, editors. Rosen's emergency medicine concepts and clinical practice. 6th edition. Philadelphia: Mosby Elsevier; 2006. p. 1710–25.
17. Chavez-Bueno S, McCracken GH Jr. Bacterial meningitis in children. Pediatr Clin North Am 2005;52:795–810.
18. Tunkel AR, Hartman BJ, Kaplan SL, et al. Practice guidelines for the management of bacterial meningitis: Infectious Disease Society of American (IDSA) guidelines. Clin Infect Dis 2004;39:1267–84.
19. Cunha BA. Central nervous system infections in the compromised host: a diagnostic approach. Infect Dis Clin North Am 2001;15(2):567–90.
20. Studahl M, Bergstrom T, Hagberg L. Acute viral encephalitis in adults – a prospective study. Scand J Infect Dis 1998;30(3):215–20.
21. Solomon T, Ooi MH, Beasley DW, et al. West Nile encephalitis. BMJ 2003; 326(7394):865–9.
22. Puxty JA, Fox RA, Horan MA. The frequency of physical signs usually attributed to meningeal irritation in elderly patients. J Am Geriatr Soc 1983;31(10):216–20.
23. Gorse GJ, Thrupp LD, Nudleman KL, et al. Bacterial meningitis in the elderly. Arch Intern Med 1984;144(8):1603–7.
24. Kulchycki LK, Edlow JA. Geriatric neurologic emergencies. Emerg Med Clin North Am 2006;24(3):273–98.
25. Adedipe A, Lowenstein R. Infectious emergencies in the elderly. Emerg Med Clin North Am 2006;24:433–48.
26. Huang DB, Schantz PM, White AC Jr. Helminthic infections. In: Scheld WM, Whitley RJ, Marra CM, editors. Infections of the central nervous system. 3rd edition. Philadelphia: Lippincott, Williams & Wilkins; 2004. p. 797–828.
27. Marra CM, Whitley RJ, Scheld WM. Approach to the patient with central nervous system infection. In: Scheld WM, Whitley RJ, Marra CM, editors. Infections of the central nervous system. 3rd edition. Philadelphia: Lippincott, Williams & Wilkins; 2004. p. 1–4.

28. Hasbrun R, Abrahams J, Jekel J, et al. Computed tomography of the head before lumbar puncture in adults with suspected meningitis. N Engl J Med 2001;345:24.
29. Kapur R, Yoder MC, Polin RA. Developmental immunology. In: Martin RJ, Fanaroff AA, Walsh MC, editors. 8th edition, Fanaroff and Martin's neonatal-perinatal medicine, vol. 2. Philadelphia: Mosby Elsevier; 2006. p. 761–90.
30. Tunkel AR, Glaser CA, Bloch KC, et al. The management of encephalitis clinical practice guidelines by the Infectious Diseases Society of America. Clin Infect Dis 2008;47:303–27.
31. Thompson RB Jr, Bertram H. Laboratory diagnosis of central nervous system infections. Infect Dis Clin North Am 2001;15(4):1047–71.
32. Polage CR, Petti CA. Assessment of the utility of viral culture of cerebrospinal fluid. Clin Infect Dis 2006;43:1578–9.
33. Mathisen GE, Johnson JP. Brain abscess. Clin Infect Dis 1997;25:763–81.
34. Carpenter J, Stapleton S, Holliman R. Retrospective analysis of 49 cases of brain abscess and review of the literature. Eur J Clin Microbiol Infect Dis 2007;26(1): 1–11.
35. Yang SY. Brain abscess: a review of 400 cases. J Neurosurg 1981;55(5):794–9.
36. Wenger JD, Hightower AW, Facklam RR, et al. Bacterial meningitis in the United States. 1986 report of a multistate surveillance study. The Bacterial Meningitis Study Group. J Infect Dis 1990;162(6):1316–22.
37. Schuchat A, Robinson K, Wenger JD, et al. Bacterial meningitis in the United States in 1995. Active surveillance team. N Engl J Med 1997;337(14):970–6.
38. Diseases transmitted by animals (zoonoses). In: Committee on Infectious Diseases American Academy of Pediatrics, editor. Redbook: 2009 report of the Committee on Infectious Diseases. 28th edition. Elk Grove Village (IL): American Academy of Pediatrics; 2009. p. 864–70.
39. *Haemophilus influenzae*. In: Committee on Infectious Diseases American Academy of Pediatrics, editor. Redbook: 2009 report of the Committee on Infectious Diseases. 28th edition. Elk Grove Village (IL): American Academy of Pediatrics; 2009. p. 314–5.
40. Pneumococcal infections. In: Committee on Infectious Diseases American Academy of Pediatrics, editor. Redbook: 2009 report of the Committee on Infectious Diseases. 28th edition. Elk Grove Village (IL): American Academy of Pediatrics; 2009. p. 524–6.
41. van de Beek D, de Gans J, McIntyre P, et al. Corticosteroids in acute bacterial meningitis. Cochrane Database Syst Rev 2007;1:CD004405.
42. Kamei S, Sekizawa T, Shiota H, et al. Evaluation of combination therapy using acyclovir and corticosteroids in adult patients with herpes simplex viral encephalitis. J Neurol Neurosurg Psychiatry 2005;76:1544–9.
43. Masson CB. The dangers of diagnostic lumbar puncture in increased intracranial pressure due to brain tumor, with a review of 200 cases in which lumbar puncture was done. Res Nerv Ment Dis Proc 1937;8:422–34.
44. Korein J, Cravioto H, Leicach M. Reevaluation of lumbar puncture; a study of 129 patients with papilledema or intracranial hypertension. Neurology 1959;9(4): 290–7.
45. Sencer W. The lumbar puncture in the presence of papilledema. J Mt Sinai Hosp N Y 1956;23(6):808–15.
46. Rennick G, Shann F, de Campo J. Cerebral herniation during bacterial meningitis in children. BMJ 1993;306(6883):953–5.
47. Oliver WJ, Shope TC, Kuhns LR. Fatal lumbar puncture: fact versus fiction–an approach to a clinical dilemma. Pediatrics 2003;222(3 Pt.):e174–6.

48. Shetty AK, Desselle BC, Craver RD, et al. Fatal cerebral herniation after lumbar puncture in a patient with a normal computed tomography scan. Pediatrics 1999;103(6 Pt.1):1284–7.
49. Nigrovic LE, Kuppermann N, Macias CG, et al. Clinical prediction rule for identifying children with cerebrospinal fluid pleocytosis at very low risk of bacterial meningitis. JAMA 2007;297(1):52–60.
50. Chavanet P, Schaller C, Levy C, et al. Performance of a predictive rule to distinguish bacterial and viral meningitis. J Infect 2007;54:328–36.
51. Michos AG, Syriopoulou VP, Hedjichristodoulou C, et al. Aseptic meningitis in children: analysis of 506 cases. PLoS One 2007;2:e674.
52. Carroll ED, Beadsworth MB, Jenkins N, et al. Clinical and diagnostic findings of an echovirus meningitis outbreak in the Northwest of England. Postgrad Med J 2006;82(963):60–4.
53. Bernit E, deLamballerie X, Zandotti C, et al. Prospective investigation of a large outbreak of meningitis due to echovirus 30 during summer 2000 in Marseilles, France. Medicine (Baltimore) 2004;83(4):245–53.
54. Kost CB, Rogers B, Oberste MS, et al. Multicenter beta of the GeneXpert enterovirus assay. J Clin Microbiol 2007;45(4):1081–6.
55. Tauber MG, Khayem-Bashi M, Sande MA, et al. Effects of ampicillin and corticosteroids on brain water content, cerebrospinal fluid pressure, and cerebrospinal fluid lactate levels in experimental pneumococcal meningitis. J Infect Dis 1985; 151:528–34.
56. Tunkel AR, Scheld WM. Acute meningitis. In: Mandell GL, Bennett JE, Dolan R, editors. Mandell, Bennett & Dolan: principles & practice of infectious diseases. 6th edition. Philadelphia: Churchill & Livingstone; 2005. p. 1083–126.
57. de Gans J, van de Beek D. Dexamethasone in adults with bacterial meningitis. N Engl J Med 2002;347(20):1549–56.
58. Lebel MH, Freij BJ. Dexamethasone therapy for bacterial meningitis: results of two double-blind, placebo-controlled trials. N Engl J Med 1988;319:964–71.
59. McIntyre PB, Berkey CS, King SM, et al. Dexamethasone as adjunctive therapy in bacterial meningitis: a meta-analysis of randomized clinical trials since 1988. JAMA 1997;278:925–31.
60. Wald ER, Kaplan ST, Mason ED Jr, et al. Dexamethasone therapy for children with bacterial meningitis – meningitis study group. Pediatrics 1995;95(1):21–8.
61. Schaad UB, Lips U, Gnehm HE, et al. Dexamethasone therapy for bacterial meningitis in children. Swiss Meningitis Study Group. Lancet 1993;342(8869): 457–61.
62. Daoud AS, Batieha A, Al-Sheyyab M, et al. Lack of effectiveness of dexamethasone in neonatal bacterial meningitis. Eur J Pediatr 1999;158(3):230–3.
63. Molyneaux EM, Walsh AL, Forsyth H, et al. Dexamethasone treatment in childhood bacterial meningitis in Malawi: a randomized control trial. Lancet 2002; 360(9328):211–8.
64. Scarborough M, Gordon SB, Whitty CJM, et al. Corticosteroids for bacterial meningitis in adults in sub-Saharan Africa. N Engl J Med 2007;357(24):2441–50.

Traumatic Alterations in Consciousness: Traumatic Brain Injury

Brian J. Blyth, MD*, Jeffrey J. Bazarian, MD, MPH

KEYWORDS

• Concussion • Trauma • Brain • Injury

The purpose of this review is to provide an overview of mild traumatic brain injury (mTBI) in a form useful for emergency physicians. mTBI is a disease with considerable public health impact and is the subject of a vast amount of current research. The authors' discussion of this disease is necessarily limited both by space constraints and the interests of their target audience. For more detailed discussions of various topics covered in this review, the reader is directed to the publications listed in **Table 1**.

DEFINITION OF TRAUMATIC BRAIN INJURY

Traumatic brain injury (TBI) is defined as any traumatically induced structural injury or physiologic disruption of brain function as a result of an external force. TBI is manifested by one or more clinical signs occurring immediately afterwards including a loss, decreased, or altered level of consciousness, amnesia, neurologic deficit, or intracranial lesion.[1] External forces may include direct impact of the head with another object, indirect forces from acceleration/deceleration, or a blast injury. The Glasgow Coma Score (GCS) has traditionally been used to classify TBI as mild (GCS 13–15), moderate (GCS 9–12), or severe (GCS 3–8). A more recent classification scheme for TBI uses length of loss of consciousness (LOC), alteration of consciousness (AOC), and posttraumatic amnesia (PTA), as well as imaging findings to categorize TBI (**Table 2**).[1] It is important to stress that mild TBI (mTBI) is clinically defined based solely on self-reported or observed symptoms, and often occurs with normal neuroimaging.

This work was supported by Grant No. 5R01HD051865-03 from the National Institutes of Health (J.J.B. and B.J.B.) and a Jahnigen Career Development Scholars Award (B.J.B).
Department of Emergency Medicine, Center for Neural Development and Disease, University of Rochester School of Medicine and Dentistry, 601 Elmwood Avenue, Box 645, Rochester, NY 14642, USA
* Corresponding author.
E-mail address: brian_blyth@urmc.rochester.edu

Emerg Med Clin N Am 28 (2010) 571–594
doi:10.1016/j.emc.2010.03.003 emed.theclinics.com
0733-8627/10/$ – see front matter

Table 1
Recommended further reading

Topic	References	Notes
Epidemiology	Summers et al[14]	Brief review of literature pertaining to the epidemiology of both military and civilian TBI
Biomechanics	LaPlaca et al[15]	Thorough review of basic biomechanics relevant to central nervous system trauma including discussion of experimental models of injury
Mechanisms to loss of consciousness	Shaw[33]	Detailed account of the historical development and current theories of altered consciousness resulting from TBI
Acute clinical management	Jagoda et al[42]	American College of Emergency Physicians and Centers for Disease Control clinical polices for the acute management of adult mTBI
Subacute and chronic clinical management	VA/DoD Clinical Practice Guideline for Management of Concussion/mTBI[1]	Definite clinical guidelines for subacute and chronic management of adult mTBI (>1 week post injury)
Long-term health effects	IOM (Institute of Medicine), Gulf War and Health, Volume 7[24]	Comprehensive review of evidence for long-term consequences of TBI

Indeed, the mTBI definition included in **Table 1** classifies TBI with positive neuroimaging as at least moderate in severity. Two older, but still commonly used mTBI definitions by the American Congress of Rehabilitation Medicine[2] and the Centers for Disease Control and Prevention[3] define patients as mild if they have positive

Table 2
Clinical criteria for TBI severity

Criteria	Mild	Moderate	Severe
Structural imaging	Definition dependent[a]	Normal or abnormal	Normal or abnormal
Loss of consciousness (LOC)	0–30 min	>30 min and <24 h	>24 h
Alteration of consciousness (AOC)[b]	A moment up to 24 h	>24 h. Severity based on other criteria	
Posttraumatic amnesia (PTA)	0–1 d	>1 and <7 d	>7 d
GCS (best score in first 24 h)	13–15	9–12	<9

[a] Patients who otherwise meet the clinical criteria for mTBI but have intracranial imaging abnormalities may be classified as complicated mTBI or moderate TBI depending on the definition used.
[b] Alteration of mental status must be immediately related to the trauma to the head. Typical symptoms may include looking or feeling dazed, confusion, difficulty thinking clearly or responding appropriately to mental status questions, or inability to describe events immediately before or after the traumatic event.

Data from IOM (Institute of Medicine). Gulf War and health, Vol. 7: Long-term consequences of traumatic brain injury. Washington, DC: The National Academies Press; 2009.

neuroimaging findings but meet all other clinical criteria for mTBI. Patients who have abnormal intracranial imaging but otherwise meet a clinical definition of mTBI are referred to as complicated mTBI.[4]

Concussion is a common term for mTBI and will be used interchangeably within this article. Our understanding of TBI remains rudimentary relative to many other medical problems of similar magnitude. A symptom-based classification uses the description of symptoms evident on history and physical examination to classify illness. This method is imprecise, often grouping disparate pathophysiological processes together as single clinical entities. This imprecision is particularly problematic in moderate and severe TBI where multiple injury processes as evidenced by heterogeneous imaging findings are often present simultaneously. As knowledge of a disease increases and diagnostic tools improve, a more sophisticated classification emerges that may include anatomic, physiologic, metabolic, immunologic, and genetic factors. TBI has been the subject of intensive research in recent years, and recommendations for improved classification of this diverse disease are beginning to appear in the literature.[5]

Epidemiology

An estimated 1.4 million Americans presented to emergency departments for medical care after TBI each year between 1995 and 2001.[6] Over 1 million of these patients had mTBI. The incidence of ED-attended concussion is 444 in 100,000 in the United States;[7] however, it is thought that nearly 40% of patients suffering mTBI do not seek hospital-based care, and 25% do not report their injuries to health care providers at all.[8] An estimated 5% to 25% of all patients with concussion have postconcussive symptoms or other cognitive deficits that persist beyond 1 year.[9–11] This number is greater than the annual incidence of multiple sclerosis, Parkinson disease, myasthenia gravis, and Huntington disease combined.[12] TBI is more common in men than women, with 60% of TBI occurring in males.[6] Young children, adolescents, and the elderly suffer the highest rates of TBI.[6] The most common mechanisms of TBI are falls, automobile accidents, being struck by or against an object, and assault. The rate of hospitalizations for TBI fell dramatically during the 1980s and 1990s.[6] Wounded veterans from the wars in Iraq and Afghanistan may represent a nontrivial increase in patients living with mTBI. Approximately 20% of troops returning from combat deployments in Iraq have clinician-confirmed mTBI. These patients typically have TBI resulting from a blast,[13] and often have comorbid posttraumatic stress disorder (PTSD) or depression.[14]

Biomechanics

Traumatic injury results from the transfer of energy from the environment to tissue that is greater than the amount that can be absorbed without dysfunction. Biomechanics is the study of the interaction of forces and physical responses in biologic systems. Traumatic insults generally occur over short periods of time and are referred to as dynamic loading. Dynamic loading includes both direct or impact loading, as well as impulsive loading whereby no physical contact occurs. The loads absorbed by the brain after trauma generally include linear and rotational components called angular loads. The rate and duration of the insult are important because loads applied at high rates tend to result in more damage.[15] For example, the force involved in punching a wall can also be applied by pressing your fist against that same wall for a few minutes: the former instance results in a boxer's fracture whereas the latter does not. Focal injury such as contusion results from direct loading and often occurs in the absence of widespread injury. In contrast, diffuse axonal injury (DAI) often occurs as a result of the rotational acceleration accompanying indirect loading.[16] Humans are particularly susceptible given their large cranium connected to the trunk by relatively weak neck musculature. Rotational acceleration produces substantial and widespread strains within the brain resulting from both acceleration and deceleration. These diffuse strains lead to differential movement of the brain relative to the skull, which can cause hemorrhage. Shear strain is most prominent after rotational injury, and brain tissue is particularly sensitive to this type of strain.[17] In animal models, rotational acceleration is required to produce concussion, whereas isolated linear acceleration produced contusions and subdural hematomas but no LOC.[18]

Pathophysiology

The initial traumatic insult results in mechanical damage including rupture of cellular and vascular membranes with release of intracellular contents, ultrastructural damage of axons, and changes in cerebral blood flow.[19,20] Subsequent metabolic derangement includes widespread release of excitatory neurotransmitters such as glutamate, severe dysregulation of calcium homeostasis, energy failure due to adenosine triphosphate depletion, free radical generation, and cell death by necrotic and apoptotic pathways.[20,21] More global consequences of the traumatic insult include increased intracranial pressure, decreased cerebral blood flow, tissue ischemia, cerebral edema, and functional blood-brain barrier dysfunction.[22,23] Following the initial damage, repair and recovery processes begin through the removal of cellular debris, glial scar formation, and plastic changes in neural networks.[24] Because of the difficulties studying human mTBI, the mechanisms described in this section were derived principally from animal studies and, to a lesser degree, from humans with severe TBI (sTBI). Similar processes are thought to occur in human mTBI.

Putative Causes of Altered Consciousness in mTBI

The definitive causes of altered consciousness are not known. LOC requires either loss of the function of both cerebral hemispheres or of the reticular activating system. Several plausible hypothetical mechanisms have been proposed for the AOC that occurs with mTBI. These hypotheses include the reticular, pontine-cholinergic system, centripetal, and convulsive hypotheses. The reticular activating system (RAS) resides in the brainstem reticular formation, which extends from the top of the spinal column to the rostral midbrain with extensions into the thalamus and hypothalamus. The RAS is excited by input from surrounding sensory tracts and transmits this excitation to the cortex to induce generalized cortical and behavioral arousal. In the absence of input from the RAS, consciousness is impaired.

Under the reticular hypothesis of concussion, LOC after brain trauma results from a disturbance or depression of the activity of polysynaptic pathways within the RAS.[25] It is not completely understood how a traumatic dysfunction of the RAS occurs; however, it is believed to result from shearing or tensile strains on RAS pathways at the craniocervical junction. Neuropathological evidence for this is limited. The hypothesis also fails to address traumatic amnesia. A further difficulty is that EEG findings do not support depression of the RAS in concussion.

The pontine-cholinergic system hypothesis differs from the reticular activating system hypothesis in that RAS dysfunction is thought to occur as a consequence of trauma-induced activation of the inhibitory cholinergic system of the dorsal pontine tegmentum.[26] In animal models, injection of cholinergic agonists into the brainstem induces unconsciousness[27,28] whereas similar injections of cholinergic antagonists reduce the duration of traumatic unconsciousness.[29] Furthermore, electroencephalographic (EEG) studies show widespread neuronal discharge after concussion, and elevated acetylcholine is found in the cerebrospinal fluid of patients after TBI. However, it is not clear that activation of this system can produce LOC due to RAS suppression.

The centripetal hypothesis posits that sudden rotational forces cause shearing strains and stresses that result in functional decoupling of nerve fibers.[18] The depth of this functional decoupling is directly related to the extent of rotational acceleration delivered to the brain. Also, with greater rotational acceleration the likelihood of mechanical injury to fibers increases. Lower inertial forces that result in functional decoupling between the subcortex or diencephalon and the cortex may result in amnesia or confusion without LOC. Furthermore, greater forces resulting in decoupling between more superficial structures and the mesencephalon result in LOC. This hypothesis nicely explains posttraumatic amnesia and dazed states; however, it also requires very high energy injuries to cause full LOC. Consequently, patients with LOC would often have accompanying structural brain injury that simply is not observed.

Patients with concussion have similar symptoms to those who have experienced generalized epileptic seizures or electroconvulsive therapy (ECT). This overlap of symptoms has led to speculation that similar pathophysiological events occur in all 3 conditions. Close observation of human patients and animal models shows that concussive injury generally causes an initial convulsive event followed by a longer and more prominent paralytic phase.[30,31] EEG recordings from concussed animals also show initial, transient epileptiform activity. According to the convulsive hypothesis the symptoms associated with concussion are due to direct injury to neurons, resulting in hyperexcitability and widespread membrane depolarization followed by neuronal exhaustion.[32] These 2 neuronal states correspond to the convulsive and paralytic phases, respectively.

The convulsive hypothesis is able to reasonably account for a broader range of postconcussive behaviors than its competitors, including LOC, amnesia, convulsive movements, autonomic disturbances, and the dazed or "dinged" state.[33] While this hypothesis does a better job than the others at providing a unified explanation for the broad range of symptoms observed as an acute result of mTBI, it does not account for the structural abnormalities that occur as a result of mTBI. In summary, none of the individual hypotheses currently available explain all the findings seen with mTBI. Given the often complementary strengths and weaknesses of the 4 hypotheses discussed above, it seems likely that the mechanisms of altered consciousness after TBI may be due to a combination of processes. For a detailed explanation of these hypotheses, the reader is directed to the excellent review by Shaw.[33]

DIAGNOSIS OF MTBI

Clinical Presentation

A 28-year-old man presents to the Emergency Department (ED) after a motor vehicle accident. He was the restrained driver in a car that skidded of the road in icy conditions and collided head-on with a tree at 50 mph. There was airbag deployment. The paramedic reports that he was unconscious initially but that he was alert and oriented during transport.

Differential Diagnosis

The diagnosis of mTBI is made clinically and relies heavily on the history obtained from the patient and any witnesses. Obtaining a reliable history is often difficult because of posttraumatic amnesia, persistent altered mental status, or intoxication, a frequent comorbid factor in mTBI patients. Diagnoses with similar presentations include seizure, syncope, intoxication, malingering, anxiety, and other psychiatric conditions.

Clinical Criteria

Several clinical criteria for the diagnosis of mTBI exist.[1–3] Concussion or mTBI is defined as a LOC of less than 30 minutes or amnesia lasting less than 24 hours, or any period of altered mental status at the time of injury. In conjunction, patients must also have a GCS of 13 to 15 and normal structural imaging to meet the criteria for mTBI. Lower GCS scores classify the patient as having moderate (GCS 9–12) or severe (GCS 3–8) TBI.

Imaging

The imaging study of choice in mTBI is noncontrast head computed tomography (CT). This study is preferred over others because it is sensitive for traumatic injuries that require neurosurgical intervention including acute bleeding, increased intracranial pressure, and skull fracture. Although as many as 15% of mTBI patients will have an acute injury detected by noncontrast head CT, only 1% of those abnormalities require neurosurgical intervention.[34–40] Other imaging modalities are of limited use for the clinical evaluation of mTBI patients and are not recommended. Although magnetic resonance imaging (MRI) is 30% more sensitive than CT for the detection of traumatic abnormalities after mTBI,[41] there is no evidence that it identifies more patients requiring neurosurgical intervention.[42] More exotic imaging modalities including functional MRI, diffusion tensor imaging MRI, magnetic resonance spectroscopy, single-photon emission computed tomography, and positron emission tomography are valuable research tools but do not have proven clinical utility.

Decision Rules

The low rate of clinically important brain injury seen on head CT obtained acutely after mTBI has resulted in efforts to minimize unnecessary studies through the application of rigorously validated clinical decision rules. Two major decision rules applying to adult mTBI patients include the Canadian CT Head Rule[43] and the New Orleans Criteria.[44] For patients with a GCS of 15, both of these rules have equivalent sensitivities for detecting injuries requiring neurosurgical intervention; however, the Canadian CT Head Rule has a higher specificity for some clinical outcomes and its use may reduce imaging rates.[45] In pediatric populations, increased concern for radiation exposure and the potential requirement for sedation make minimizing unnecessary CT after mTBI even more compelling than in adult populations. Kuppermann and colleagues[46] recently reported a very sensitive decision rule that identifies low-risk children who do not require a head CT after mTBI. Indications for obtaining head CT after mTBI based on these decision rules are summarized in **Fig. 1**.

Biomarkers

There is substantial interest in developing protein biomarkers obtained from serum to aid the diagnosis and guide the treatment of TBI of all severities. Although several potential biomarkers have been studied,[47–53] to date only serum S100B has accepted clinical utility for mTBI. Specifically, elevated S100B has a high negative predictive value for clinically important injury on head CT after mTBI. In a large cohort, elevated S100B was 99% sensitive for the detection of injury on CT scan,[54] prompting the use of this test as the clinical standard of care in several European countries. The test has the added advantage of not being affected by concomitant alcohol intoxication.[55] Although not yet approved by the Food and Drug Administration (FDA) in the United

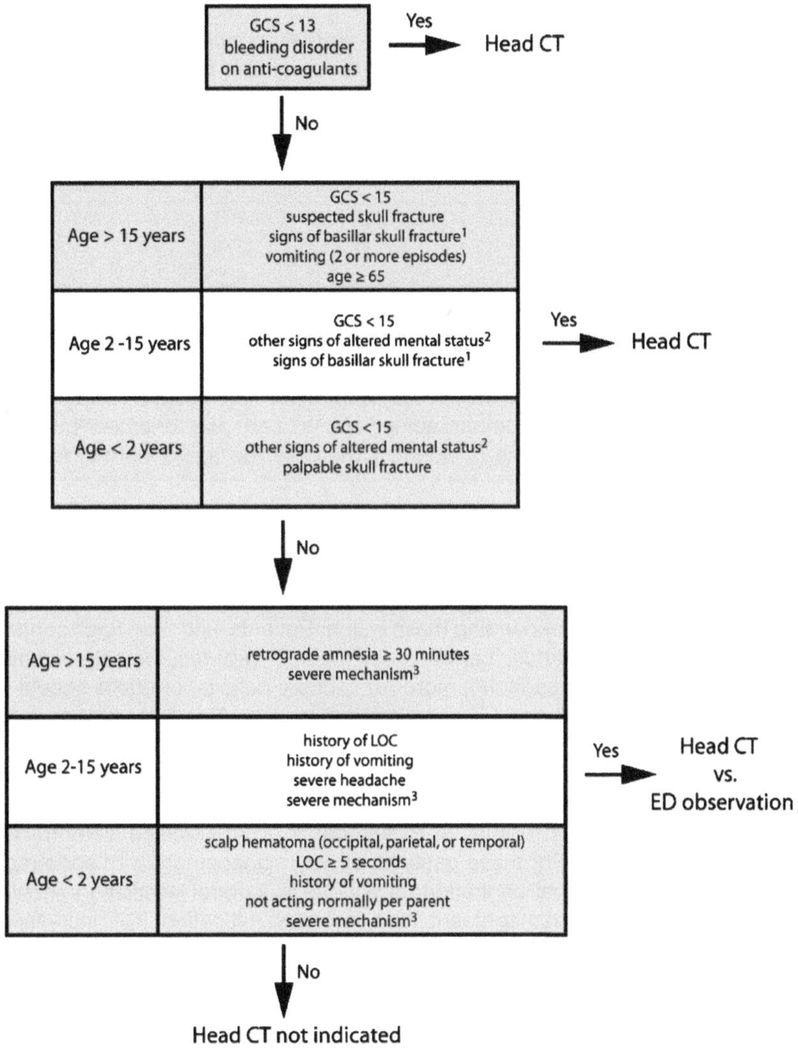

1. hemotympanum, racoon eyes, CSF otorhea or rinorrhea, Battle's Sign
2. agitation, somnolence, repetitive questioning, slow respons to verbal communication
3. severe mechanisms include:
   a. motor vehicle accident with ejection, rollover, or death of another occupant
   b. falls of > 3 feet (ages 2 and over), or >1.5 feet (under age 2)
   c. pedestrian or bicyclist struck by motor vehicle
   d. head struck by high-impact object.

Fig. 1. Indications for obtaining noncontrast head CT after TBI. Noncontrast head CT is the study of choice to evaluate TBI patients for clinically important neurotrauma. Clinically important neurotrauma is defined as any traumatically induced intracranial injury that requires neurosurgical intervention or requires hospital admission and neurosurgical follow-up. Clinically important TBI occurs rarely after mTBI, therefore minimizing unnecessary head CT scans is desirable. This figure integrates validated decision rules for both adult[45] and pediatric patients[46] designed to minimize unnecessary CT scans after mTBI.

States, the American College of Emergency Physicians recently issued a guideline stating that for mTBI patients with serum S100B concentrations of less than 0.1 μg/mL measured within 4 hours of injury, it is reasonable to consider not obtaining a head CT.[42] Multicenter studies to evaluate the accuracy of this test in United States patient populations are currently underway and may provide the data necessary for FDA approval.

TREATMENT OF MTBI

Clinical Presentation

After receiving the prehospital provider's report, you note that the patient is complaining of headache, back pain, and abdominal pain. He has no significant medical history and takes no medications. Pertinent findings on examination include a slight tachycardia, an abrasion on his forehead, mild tenderness in his upper abdomen, and diffuse tenderness over his lumbar spine. He is alert and oriented but cannot remember any events since the accident. Otherwise, he has a normal neurologic examination.

ED Priorities

Initial assessment of the mTBI patient in the ED is focused on identifying patients who may require medical or neurosurgical intervention for the treatment of increased intracranial pressure or an expanding mass lesion. Patients with "red flag" conditions such as altered mental status, papillary asymmetry, seizures, repeated vomiting, double vision, worsening headache, motor or sensory deficits, or ataxia should have an emergent noncontrast head CT scan performed. See **Fig. 1** for further imaging recommendations.

Patients with intracranial imaging abnormalities or declining mental status require immediate neurosurgical consultation. Worsening mental status is typically caused by increasing intracranial pressure (ICP) leading to compromised cerebral blood flow and oxygen delivery. For these patients, airway management with endotracheal intubation to protect against aspiration as well as to control ventilation should be considered. Nonsurgical management also includes mitigating ICP increases by raising the head of the bed to 30° and treatment with hyperosmolar agents such as intravenous mannitol. Finally, brief periods of hyperventilation can also reduce dangerous ICP increases. Mechanistically, hyperventilation causes vasoconstriction and reduces ICP by decreasing cerebral blood flow. Overaggressive hyperventilation can result in ICP decreases at the expense of adequate tissue perfusion. Therefore, prolonged hyperventilation should be used only when other therapies have failed.

Clinical Presentation

You obtain imaging studies, including CT of head, neck, abdomen, and pelvis, which reveal no traumatic injuries. After returning from radiology, the patient does not recall meeting you. Although his head CT did not reveal a traumatic injury, he is admitted for observation overnight due to his persistent anterograde amnesia. He has an uneventful night and his amnesia resolves. He receives detailed discharge instructions that include a description of "red flag conditions," common postconcussive symptoms, and reassurance that the vast majority of patients recover completely from concussion. He is advised to avoid activities that exacerbate his symptoms, to take acetaminophen as needed for headache, and to follow up with a visit to a local concussion clinic in 1 week if he is having any persistent discomfort from his concussion. He is accompanied home by his fiancée who will stay with him over the next 24 hours.

Acute Phase: Within 1 Week of Injury

After evaluating for "red flag" signs and symptoms (see ED Priorities), a thorough history of symptoms including loss or alteration of consciousness, headache, irritability, unsteadiness, vertigo, photophobia, or phonophobia should be obtained. The physical examination includes a focused neurologic examination including assessment of cranial nerves, postural instability, visual function, and mental status. Noncontrast head CT should be obtained when indicated (see **Fig. 1**). Neurosurgical consultation is necessary for patients with imaging abnormalities. These patients are often admitted for 24 hours for ongoing mental status monitoring and repeat head CT prior to discharge. Patients in whom imaging is not indicated or who have a normal head CT may be safely discharged.[56–58]

Discharge instructions for mTBI patients include 2 principal elements: symptoms requiring immediate reevaluation (see ED Priorities) and postconcussive symptom education. Postconcussive symptoms include headache, sleep disturbances, vertigo, nausea, fatigue, sensitivity to light or noise, attention and concentration problems, depression, and emotional lability. The vast majority of adults with postconcussive symptoms recover within 3 to 12 months.[59] Early patient education that includes likely postconcussive symptoms and reassurance about an expected positive recovery has been shown to speed recovery and decrease postconcussive symptoms.[60–62] Headache should be managed with acetaminophen. Nonsteroidal anti-inflammatory drugs (NSAIDs) may be used in patients with negative neuroimaging but should be deferred until 48 hours after injury if imaging was not obtained. In addition, narcotics should be avoided in the treatment of posttraumatic headache.

Pharmacologic treatment of other postconcussive symptoms is not recommended in the acute phase. Rather, patients with symptoms other than headache should be advised to rest and encouraged to return to normal activity as soon as possible. However, individuals whose normal activity includes a high risk for re-injury should have careful evaluation of their symptoms and examination findings with consideration of their specific activities that result in a high injury risk. Specific limitations on activity may be recommended for these patients to mitigate their individual risk. Patients reporting fatigue may be given a graded return to work or activity. For patients with normal activities involving significant physical activity, exertional testing may be performed. If this results in a return of symptoms, a monitored progressive return to these activities as tolerated should be recommended.[1]

Clinical Presentation

Two weeks after the initial injury, the patient continues to suffer from frequent headaches that are only slightly relieved by acetaminophen. He also complains of increased irritability, sleepiness, and difficulty concentrating. During an initial follow-up visit, a detailed history and physical examination fails to reveal comorbid psychiatric or physical problems including PTSD, depression, substance abuse, hypertension, cervical spine abnormalities, sinus infections, or visual acuity deficits. However, the patient indicates that he has not been sleeping well due to persistent headache. He is started on an NSAID for his headaches, and provided with education regarding good sleep hygiene and relaxation techniques. He is also advised to begin a regular exercise program. A follow-up appointment is scheduled in 4 weeks.

Initial Management of Postconcussive Symptoms

This section provides an overview of therapy for the initial treatment of patients with mTBI and symptoms lasting more than 1 week after injury. Patients with a delayed initial presentation should also be treated according to these guidelines. Detailed recommendations for the evaluation and treatment of specific symptoms can be found in the VA/DoD Clinical Practice Guideline for Management of Concussion/ mTBI.[1]

Symptom classification and goals of therapy

Postconcussive symptoms generally fall into 3 categories: physical, cognitive, and behavioral or emotional. Typical physical symptoms include headache, nausea, vomiting, dizziness, fatigue, blurred vision, sleep disturbances, light or noise sensitivity, balance problems, and transient neurologic abnormalities. Cognitive symptoms may occur with attention, concentration, memory, processing speed, judgment, and executive functioning. Behavioral/emotional symptoms include depression, anxiety, agitation, irritability, and aggression.

Because there is an incomplete understanding of the etiology of symptoms after mTBI, the goal of intervention for postconcussive symptoms is to improve identified problems rather than affect a cure. It is believed that symptoms resulting from mTBI are interrelated, and alleviation of one symptom often leads to improvement in others. Postconcussive symptoms are also common to many other psychiatric ailments including depression, anxiety disorders, PTSD, and substance abuse disorders. Indeed, there is substantial evidence that affective disorders, PTSD, and substance abuse disorders are often associated with mTBI.[59,63,64] These disorders are also associated with higher rates of persistent postconcussive symptoms.[65,66] Consequently, aggressive treatment of any comorbid psychiatric illness may help to improve postconcussive symptoms.

Patient evaluation

Patient evaluation should include a thorough history, physical examination, and review of the medical record. A review of sleep habits is particularly important as poor sleep may contribute to symptoms including headache, fatigue, anxiety, irritability, depressive thoughts, poor concentration, memory difficulties, and poor decision making. TBI patients should also be screened for psychiatric conditions including PTSD, depression, and substance abuse disorders. Low-yield diagnostic testing should be minimized. There is limited evidence to support the utility of comprehensive neuropsychological/cognitive testing within the first 30 days of mTBI, and a focused clinical interview is sufficient to assess for cognitive difficulties.[67] Laboratory studies including electrolytes, a complete blood count, and thyroid function testing may be useful, particularly when evaluating behavioral and cognitive symptoms. Imaging studies are of limited use.

Physical symptoms should prompt a search for treatable causes. Screening patients with headaches for preexisting headache conditions, hypertension, cervical spine abnormalities, sinus infections, and visual acuity deficits may provide useful avenues of treatment. Symptoms related to dizziness including poor coordination, unsteadiness, vertigo, or loss of balance may be due to medication effects, orthostatic hypotension, or peripheral vertigo. Nausea may be caused by medications or gastroesophageal reflux disease. Nasal polyps, sinus infection, and traumatic injury to the lingual or olfactory nerves may cause appetite changes. Physical injuries to the eye including corneal abrasions, lens dislocation, retinal detachment, and optic nerve injury should be considered in the evaluation of postconcussive visual complaints. Ear abnormalities including infection, tympanic membrane rupture, and auditory nerve injury may lead to phonophobia.

GENERAL TREATMENT GUIDELINES

Treatment of physical symptoms includes treating the underlying causative or contributory conditions. Interventions targeting specific patient complaints such as sleep hygiene education, physical therapy, relaxation, and modification of the environment should be used. Moreover, medications may be used to relieve pain, enable sleep, and reduce stress.[1] Cognitive deficits are often measurable within 30 days of mTBI but generally return to normal within the same period.[68–70] Unfortunately, many patients continue to have subjective cognitive complaints.[9,71–75] Educational and cognitive-behavioral interventions consistently improve subjective cognitive complaints.[61,76–79] Behavioral symptoms may improve with psychotherapeutic and pharmacologic interventions. Treatment should be based on severity and nature of the symptom presentation. Patients with atypical symptoms or with significant suspected or confirmed comorbid illnesses may benefit from specialty referral or consultation. Finally, "red flag" conditions indicating an acute neurologic condition requiring urgent neurologic or neurosurgical intervention should prompt emergent transfer to a medical facility with an appropriate level of care.

The primary goal of pharmacologic therapies for mTBI is symptomatic improvement. At present, disease-altering therapies are not available. Drug therapy for mTBI symptoms should follow several general principles. Medications that lower the seizure threshold such as buproprion and some antipsychotic medicines should be avoided. Similarly, medications such as lithium, anticholinergic agents, benzodiazepines, and others can cause altered mental status and should also be avoided. Starting doses should be as low as possible and titrated to effect under close monitoring. By contrast, maximal tolerated dosing should be trialed before switching to a new agent to avoid undertreatment. Patients should be advised to avoid alcohol, caffeine, and herbal supplements. Limited doses of medications with significant toxicity in intentional overdoses such as tricyclic antidepressants should also be considered because suicide risk is high in brain-injured patients. Finally, patients should be monitored closely for medication interactions and toxicity.

Medication therapy for patients in the first week after injury should be reserved for the treatment of headache only. Acetaminophen is the agent of choice. NSAIDs should not be used until 48 hours after injury unless there is normal neuroimaging data for the patient. Other immediate postconcussive symptoms should not be treated as they typically resolve spontaneously within the first week of injury.

Headache

Headache is the most common symptom after mTBI, affecting more than 90% of patients. Posttraumatic headaches commonly fall into 1 of 3 categories: tension, migraine, or a combination of the 2. The evaluation of posttraumatic headache should include assessment for neurologic findings suggestive of serious intracranial abnormalities. Focal neurologic deficits should prompt additional urgent investigation with appropriate neuroimaging. A medication review for patients with symptoms lasting more than 2 weeks is also important, as rebound headaches are common in with daily acetaminophen or NSAID use. Similarly, withdrawal from caffeine or nicotine may also result in headache. Patients who state that their headache improves only with opiates should be referred to a pain or headache specialist. Headache symptoms often improve after treatment of comorbid conditions such as sleep disturbances, anxiety, and depression.

Pharmacologic treatment should be selected based on the type of headache suspected. Similar to opiate-dependent patients, those with symptoms that do not improve within 3 months of initiating therapy should be referred to a headache or pain specialist. Episodic tension type headaches may be treated with aspirin, acetaminophen, or NSAIDs. These medications typically work best when combined with other treatment modalities such as a regular exercise program, relaxation techniques, or biofeedback. Combination medications that include caffeine or a sedative may be more effective but also have a greater likelihood of rebound headache.

Migraine treatment is divided into the prevention and management of acute episodes. Awareness and avoidance of precipitating events should be encouraged. Abortive medications for acute episodes include sumatriptan and zolmatriptan. These medications are most effective when used early in the course of the episode. Some patients with established migraines may require rescue medications to break their headache. Examples of effective rescue medications include ketorolac, butorphanol, opioids, prochlorparazine, and promethazine. Patients with migraine headaches that occur more than once a month should be placed on prophylaxis. First-line agents for prophylaxis include metroprolol and toprimate. Prophylactic agents may take as long as 3 months to become maximally effective. Finally, mixed headache types may require separate agents for treatment of the tension and migraine components.

Disequilibrium and Vertigo

Up to 30% of patients with mTBI complain of disturbed equilibrium or vertigo.[80] Despite this, symptoms do not correlate with objective evidence after the first week after injury.[81] A thorough medication review should be performed for all mTBI patients complaining of dizziness. Medications such as stimulants, benzodiazepines, tricyclics, monoamine oxidase inhibitors, tetracyclics, neuroleptics, selective serotonin reuptake inhibitors, β-blockers, and cholinesterase inhibitors may cause or exacerbate dizziness. Vestibular suppression may be useful in the acute phase but has not proven effective for persistent symptoms.[82] Vestibular suppressants should only be used if the symptoms significantly limit the patient's functional activities as they may result in delayed improvement.[83,84] Meclizine is the first agent recommended. Scopolamine and dimenhydrinate may be used if meclizine fails. Benzodiazepines should only be used after careful consideration of their sedating and habit-forming properties. Trials should be limited to 2 weeks' duration.

Fatigue and Sleep Disturbances

Another common symptom after mTBI is fatigue, which may be due to central nervous system dysfunction, sleep disturbances, or depression. Proper assessment of this symptom requires a thorough history of pre- and postinjury levels of activity. There are also several validated instruments to objectively measure fatigue.[85,86] Physical causes of fatigue may also be assessed with laboratory testing including metabolic panel, a complete blood count, and thyroid function testing. Review of the patient's medication history, alcohol, caffeine, and illicit drug use should also be performed, as all of these may result in fatigue. Before initiating medications for fatigue, conservative measures such as education of the patient, initiating an exercise program, and referring the patient for physical or cognitive-behavioral therapy should be trialed. There is limited evidence for the efficacy of stimulant treatment for fatigue after mTBI. Commonly used agents include modafanil, methylphenidate, and amantadine. These medications should only be used if symptoms have lasted more than 4 weeks, the patient does not have substance abuse issues, and addressing other factors mentioned in this section have failed to improve symptoms. Trials of these medications should last at least 3 months.

Sleep disturbances are common after mTBI. The goal of therapy is to restore a regular, unbroken night-time sleep pattern and improve the perception of sleep quality. Any drug therapy for sleep disturbances should be accompanied by education regarding good sleep hygiene. Furthermore, concomitant primary sleep disorders such as obstructive sleep apnea, restless legs syndrome, and narcolepsy should be appropriately treated. In the acute phase, short-term treatment with nonbenzodiazepine sleep medications such as zolpidem may be helpful. Prazosin may be used in patients with nightmares or agitation during sleep.

Clinical Presentation

The patient returns to the concussion clinic 4 weeks after his initial visit and 6 weeks after his accident. He reports that he instituted the sleep hygiene recommendations given to him on the prior visit and that his headaches, sleepiness, irritability, and concentration difficulties subsequently resolved. He has required NSAIDs with decreasing frequency and has not had a headache in the last 2 weeks. The patient is sent home with instructions to contact the clinic for a future appointment if symptoms return.

FOLLOW-UP

All patients require a follow-up assessment within 4 to 6 weeks of initiation of therapy. Patients can be grouped into 3 categories at this second assessment: those with complete symptom resolution, those with partial resolution, and those with no improvement or worsened symptoms. Patients whose symptoms completely resolve should be given contact information to make a future appointment if symptoms return. Patients with a partial response may benefit from augmentation or adjustment of their current therapy. Those patients whose symptoms are refractory to initial treatment should be considered to have persistent postconcussive symptoms and treated according to the following guidelines.

Management of Persistent Postconcussive Symptoms

This section is relevant for patients who have had an initial evaluation and failed a trial of treatment for mTBI-related symptoms. Patients with delayed presentation for mTBI symptoms should first be treated according to the section Initial Management of Postconcussive Symptoms, regardless of the interval since injury. The definitive reference is the VA/DoD Clinical Practice Guideline for Management of Concussion/mTBI.[1]

Patients with persistent postconcussive symptoms often have concomitant behavioral health, psychosocial support, or compensation and litigation issues. Attention should be given to addressing these issues, as this may help mitigate symptoms refractory to initial treatment. The evaluation of the patient with persistent postconcussive symptoms should include an assessment of available support systems, a mental health history including premorbid conditions, co-occurring symptoms such as chronic pain or personality disorders, substance abuse disorders, secondary gain issues, job status, and other financial or legal difficulties.[1] Finally, all patients presenting with persistent postconcussive symptoms should be assessed for any potential danger to themselves or others.

Less than 5% of patients have persistent symptoms 1 year or more after injury.[11] Patients typically have more physical complaints within 4 weeks of injury after which emotional complaints predominate.[87] Once a thorough assessment has been obtained, the principal goal is to identify appropriate referrals for management of the persistent symptoms. Patients with behavioral symptoms and possible comorbid psychiatric conditions may benefit from referral to mental health professionals. Persistent physical symptoms should be evaluated by appropriate specialists. Persistent cognitive symptoms are rare and are frequently accompanied by comorbid conditions such as mood disorders, poor physical health, poor psychosocial support, or chronic pain. In addition to addressing these comorbid conditions, these patients should be referred for neuropsychiatric evaluation to determine appropriate treatment options. Cognitive rehabilitation may be helpful for patients with persistent difficulties in memory, executive function, or attention.[88–90] A social work referral is appropriate for patients with poor psychosocial support, legal difficulties, or financial problems. Although there is consistent evidence of an association between mTBI-related compensation or litigation and increased symptom reporting and poor outcome,[59,91–93] there is no evidence to support a therapeutic benefit of attributing persistent symptoms to these secondary gain issues.[1] Consequently, clinicians should not allow symptom exaggeration by patients seeking compensation to alter their care plans.

Given the diverse group of health professionals involved in the treatment of persistent postconcussive symptoms, a multidisciplinary team approach with the referring provider as the coordinator of care is required. A designated case manager can be very helpful for coordinating care. Typical tasks benefiting from case management includes coordination of referrals, ensuring appropriate patient and family education, participation in short- and long-term goal setting, ensuring that appropriate social service and mental health screening is performed, and coordination with the multidisciplinary team. Ongoing follow-up visits should occur regularly with goals of monitoring symptom severity, reviewing symptom impact on activities, and the effectiveness of treatments.

Return to Play after Sports Injury

Guidelines for returning to play in an athlete differ from general instructions for return to normal activities after mTBI in that they are designed to prevent a repeat mTBI while the patient is recovering from the initial injury. In general, the risks of suffering a second and third TBI are threefold and 8- to 9-fold greater than the risk of a first TBI, respectively.[94] Furthermore, case reports suggest that athletes are at increased risk for concussion in the period immediately after their initial injury.[95] Therefore, consideration of the concussion risk in a sports-specific manner is important.[96] Return to play guidelines are consensus rather than evidence based. The most commonly used guidelines include those by the American Academy of Neurology (AAN) and by Cantu.[97,98] Both sets of guidelines use severity of the concussion and presence of postconcussive symptoms as the criteria for return to play decision making. The Cantu guidelines allow a player to return once he or she is asymptomatic for 1 week if posttraumatic amnesia lasted less than 24 hours and the initial loss of unconsciousness was less than 5 minutes. Players with more severe symptoms at the time of their concussion should not play for 1 month, and then can return after an additional 1 week without symptoms. In players with a history of multiple concussions, consideration should be given to sitting out for the remainder of the season.

Although the consensus-based back to play guidelines referenced in this section are clinically accepted as the standard of care, they are not infallible. A recent example of a second injury despite scrupulous application of these guidelines is seen with Brian Westbrook, a professional football player in the National Football League (NFL). Mr Westbrook suffered the first concussion of his 8-year NFL career on October 26, 2009, suffering a brief LOC with associated retrograde amnesia after being tackled in a game. He was held from play for 3 weeks due to lingering headache and then suffered a second concussion in his first game back from injury. While there was widespread speculation that he might not return that season or even that his football career was over, he did play the final 2 games of the season without further injury after being out for a total of 5 weeks. Although no guideline can prevent all adverse events, it is possible that improved guidelines could result in fewer repeat injuries. Prospectively validated, evidence-based return to play guidelines are needed.

SEQUELAE OF MTBI

Postconcussive Symptoms and Cognitive Deficits

Common postconcussive symptoms include headache, dizziness, fatigue, sleep disturbances, memory problems, balance problems, sensitivity to sound or tinnitus, concentration difficulties, and irritability. These symptoms are notably nonspecific and are associated with many other diseases. Nonetheless, several studies have reported higher rates of these symptoms in patients after mTBI than in patients with no injury or extracranial trauma without TBI.[64,99,100] The percentage of patients who suffer from persistent postconcussive symptoms diminishes with time after injury. Less than 25% of patients are likely to have problems lasting more than 12 months after injury.[11] Although cognitive complaints are fairly common after mTBI, measurable cognitive deficits are generally only present after severe or moderate TBI.[101,102] There is little evidence of objective cognitive deficits after mTBI.[103]

Motor, Balance, and Cranial Nerve Abnormalities

In general, objective findings after mTBI are absent. Balance problems are emerging as a promising exception to this rule. In one study of 37 mTBI patients, testing of saccades, oculomotor smooth pursuit, upper limb visuomotor function, and neuropsychologic domains was performed, and the results compared with uninjured control patients. At 1 year after injury, eye and upper limb movement, but not cognitive function, remained impaired in the mTBI patients.[104] In a more recent study, the same group found that eye movement impairment was significantly worse in mTBI patients suffering from postconcussive syndrome relative to mTBI patients with good recovery.[105]

Psychiatric Diagnoses

Many studies have found an association between TBI of all severities and major depressive disorder.[63,106,107] This observed association was not likely to be explained by depression prior to injury; however, prior mood disorder may be an increased risk for TBI.[108,109] While there are few studies of a relationship between mania or bipolar disorder and TBI, the existing evidence suggests that there is not a strong relationship between them.[110–112] There is limited evidence supporting an association between mTBI and PTSD in military populations. In a study of 2525 soldiers returning after a 1-year deployment to Iraq, researchers identified a clear association between PTSD and mild TBI with LOC (odds ratio, 2.98; 95% confidence interval [CI], 1.70–5.24).[64] A second cross-sectional study of 2235 Afghanistan and Iraq war veterans also found an association between PTSD and mTBI.[113] However, 2 studies of civilian populations found no relationship between mTBI and PTSD.[114,115]

Second Impact Syndrome

Second impact syndrome (SIS) is a dreaded, rare complication of mTBI that occurs after a patient suffers a second mTBI while remaining symptomatic from the first. A patient typically will suffer a head injury during play resulting in postconcussive symptoms. After returning to play while still suffering symptoms the patient sustains a second, apparently minor head trauma, and rapidly suffers depressed mental status resulting in death or a persistent vegetative state. It is postulated that this disorder is caused by disordered cerebral autoregulation resulting from the initial TBI. The condition has mainly been reported in young men who play contact sports. The term SIS was first coined by Saunders and Harbaugh;[116] however, a similar syndrome was previously described by Schneider.[117]

While SIS has become firmly fixed in the minds of clinicians as an important complication of mTBI, there is some question regarding whether it is a true clinical entity.[118] A critical review of reported cases of SIS found that most did not meet a reasonable clinical definition of SIS. Cases often lacked neuropathologic evidence of unexplained cerebral swelling.[119] Even more problematic, most of the reported cases of precipitous neurologic collapse after a seemingly minor trauma occurred in the absence of any documented "first impact." Of the 17 cases reviewed, only 5 were classified as "probable SIS." Given this analysis it is reasonable to conclude that the term SIS is inaccurate. Diffuse cerebral swelling can very rarely occur after mTBI, principally in children and adolescents; however, a second mTBI is not required.

Seizures

Although there is sufficient evidence to support a causal relationship between moderate or severe TBI and the development of unprovoked seizures, the evidence is limited for an association between seizures and mTBI.[24] In nonmilitary TBI populations, there is a 3.6-fold increase in the incidence of seizures relative to noninjured patients after TBI of all severities. After severe TBI there was a 17-fold increase in seizure incidence, which declined to 2.9-fold in moderate TBI patients. For mTBI patients with LOC or posttraumatic amnesia, the incidence of seizures was 1.5 times that of controls (95% CI 1.0–2.2).[94,120] These studies were limited in that pediatric patients, who have a higher baseline incidence of seizures than adults, were not analyzed separately from adults. Posttraumatic seizure risk is greatest in the first year after injury. After 4 years, TBI patients are no longer at increased risk relative to uninjured subjects.[121]

Dementia and Neurodegeneration

Alzheimer disease is the most common neurodegenerative disease, resulting in progressive dementia and eventual death. Familial or early-onset Alzheimer disease is caused by specific mutations and comprises approximately 10% of cases. The remaining 90% of cases are referred to as sporadic. Although the mechanisms of disease progression in sporadic Alzheimer disease are not known, it likely results from a combination of genetic and environmental factors. TBI is the strongest known environmental exposure associated with subsequent development of sporadic Alzheimer disease. A retrospective cohort study of World War II veterans with documented closed head injury demonstrated an increase risk of Alzheimer type dementia relative to nonhead-injured controls (hazard ratio 2.00, 95% CI 1.03–3.90).[122] A meta-analysis of 7 case-control studies revealed similar results.[123]

Dementia pugilistica, also known as chronic traumatic encephalopathy, is a neurodegenerative condition that affects athletes in sports that involve repeated head trauma such as boxing and mixed martial arts.[124] Characteristic neuropathologic changes include cerebellar damage, cortical damage, and other scarring of the brain; substantia nigral degeneration; neurofibrillary tangles in the cerebral cortex and temporal horn areas; and abnormalities of the septum pellucidum. Autopsy of professional football players who died in their forties after developing dementia also showed neurodegenerative changes consistent with chronic traumatic encephalopathy.[125–127]

Neuropsychologic deficits associated with dementia pugilistica have been found in some studies[128,129] but not others.[130,131]

Parkinsonism is a constellation of symptoms including tremor, rigidity, bradykinesia, and postural instability, and is caused by loss of central dopamine. Very little has been reported regarding association between TBI and parkinsonism; however, several case-control studies have shown an increased risk after mTBI with LOC or posttraumatic amnesia.[132,133] The risk for the development of parkinsonism seems to increase with severity of TBI.[132,134]

SUMMARY

mTBI is a widespread problem. Because of our limited understanding of the injury pathophysiology, the diagnosis of mTBI is based entirely on clinical symptoms, and often occurs in the absence of objective findings. The central feature of mTBI is a transiently altered state of consciousness after a traumatic injury to the head. The priority of emergency care is to identify potentially life-threatening intracranial injuries through the judicious application of appropriate imaging studies and neurosurgical consultation. Although post-mTBI symptoms quickly and completely resolve in the vast majority of cases, a significant number of patients will complain of lasting problems. Postconcussive complaints tend to be interrelated, and relief of one may have beneficial effects on others. Although the evidence is not definitive, longer-term sequelae of mTBI may include seizure disorders and neurodegeneration. Recognizing the potentially life-changing aspects of mTBI should be an important priority for the emergency physician because simple, early interventions, such as education regarding the expected positive outcome from the injury and prompt treatment, can prevent chronic symptoms from occurring.

REFERENCES

1. The Concussion/mTBI Working Group. VA/DoD clinical practice guideline for management of concussion/mTBI. Available at: http://www.dvbic.org/images/pdfs/Providers/VADoD-CPG-Concussion-mTBI.aspx. Accessed October 1, 2009.
2. ACRM. American Congress of Rehabilitation Medicine Mild Traumatic Brain Injury Committee of the Head Injury Interdisciplinary Special Interest Group. Definition of mild traumatic brain injury. J Head Trauma Rehabil 1993;8(3):86–7.
3. National Center for Injury Prevention and Control. Report to congress on mild traumatic brain injury in the United States: steps to prevent a serious public health problem. Atlanta (GA): Centers for Disease Control and Prevention; 2003.
4. Lange RT, Iverson GL, Franzen MD. Neuropsychological functioning following complicated vs. uncomplicated mild traumatic brain injury. Brain Inj 2009;23(2):83–91.
5. Saatman KE, Duhaime AC, Bullock R, et al. Classification of traumatic brain injury for targeted therapies. J Neurotrauma 2008;25(7):719–38.
6. Langlois JA, Rutland-Brown W, Thomas KE. Traumatic brain injury in the United States: emergency department visits, hospitalizations, and deaths. Atlanta (GA): Centers for Disease Control and Prevention, National Center for Injury Prevention and Control; 2006.
7. Jager TE, Weiss HB, Coben JH, et al. Traumatic brain injuries evaluated in U.S. emergency departments, 1992–1994. Acad Emerg Med 2000;7(2):134–40.
8. Sosin DM, Sniezek JE, Thurman DJ. Incidence of mild and moderate brain injury in the United States, 1991. Brain Inj 1996;10(1):47–54.

9. Alves WM, Macciocchi SN, Barth JT. Postconcussive symptoms after uncomplicated mild head injury. J Head Trauma Rehabil 1993;8(3):48–59.
10. Middleboe T, Andersen HS, Birket-Smith M, et al. Minor head injury: impact on general health after 1 year. A prospective follow-up study. Acta Neurol Scand 1992;85(1):5–9.
11. Iverson GL. Post-concussive disorder. New York: Demos Medical Publishing LLC; 2007.
12. Alexander MP. Mild traumatic brain injury: pathophysiology, natural history, and clinical management. Neurology 1995;45(7):1253–60.
13. Gondusky JS, Reiter MP. Protecting military convoys in Iraq: an examination of battle injuries sustained by a mechanized battalion during Operation Iraqi Freedom II. Mil Med 2005;170(6):546–9.
14. Summers CR, Ivins B, Schwab KA. Traumatic brain injury in the United States: an epidemiologic overview. Mt Sinai J Med 2009;76(2):105–10.
15. LaPlaca MC, Simon CM, Prado GR, et al. CNS injury biomechanics and experimental models. Prog Brain Res 2007;161:13–26.
16. Gennarelli TA, Thibault LE, Adams JH, et al. Diffuse axonal injury and traumatic coma in the primate. Ann Neurol 1982;12(6):564–74.
17. Holbourn AH. Mechanics of head injuries. Lancet 1943;242(6267):438–41.
18. Ommaya AK, Gennarelli TA. Cerebral concussion and traumatic unconsciousness. Correlation of experimental and clinical observations of blunt head injuries. Brain 1974;97(4):633–54.
19. McIntosh TK. Neurochemical sequelae of traumatic brain injury: therapeutic implications. Cerebrovasc Brain Metab Rev 1994;6(2):109–62.
20. Werner C, Engelhard K. Pathophysiology of traumatic brain injury. Br J Anaesth 2007;99(1):4–9.
21. Thompson HJ, Lifshitz J, Marklund N, et al. Lateral fluid percussion brain injury: a 15-year review and evaluation. J Neurotrauma 2005;22(1):42–75.
22. Statler KD, Jenkins LW, Dixon CE, et al. The simple model versus the super model: translating experimental traumatic brain injury research to the bedside. J Neurotrauma 2001;18(11):1195–206.
23. Marklund N, Bakshi A, Castelbuono DJ, et al. Evaluation of pharmacological treatment strategies in traumatic brain injury. Curr Pharm Des 2006;12(13):1645–80.
24. Institute of Medicine (IOM). Gulf War and Health, vol. 7: Long-term consequences of traumatic brain injury. Washington, DC: The National Academies Press; 2009.
25. Adams RD, Victor M, Ropper AH. Principles of neurology. 6th edition. New York: McGraw-Hill; 1997.
26. Hayes RL, Lyeth BG, Jenkins LW. Neurochemical mechanisms of mild and moderate head injury: implications for treatment. In: Levin HS, Eisenberg HM, Benton AL, editors. Mild head injury. Oxford (UK): Oxford University Press; 1989. p. 54–79.
27. Katayama Y, Watkins LR, Becker DP, et al. Evidence for involvement of cholinoceptive cells of the parabrachial region in environmentally induced nociceptive suppression in the cat. Brain Res 1984;299(2):348–53.
28. Hayes RL, Pechura CM, Katayama Y, et al. Activation of pontine cholinergic sites implicated in unconsciousness following cerebral concussion in the cat. Science 1984;223(4633):301–3.
29. Lyeth BG, Dixon CE, Hamm RJ, et al. Effects of anticholinergic treatment on transient behavioral suppression and physiological responses following concussive brain injury to the rat. Brain Res 1988;448(1):88–97.

30. Ishige N, Pitts LH, Hashimoto T, et al. Effect of hypoxia on traumatic brain injury in rats: Part 1. Changes in neurological function, electroencephalograms, and histopathology. Neurosurgery 1987;20(6):848–53.
31. Marmarou A, Foda MA, van den Brink W, et al. A new model of diffuse brain injury in rats. Part I: pathophysiology and biomechanics. J Neurosurg 1994; 80(2):291–300.
32. Walker AE, Kollros JJ, Case TJ. The physiological basis of concussion. J Neurosurg 1944;1(2):103–16.
33. Shaw NA. The neurophysiology of concussion. Prog Neurobiol 2002;67(4): 281–344.
34. Stein SC, Ross SE. The value of computed tomographic scans in patients with low-risk head injuries. Neurosurgery 1990;26(4):638–40.
35. Nagurney JT, Borczuk P, Thomas SH. Elder patients with closed head trauma: a comparison with nonelder patients. Acad Emerg Med 1998;5(7): 678–84.
36. Miller EC, Holmes JF, Derlet RW. Utilizing clinical factors to reduce head CT scan ordering for minor head trauma patients. J Emerg Med 1997;15(4):453–7.
37. Jeret JS, Mandell M, Anziska B, et al. Clinical predictors of abnormality disclosed by computed tomography after mild head trauma. Neurosurgery 1993;32(1):9–15 [discussion: 15–6].
38. Jennett B, Teasdale G, Galbraith S, et al. Severe head injuries in three countries. J Neurol Neurosurg Psychiatr 1977;40(3):291–8.
39. Harad FT, Kerstein MD. Inadequacy of bedside clinical indicators in identifying significant intracranial injury in trauma patients. J Trauma 1992;32(3):359–61 [discussion: 61–3].
40. Borczuk P. Predictors of intracranial injury in patients with mild head trauma. Ann Emerg Med 1995;25(6):731–6.
41. Mittl RL, Grossman RI, Hiehle JF, et al. Prevalence of MR evidence of diffuse axonal injury in patients with mild head injury and normal head CT findings. AJNR Am J Neuroradiol 1994;15(8):1583–9.
42. Jagoda AS, Bazarian JJ, Bruns JJ Jr, et al. Clinical policy: neuroimaging and decision making in adult mild traumatic brain injury in the acute setting. Ann Emerg Med 2008;52(6):714–48.
43. Stiell IG, Wells GA, Vandemheen K, et al. The Canadian CT head rule for patients with minor head injury. Lancet 2001;357(9266):1391–6.
44. Haydel MJ, Preston CA, Mills TJ, et al. Indications for computed tomography in patients with minor head injury. N Engl J Med 2000;343(2):100–5.
45. Stiell IG, Clement CM, Rowe BH, et al. Comparison of the Canadian CT head rule and the New Orleans criteria in patients with minor head injury. JAMA 2005;294(12):1511–8.
46. Kuppermann N, Holmes JF, Dayan PS, et al. Identification of children at very low risk of clinically-important brain injuries after head trauma: a prospective cohort study. Lancet 2009;374(9696):1160–70.
47. Tasci A, Okay O, Gezici AR, et al. Prognostic value of interleukin-1 beta levels after acute brain injury. Neurol Res 2003;25(8):871–4.
48. Ringger NC, O'Steen BE, Brabham JG, et al. A novel marker for traumatic brain injury: CSF alphaII-spectrin breakdown product levels. J Neurotrauma 2004; 21(10):1443–56.
49. Pelinka LE, Kroepfl A, Schmidhammer R, et al. Glial fibrillary acidic protein in serum after traumatic brain injury and multiple trauma. J Trauma 2004;57(5): 1006–12.

50. Olsson A, Csajbok L, Ost M, et al. Marked increase of beta-amyloid(1-42) and amyloid precursor protein in ventricular cerebrospinal fluid after severe traumatic brain injury. J Neurol 2004;251(7):870–6.
51. Missler U, Wiesmann M, Wittmann G, et al. Measurement of glial fibrillary acidic protein in human blood: analytical method and preliminary clinical results. Clin Chem 1999;45(1):138–41.
52. Berger RP, Heyes MP, Wisniewski SR, et al. Assessment of the macrophage marker quinolinic acid in cerebrospinal fluid after pediatric traumatic brain injury: insight into the timing and severity of injury in child abuse. J Neurotrauma 2004;21(9):1123–30.
53. Papa L, Akinyi L, Liu MC, et al. Ubiquitin C-terminal hydrolase is a novel biomarker in humans for severe traumatic brain injury. Crit Care Med 2009;38(1):318–9.
54. Biberthaler P, Linsenmeier U, Pfeifer KJ, et al. Serum S-100B concentration provides additional information for the indication of computed tomography in patients after minor head injury: a prospective multicenter study. Shock 2006; 25(5):446–53.
55. Biberthaler P, Mussack T, Wiedemann E, et al. Elevated serum levels of S-100B reflect the extent of brain injury in alcohol intoxicated patients after mild head trauma. Shock 2001;16(2):97–101.
56. Nagy KK, Joseph KT, Krosner SM, et al. The utility of head computed tomography after minimal head injury. J Trauma 1999;46(2):268–70.
57. Livingston DH, Loder PA, Hunt CD. Minimal head injury: is admission necessary? Am Surg 1991;57(1):14–7.
58. Dunham CM, Coates S, Cooper C. Compelling evidence for discretionary brain computed tomographic imaging in those patients with mild cognitive impairment after blunt trauma. J Trauma 1996;41(4):679–86.
59. Carroll LJ, Cassidy JD, Peloso PM, et al. Prognosis for mild traumatic brain injury: results of the who collaborating centre task force on mild traumatic brain injury. J Rehabil Med 2004;(43 Suppl):84–105.
60. Holm L, Cassidy JD, Carroll LJ, et al. Summary of the WHO collaborating centre for neurotrauma task force on mild traumatic brain injury. J Rehabil Med 2005; 37(3):137–41.
61. Comper P, Bisschop SM, Carnide N, et al. A systematic review of treatments for mild traumatic brain injury. Brain Inj 2005;19(11):863–80.
62. Borg J, Holm L, Peloso PM, et al. Nonsurgical intervention and cost for mild traumatic brain injury: results of the WHO Collaborating centre task force on mild traumatic brain injury. J Rehabil Med 2004;(43 Suppl):76–83.
63. Fann JR, Burington B, Leonetti A, et al. Psychiatric illness following traumatic brain injury in an adult health maintenance organization population. Arch Gen Psychiatry 2004;61(1):53–61.
64. Hoge CW, McGurk D, Thomas JL, et al. Mild traumatic brain injury in U.S. Soldiers returning from Iraq. N Engl J Med 2008;358(5):453–63.
65. Mooney G, Speed J. The association between mild traumatic brain injury and psychiatric conditions. Brain Inj 2001;15(10):865–77.
66. Rapoport MJ, Kiss A, Feinstein A. The impact of major depression on outcome following mild-to-moderate traumatic brain injury in older adults. J Affect Disord 2006;92(2–3):273–6.
67. Cassidy JD, Carroll LJ, Peloso PM, et al. Incidence, risk factors and prevention of mild traumatic brain injury: results of the WHO Collaborating centre task force on mild traumatic brain injury. J Rehabil Med 2004;(43 Suppl):28–60.

68. Belanger HG, Curtiss G, Demery JA, et al. Factors moderating neuropsychological outcomes following mild traumatic brain injury: a meta-analysis. J Int Neuropsychol Soc 2005;11(3):215–27.
69. Belanger HG, Vanderploeg RD. The neuropsychological impact of sports-related concussion: a meta-analysis. J Int Neuropsychol Soc 2005;11(4):345–57.
70. Schretlen DJ, Shapiro AM. A quantitative review of the effects of traumatic brain injury on cognitive functioning. Int Rev Psychiatry 2003;15(4):341–9.
71. Deb S, Lyons I, Koutzoukis C. Neurobehavioural symptoms one year after a head injury. Br J Psychiatry 1999;174:360–5.
72. Dikmen S, McLean A, Temkin N. Neuropsychological and psychosocial consequences of minor head injury. J Neurol Neurosurg Psychiatr 1986;49(11):1227–32.
73. Hartlage LC, Durant-Wilson D, Patch PC. Persistent neurobehavioral problems following mild traumatic brain injury. Arch Clin Neuropsychol 2001;16(6):561–70.
74. Luis CA, Vanderploeg RD, Curtiss G. Predictors of postconcussion symptom complex in community dwelling male veterans. J Int Neuropsychol Soc 2003;9(7):1001–15.
75. Powell TJ, Collin C, Sutton K. A follow-up study of patients hospitalized after minor head injury. Disabil Rehabil 1996;18(5):231–7.
76. Anson K, Ponsford J. Evaluation of a coping skills group following traumatic brain injury. Brain Inj 2006;20(2):167–78.
77. Bedard M, Felteau M, Mazmanian D, et al. Pilot evaluation of a mindfulness-based intervention to improve quality of life among individuals who sustained traumatic brain injuries. Disabil Rehabil 2003;25(13):722–31.
78. Hinkle JL, Alves WM, Rimell RW, et al. Restoring social competence in minor head-injury patients. J Neurosci Nurs 1986;18(5):268–71.
79. Mittenberg W, Tremont G, Zielinski RE, et al. Cognitive-behavioral prevention of postconcussion syndrome. Arch Clin Neuropsychol 1996;11(2):139–45.
80. Cicerone KD, Kalmar K. Persistent postconcussion syndrome: the structure of subjective complaints after mild traumatic brain injury. J Head Trauma Rehabil 1995;10(3):1–17.
81. Gottshall KR, Gray NL, Drake AI, et al. To investigate the influence of acute vestibular impairment following mild traumatic brain injury on subsequent ability to remain on activity duty 12 months later. Mil Med 2007;172(8):852–7.
82. Zee DS. Perspectives on the pharmacotherapy of vertigo. Arch Otolaryngol 1985;111(9):609–12.
83. Pyykko I, Magnusson M, Schalen L, et al. Pharmacological treatment of vertigo. Acta Otolaryngol Suppl 1988;455:77–81.
84. Hain TC, Yacovino D. Pharmacologic treatment of persons with dizziness. Neurol Clin 2005;23(3):831–53, vii.
85. Krupp LB, LaRocca NG, Muir-Nash J, et al. The fatigue severity scale. Application to patients with multiple sclerosis and systemic lupus erythematosus. Arch Neurol 1989;46(10):1121–3.
86. Chalder T, Berelowitz G, Pawlikowska T, et al. Development of a fatigue scale. J Psychosom Res 1993;37(2):147–53.
87. Yang CC, Tu YK, Hua MS, et al. The association between the postconcussion symptoms and clinical outcomes for patients with mild traumatic brain injury. J Trauma 2007;62(3):657–63.
88. Cicerone KD. Remediation of "working attention" in mild traumatic brain injury. Brain Inj 2002;16(3):185–95.

89. Cicerone KD, Dahlberg C, Malec JF, et al. Evidence-based cognitive rehabilitation: updated review of the literature from 1998 through 2002. Arch Phys Med Rehabil 2005;86(8):1681–92.
90. Tiersky LA, Anselmi V, Johnston MV, et al. A trial of neuropsychologic rehabilitation in mild-spectrum traumatic brain injury. Arch Phys Med Rehabil 2005;86(8): 1565–74.
91. Binder LM, Rohling ML. Money matters: a meta-analytic review of the effects of financial incentives on recovery after closed-head injury. Am J Psychiatry 1996; 153(1):7–10.
92. Kashluba S, Paniak C, Casey JE. Persistent symptoms associated with factors identified by the WHO task force on mild traumatic brain injury. Clin Neuropsychol 2008;22(2):195–208.
93. Suhr JA, Gunstad J. Postconcussive symptom report: the relative influence of head injury and depression. J Clin Exp Neuropsychol 2002;24(8): 981–93.
94. Annegers JF, Grabow JD, Kurland LT, et al. The incidence, causes, and secular trends of head trauma in Olmsted County, Minnesota, 1935-1974. Neurology 1980;30(9):912–9.
95. Kelly JP, Nichols JS, Filley CM, et al. Concussion in sports. Guidelines for the prevention of catastrophic outcome. JAMA 1991;266(20):2867–9.
96. Kissick J, Johnston KM. Return to play after concussion: principles and practice. Clin J Sport Med 2005;15(6):426–31.
97. Anonymous. Practice parameter: the management of concussion in sports (summary statement). Neurology 1997;48(3):581–5.
98. Cantu RC. Return to play guidelines after a head injury. Clin Sports Med 1998; 17(1):45–60.
99. Gerber DJ, Schraa JC. Mild traumatic brain injury: searching for the syndrome. J Head Trauma Rehabil 1995;10(4):28–40.
100. Masson F, Maurette P, Salmi LR, et al. Prevalence of impairments 5 years after a head injury, and their relationship with disabilities and outcome. Brain Inj 1996;10(7):487–97.
101. Incoccia C, Formisano R, Muscato P, et al. Reaction and movement times in individuals with chronic traumatic brain injury with good motor recovery. Cortex 2004;40(1):111–5.
102. Ruff RM, Evans R, Marshall LF. Impaired verbal and figural fluency after head injury. Arch Clin Neuropsychol 1986;1(2):87–101.
103. Vanderploeg RD, Curtiss G, Belanger HG. Long-term neuropsychological outcomes following mild traumatic brain injury. J Int Neuropsychol Soc 2005; 11(3):228–36.
104. Heitger MH, Jones RD, Dalrymple-Alford JC, et al. Motor deficits and recovery during the first year following mild closed head injury. Brain Inj 2006;20(8): 807–24.
105. Heitger MH, Jones RD, Macleod AD, et al. Impaired eye movements in post-concussion syndrome indicate suboptimal brain function beyond the influence of depression, malingering or intellectual ability. Brain 2009; 132(Pt 10):2850–70.
106. Jorge RE, Robinson RG, Moser D, et al. Major depression following traumatic brain injury. Arch Gen Psychiatry 2004;61(1):42–50.
107. Vanderploeg RD, Curtiss G, Luis CA, et al. Long-term morbidities following self-reported mild traumatic brain injury. J Clin Exp Neuropsychol 2007;29(6): 585–98.

108. Fann JR, Leonetti A, Jaffe K, et al. Psychiatric illness and subsequent traumatic brain injury: a case control study. J Neurol Neurosurg Psychiatr 2002;72(5): 615–20.
109. Vassallo JL, Proctor-Weber Z, Lebowitz BK, et al. Psychiatric risk factors for traumatic brain injury. Brain Inj 2007;21(6):567–73.
110. Koponen S, Taiminen T, Portin R, et al. Axis I and II psychiatric disorders after traumatic brain injury: a 30-year follow-up study. Am J Psychiatry 2002;159(8): 1315–21.
111. Sagduyu K. Association of mild traumatic brain injury with bipolar disorder. J Clin Psychiatry 2002;63(7):594.
112. Silver JM, Kramer R, Greenwald S, et al. The association between head injuries and psychiatric disorders: findings from the New Haven NIMH epidemiologic catchment area study. Brain Inj 2001;15(11):935–45.
113. Schneiderman AI, Braver ER, Kang HK. Understanding sequelae of injury mechanisms and mild traumatic brain injury incurred during the conflicts in Iraq and Afghanistan: persistent postconcussive symptoms and posttraumatic stress disorder. Am J Epidemiol 2008;167(12): 1446–52.
114. Bryant RA, Harvey AG. The influence of traumatic brain injury on acute stress disorder and post-traumatic stress disorder following motor vehicle accidents. Brain Inj 1999;13(1):15–22.
115. Creamer M, O'Donnell ML, Pattison P. Amnesia, traumatic brain injury, and post-traumatic stress disorder: a methodological inquiry. Behav Res Ther 2005; 43(10):1383–9.
116. Saunders RL, Harbaugh RE. The second impact in catastrophic contact-sports head trauma. JAMA 1984;252(4):538–9.
117. Schneider RC. Head and neck injuries in football: mechanisms, treatment and prevention. Baltimore (MD): Williams and Wilkins; 1973. p. 35–43.
118. McCrory PR, Berkovic SF. Second impact syndrome. Neurology 1998;50(3): 677–83.
119. McCrory P. Does second impact syndrome exist? Clin J Sport Med 2001;11(3): 144–9.
120. Annegers JF, Hauser WA, Coan SP, et al. A population-based study of seizures after traumatic brain injuries. N Engl J Med 1998;338(1):20–4.
121. Singer RB. Incidence of seizures after traumatic brain injury—a 50-year population survey. J Insur Med 2001;33(1):42–5.
122. Plassman BL, Havlik RJ, Steffens DC, et al. Documented head injury in early adulthood and risk of Alzheimer's disease and other dementias. Neurology 2000;55(8):1158–66.
123. Van Duijn CM, Clayton DG, Chandra V, et al. Interaction between genetic and environmental risk factors for Alzheimer's disease: a reanalysis of case-control studies. EURODEM Risk Factors Research Group. Genet Epidemiol 1994; 11(6):539–51.
124. Corsellis JA, Bruton CJ, Freeman-Browne D. The aftermath of boxing. Psychol Med 1973;3(3):270–303.
125. Omalu BI, DeKosky ST, Minster RL, et al. Chronic traumatic encephalopathy in a National Football League player. Neurosurgery 2005;57(1):128–34 [discussion: 28–4].
126. Omalu BI, DeKosky ST, Hamilton RL, et al. Chronic traumatic encephalopathy in a National Football League player: part II. Neurosurgery 2006;59(5):1086–92 [discussion: 92–3].

127. McKee AC, Cantu RC, Nowinski CJ, et al. Chronic traumatic encephalopathy in athletes: progressive tauopathy after repetitive head injury. J Neuropathol Exp Neurol 2009;68(7):709–35.
128. Drew RH, Templer DI, Schuyler BA, et al. Neuropsychological deficits in active licensed professional boxers. J Clin Psychol 1986;42(3):520–5.
129. Roberts AJ. Brain damage in boxers. London (UK): Pitman Medical Scientific Publications; 1969.
130. Porter MD. A 9-year controlled prospective neuropsychologic assessment of amateur boxing. Clin J Sport Med 2003;13(6):339–52.
131. Porter MD, Fricker PA. Controlled prospective neuropsychological assessment of active experienced amateur boxers. Clin J Sport Med 1996;6(2):90–6.
132. Bower JH, Maraganore DM, Peterson BJ, et al. Head trauma preceding PD: a case-control study. Neurology 2003;60(10):1610–5.
133. Goldman SM, Tanner CM, Oakes D, et al. Head injury and Parkinson's disease risk in twins. Ann Neurol 2006;60(1):65–72.
134. Taylor CA, Saint-Hilaire MH, Cupples LA, et al. Environmental, medical, and family history risk factors for Parkinson's disease: a New England-based case control study. Am J Med Genet 1999;88(6):742–9.

Psychiatric Considerations in Patients with Decreased Levels of Consciousness

James L. Young, MD[a,*], Douglas Rund, MD[b]

KEYWORDS

- Altered level of consciousness • Catatonia
- Malignant catatonia • Neuroleptic malignant syndrome
- Serotonin syndrome • Pseudo seizures
- Psychogenic nonepileptic seizures • Psychogenic coma

In most cases, a decreased level of consciousness is not typical of a primary psychiatric illness. In any patient with a decreased level of consciousness, including those with current or a past history of psychiatric illness, consideration of medical causes, such as systemic illness, intoxication, acute drug reactions, and trauma is the first priority. In the absence of an underlying medical problem or intoxication, patients with psychiatric illness are usually fully alert.

This article discusses how patients with psychiatric illness may present with altered levels of consciousness. Ways in which severe cases of psychotic disorders, mood disorders, and somatoform disorders can present in this fashion are discussed. The often misunderstood syndrome of catatonia is also presented. Adverse drug reactions that can occur with medications used to treat psychiatric illness are also considered.

Evaluation of patients with psychiatric issues that present with decreased levels of consciousness are discussed first.

APPROACH TO THE PATIENT

Patient Interview

All patients suspected of having a psychiatric illness who present to the emergency department with altered levels of consciousness need to be thoroughly screened for medical causes, including an initial assessment to determine the acuity of their illness. Extra vigilance is warranted in the evaluation of children and patients older than 40 years

[a] Department of Psychiatry, OSU Harding Hospital, Ohio State University Medical Center, 1670 Upham Drive, Columbus, OH 43210, USA
[b] Department of Emergency Medicine, Ohio State University Medical Center, Ohio State University, 456 West 10th Avenue, Columbus, OH 43210, USA
* Corresponding author.
E-mail address: james.young@osumc.edu

Emerg Med Clin N Am 28 (2010) 595–609
doi:10.1016/j.emc.2010.03.010 emed.theclinics.com

with no previous history of psychiatric illness who present with an altered level of consciousness.

Once stability is ensured, a thorough interview can be performed. The interview should be nonthreatening and nonjudgmental, and should contain key elements such as introductions, open-ended and specific questions about the chief complaint, past psychiatric history, substance abuse history, history of trauma, and a social history. The interview should serve to elicit information, establish a positive patient-physician relationship, and allow for observation of the patient's behavior.[1]

The patient's past psychiatric history, including past history of suicide attempts, drug or alcohol use, hospitalizations, or other psychiatric treatments is important. It is necessary to note the patient's past psychiatric evaluations and adherence to prescribed medications, psychiatric or otherwise. As discussed later in this article, reactions to medication, including psychotropic medications, can cause altered levels of consciousness.

In patients with a suspected psychiatric illness, a thorough social history is essential. It is vital to understand the patient's living environment and how this environment may affect their current condition. Time should be spent reviewing any history of abuse or trauma. Any of these conditions can be exacerbated by recent difficult situations, so it is necessary to gather information about recent stressors and the environment in which patients are living.

In patients with severe psychiatric illness and an altered level of consciousness the interview can be limited. Contacting corroborating sources such as family members and medical records from previous providers or treatment facilities can provide useful diagnostic information.

Mental Status Examination

The mental status examination is an essential element in the evaluation of any patient, especially those with altered levels of consciousness. Mental status abnormalities can indicate serious underlying medical pathology. It is a snapshot of the patient's current level of alertness, emotional state, the content of thoughts, and current cognitive functioning. It is important to be aware that the patient's mental state can change, and they may require periodic re-evaluation.

The relevance of the mental status examination in making an accurate diagnosis is illustrated in a study done by Reeves and colleagues.[2] In this study, a chart review was performed of 64 patients who were initially admitted to a psychiatric unit, later identified as medical emergencies and then transferred to a general medical service. The single most important error identified was failure to perform an adequate mental status examination. Other reasons cited were failure to perform an adequate physical examination, failure to obtain indicated laboratory and radiologic studies, and failure to obtain an adequate history. The most common missed diagnosis was delirium, which was most readily detected by an adequate mental status examination. Delirium always requires a search for an underlying medical cause, especially in a person with no psychiatric history.

The mental status examination is best done in a systematic fashion, and should be comprehensive. It is a wise investment of time. Information and observations made while conducting the mental status examination further guide the diagnostic hypotheses made through the rest of the evaluation.[3]

Common elements of the mental status examination are listed in **Table 1**.[4]

Physical Examination

A complete physical examination is essential to thoroughly assess for medical causes for altered levels of consciousness. Areas that may require focused attention are

Table 1
Elements of the mental status examination

Appearance	The overall appearance of the patient, including the nature and appropriateness of their attire and if they seem either sick versus healthy or calm versus distressed, and so forth
Alertness	The ability of the patient to maintain interest and attention to their environment (**Table 2**)
Orientation	A patient's awareness of self, place, and time
Attitude	The patient's general attitude toward answering questions, cooperation and seeking help
Mood	The patient's current pervasive and sustained emotional state
Affect	The present level of emotional responsiveness including the amount and the range of expressive behavior; it should be noted how congruent the affect is to the mood
Thought process	The patient's reasoning ability and soundness of their logic
Thought content	What the patient is thinking about, including suicidal, homicidal, or delusional ideation
Insight	A patient's ability to identify and understand their situation
Judgment	The ability to make good decisions that will maintain safety
Impulse control	The ability to delay gratification, follow a plan, and to think of consequences before acting

Data from Howieson DB. The neuropsychiatric evaluation. In: Yudofsky SC, Hales RE, editors. Essentials of neuropsychiatry and clinical neurosciences. Arlington (VA): American Psychiatric Publishing; 2004. p. 55–80.

examination of the head and neck for evidence of trauma, and a comprehensive neurologic examination to assess for central nervous system (CNS) pathology. In addition, vital signs are a critical component of the examination. Abnormal vital signs in a patient with diminished consciousness indicate an increased need to search for medical pathology. A diminished level of consciousness should also suggest the need for pulse oximetry and a finger stick glucose test in the vital sign assessment.

Laboratory Testing

Laboratory testing required in the assessment of patients with psychiatric illness is somewhat controversial but ultimately depends on the clinical assessment. If the

Table 2
Levels of consciousness

Alert	An alert patient is fully conscious and aware of their environment
Drowsy or lethargic	A patient who is drowsy is awake, but is fatigued and may fall asleep if not stimulated
Obtunded	An obtunded patient has an even further reduced alertness along with decreased responsiveness and decreased interest in their environment
Stuporous	When a patient is stuporous, they are generally not responsive, except to vigorous stimulation
Comatose	A comatose patient is not arousable

Data from Sadock BJ, Sadock VA. Kaplan & Sadock's comprehensive textbook of psychiatry. 7th edition. Philadelphia: Lippincott Williams & Wilkins; 2000.

patient is admitted to a psychiatric facility, medical evaluation may be limited as psychiatric assessment and treatment become priorities. In a literature review and clinical policy guideline published by the American College of Emergency Physicians in 2006, the authors concluded "in adult ED patients with primary psychiatric complaints, diagnostic evaluation should be directed by the history and physical examination."[5] Routine preset laboratory testing is not recommended for all patients. Patients with diminished level of consciousness do not belong in this category, as diminished levels of consciousness may well be the presenting feature of a medical illness.

PSYCHIATRIC PRESENTATIONS OF ALTERED LEVEL OF CONSCIOUSNESS

Various psychiatric conditions and situations that may be at issue when a patient presents with altered levels of consciousness are now described, including psychotic disorders, mood disorders, somatoform disorders, and adverse drug reactions to psychiatric medications.

Psychotic Disorders

The *Diagnostic and Statistical Manual of Mental Disorders* (4th edition) (DSM-IV) lists several types of psychotic disorders that are differentiated by type of symptoms, severity of illness, and time course. Here the focus is on schizophrenia, but many of these concepts can be generalized to the other psychotic disorders.

Schizophrenia is unfortunately a chronic life-long condition. A prodromal phase including social isolation or eccentric behavior typically precedes the first psychotic break for several years, and is usually only recognized in retrospect. The first episode of psychosis usually occurs between late adolescence and the mid-thirties. A new onset psychotic symptom in general, especially when the patient is outside of this age range, warrants further investigation for a neurologic or medical illness.

Patients with schizophrenia have 3 primary types of symptoms: positive symptoms, negative symptoms, and cognitive symptoms. The positive symptoms are predominately psychotic symptoms, which include delusions and hallucinations. Delusions have a variety of themes and persecutory delusions are most common. Hallucinations are typically auditory in schizophrenia, whereas visual symptoms are more suggestive of medical illness. A presentation of psychotic symptoms may have the appearance of a decreased level of consciousness. For example, patients may be too paranoid to talk and thus seem functionally mute. Negative symptoms include affective flattening, alogia, and avolition. Alogia refers to diminished speech (in brief replies to questions, for instance) and apparent diminished thought processes. Avolition refers to diminished initiative or goal-directed activity. Cognitive symptoms manifest as decreased ability to problem solve and organize. Many patients with schizophrenia have difficulty with performing basic activities of daily living, such as budgeting, making and keeping appointments, and shopping for groceries. Patients with schizophrenia are usually alert and oriented. It is possible that those with extremes of the negative and cognitive symptoms can appear with an altered mental state.

Catatonia

The syndrome of catatonia was first described by Karl Ludwig Kahlbaum in 1874 and has been a misunderstood clinical entity. Throughout the twentieth century, there has been a tendency to associate catatonia with schizophrenia. This may be an artifact of the early writings of Emil Kraepelin and Eugen Bleuler and their conception of dementia precox. It has been clearly shown that catatonia is most often associated with mood disorders, especially the manic and mixed episodes of bipolar disorder.

Up to 20% of patients with mania exhibit catatonia[6] compared with less than 5% in schizophrenia.[7] DSM-IV criteria for catatonia are listed in **Box 1**.

Although usually a manifestation of a primary psychiatric condition, there are some medical conditions that can cause the syndrome of catatonia. The medical causes of catatonia are varied and similar to the causes of delirium. Endocrinopathies such as hypoparathyroidism with resulting hypocalcemia, thyrotoxicosis, and pheochromocytoma can present with catatonic features. Neurologic pathology such as frontotemporal lesions, strokes in anterior brain regions, traumatic brain injury, and epilepsy may also be associated with catatonia. Catatonia can also be caused by exposure to salicylates, inhalation anesthesia, strychnine, and fluoride. There are also some infectious causes such as human immunodeficiency virus, typhoid fever, tetanus, and staphylococcus.[8] Some medications may induce or facilitate catatonia. These include antipsychotics, corticosteroids, ketamine, and disulfiram. Catatonia may also be caused by the withdrawal of benzodiazepines. In addition, patients abusing phencyclidine (PCP) can also become catatonic.[9]

There have been many recent advances in the understanding of the pathophysiology of catatonia. The syndrome is likely caused by several different neurochemical abnormalities in different areas of the brain, including decreased γ-aminobutyric acid (GABA) and dopamine activity, and increased glutamate activity. Abnormal functioning of these neurochemical circuits in different regions of the brain results in manifestations of the different catatonic symptoms. Increased glutamate activity at *N*-methyl-D-aspartate (NMDA) receptors in the posterior parietal lobe results in anosognosia of position, seen as bizarre and mundane posturing behavior.[10] Abnormal activity in the posterior parietal lobe may influence GABA and dopamine activity in areas such as the supplemental motor area and the medial orbital gyrus resulting in bradykinesia and rigidity. Involvement of the anterior cingulate-medial orbitofrontal circuit may result in diminished arousal, mutism, and akinesia.[11] If the anterior hypothalamus is involved, malignant catatonia, a life-threatening type of catatonia can occur.[9] Malignant catatonia is further explored in the next section.

Box 1
DSM-IV criteria for catatonia

DSM-IV criteria for catatonia include a clinical picture that is dominated by at least 2 of the following:

1. *Motor immobility* as shown by catalepsy (including waxy flexibility) or stupor
2. *Excessive motor activity* (that is apparently purposeless and not influenced by external stimuli)
3. *Extreme negativism* (apparently motiveless resistance to all instructions or maintenance or present posture against attempts to be moved) or mutism
4. *Peculiarities of voluntary movement* as shown by posturing (voluntary assumption of inappropriate or bizarre postures) stereotyped movements, prominent mannerisms, or prominent grimacing
5. *Echophenomenon*: The automatic mimicking of the actions of another. Echolalia is the mimicry of speech and echopraxia is mimicry of movements.

Data from American Psychiatric Association Task Force on DSM-IV. Diagnostic and statistical manual of mental disorders: DSM-IV-TR. 4th edition. Washington, DC: American Psychiatric Association; 2000.

There are several different clinical entities that may present with symptoms similar to catatonia. Some patients who have been recently traumatized or who suffer from a personality disorder may present with elective mutism. In this case, the symptom of mutism would occur in isolation, and should not be confused with catatonia.[8] Patients with Parkinson disease may present with mutism and rigidity in the form of assuming peculiar and abnormal postures. This may pose a diagnostic dilemma, but patients with Parkinson disease usually present with cogwheel rigidity and tremor. This is especially difficult to distinguish in early onset Parkinson disease, which tends to develop more quickly with a predominance of akinesia, mutism, and often the absence of tremor and cogwheel rigidity. Relief of symptoms with an anticholinergic agent such as benztropine may aid in the diagnosis.[8] Obsessive compulsive disorder may present with repetitive and stereotypic behavior, as well as grimacing and tics that may bear a resemblance to catatonia. This is especially true in patients with autism and mental retardation.[8] The locked-in syndrome that results from bilateral pontine lesions renders a patient immobile except for eye movements and blinking. Cortical functioning, including consciousness is preserved, demonstrated by voluntary eye blinking in response to questions.[8]

The definitive treatment of catatonia is to treat the underlying cause. In all patients with catatonia, potential toxic precipitants should be eliminated and any precipitating general medical or neurologic conditions should be treated. Treatment of an underlying psychiatric disorder should also be initiated. As stated earlier, there is a tendency to associate catatonia with schizophrenia when in fact it most commonly occurs with mood disorders. The use of antipsychotic medications in a catatonic patient is generally discouraged because they may worsen the catatonic symptoms, and they also place the patient at higher risk for malignant catatonia or neuroleptic malignant syndrome (NMS).[12]

Patients with a retarded catatonia and a body temperature less than 39°C should be given lorazepam parenterally or orally at 3 mg per day, and the dose should be increased rapidly until resolution is achieved. Doses of up to 20 to 30 mg/d may be necessary. Remission of catatonia with lorazepam has been reported in 80% to 100% of patients.[12]

Electroconvulsive therapy (ECT) has been shown to be an effective treatment of catatonia. Bilateral ECT is more effective than unilateral ECT in patients who are febrile, delirious, do not respond to lorazepam, or are otherwise at physiologic risk. ECT can be done daily for 2 to 5 days and remission of catatonia has been reported from 82% to 96%.[12]

Malignant Catatonia and Neuroleptic Malignant Syndrome

Malignant catatonia (MC) is a severe and potentially life-threatening form of catatonia. MC that develops as a complication of antipsychotic and other dopamine blocking medication administration is called NMS. NMS is considered to be a drug-induced MC. MC can present with altered levels of consciousness ranging from confusion to coma. Although it is difficult to predict who will develop MC, there are certain risk factors for the disease such as underlying CNS pathology and dementia. Increased ambient heat and dehydration may increase the risk.[13] This is important to consider when treating a severely psychotic patient who exhibits poor judgment and self-care. Care should be taken that restrained patients are in well-ventilated climate-controlled areas and are adequately hydrated.

MC is most commonly recognized as severe muscle rigidity and hyperthermia. In addition, patients often present with autonomic dysfunction such as tachycardia, hypertension, and tachypnea, and mental status changes including delirium.[14]

Serum creatine kinase (CK) levels may be as high as 60,000 IU/L and leukocytosis can range from 10,000 to 40,000 cells/mm^3 with a left shift.[15] An increased CK level is nonspecific and can also be seen in trauma, intramuscular injection, acute psychosis, exposure to neuroleptics, and various other neuromuscular disorders. The level of CK does not correlate with the degree or duration of muscle rigidity or increase in temperature. Evaluating and monitoring CK levels may help make the diagnosis of MC, monitor for improvement or relapse, and serve as a marker for risk of renal failure. Leukocytosis is also a nonspecific finding and may occur in several physiologic conditions such as infection, lithium therapy, stress, excitement, and vigorous exercise.[16]

It has also been shown that serum iron levels are decreased in MC. The mechanism for this finding is not clear, but the severity of MC has been correlated to the degree of decrease in serum iron. Conversely, it has been shown that iron levels improve as MC symptoms improve.[16]

MC can also present atypically. For example, MC can occur with no muscle rigidity or hyperthermia. This poses a true diagnostic dilemma because of the unpredictability of symptom onset related to starting or withdrawing neuroleptic medicines.

The mortality from MC is estimated to be 12% to 20%. The most common cause of death is renal failure secondary to myoglobinuria. The second most common cause of death is aspiration pneumonia caused by decreased levels of consciousness and dysphagia. Mortality can be caused by cardiovascular events such as myocardial infarction exacerbated by autonomic instability or fatal dysrhythmias exacerbated by electrolyte abnormalities. Deaths in patients with MC have also been attributed to thrombocytopenia and disseminated intravascular coagulation.[13]

The pathophysiology of MC has not been firmly established, however it is likely a complex dysregulation of different systems resulting in a hypermetabolic state resulting from lowered dopaminergic activity.[17]

NMS is a medication-induced MC caused by dopamine antagonist medications. In addition to antipsychotic medications, the syndrome can occur with other dopamine blocking agents such as metoclopramide and amoxapine. NMS has also been seen in patients with extrapyramidal disorders such as Parkinson disease, Wilson disease, Huntington chorea, and striatonigral degeneration. In such conditions dopamine agonists such as L-3,4-dihydroxyphenylalanine (L-Dopa) may have been abruptly withdrawn or decreased.[15] Amantadine may be of some benefit in treating NMS because of its NMDA glutamate receptor antagonist properties.[13] The incidence of NMS may be as high as 1.0% of patients treated with neuroleptics. High-potency conventional antipsychotics such as haloperidol and thiothixene are believed to have a higher risk of NMS than lower-potency neuroleptics, such as chlorpromazine and mesoridizine. NMS has been reported with the newer atypical antipsychotic medications such as olanzapine; risperidone, and even clozaril. NMS commonly occurs soon after initiation, or a recent dose increase of a neuroleptic, but can occur at any time during the treatment course. The syndrome is not clearly dose dependent but more likely occurs in individuals taking high doses of neuroleptics and those who are neuroleptic naive. There is a likely genetic component to an individual's susceptibility. Although extremely rare, NMS has been reported after only 1 dose.

Another condition that can be considered as a medication-induced MC is malignant hyperthermia. Malignant hyperthermia is a rare autosomal dominant disorder that renders susceptibility to inhalation anesthetics and succinylcholine. These patients show a hypermetabolic response to these agents resulting in muscle rigidity, increased creatinine kinase level, tremor, and fever. This condition has considerable symptom overlap with NMS and MC.[8]

MC is a potentially life-threatening condition that warrants intensive and timely treatment. The first step is to discontinue all antipsychotic and other agents with dopamine antagonism. If the patient is agitated or delirious, steps should be taken to ensure the patient's safety.[8] Hyperthermia should be treated with nonsteroidal antiinflammatory drugs or acetaminophen. More aggressive measures such as cooling blankets or gastric lavage with ice water may need to be used. If dehydrated, patients should receive appropriate intravenous (IV) fluids. The patient's blood pressure and heart rate should be monitored. β-Blockers and vasopressors may be given as necessary. Oxygen saturation must also be monitored with supplemental oxygen given as needed.[8] Patients also require frequent monitoring of their renal function via serum CK, creatinine, and urea nitrogen levels. Dialysis may be required if the symptoms do not resolve quickly. MC often presents similarly to an acute infectious process. Moreover, infection should be ruled out with blood cultures, a chest radiograph, and cerebrospinal fluid (CSF) examination.

Mood Disorders

The mood disorders consist mainly of major depressive disorder and bipolar disorder. Because mania generally presents with a heightened level of consciousness, except when the patient is catatonic, it is not discussed here. A patient experiencing a depressive episode, caused by major depressive disorder or bipolar disorder, may in some extreme circumstances present with decreased levels of consciousness.

When a patient presents with an altered mental state caused by depression or severe psychotic depression, it is extremely important to first rule out medical problems such as drug overdose, severe dehydration, or malnutrition. Psychiatric consultants will typically recommend blood chemistry analysis (including electrolytes, calcium, magnesium, blood urea nitrogen, and creatinine), liver function studies, thyroid function studies, complete blood count, and a comprehensive urine drug screen.

A depressed episode is characterized by a syndrome of symptoms including depressed mood, alterations in sleeping and eating patterns, anhedonia, excessive guilt, poor concentration, psychomotor slowing, and suicidal thoughts. The symptomatology and level of dysfunction caused by a depressed episode can range from mild to severe. Altered levels of consciousness would be atypical and should alert the clinician to possible complications, such as a comorbid medical illness or drug toxicity/overdose. Only in severe cases is the patient's level of consciousness altered by the mood disorder itself.

A patient experiencing a severe depressive episode can also present with psychotic features such as delusional thinking or auditory hallucinations. As discussed in the section on psychotic disorders, these symptoms can mimic a decreased level of consciousness. In rare cases, these patients may present as lethargic or obtunded. Mood congruent delusions include guilt, deserved punishment, sickness, or delusions of poverty. An example of a delusion that is congruent with the state of depression is Cotard syndrome. A person with Cotard syndrome (also known as negation delusion or nihilistic delusion) is when the person holds the belief that they do not exist or that they are dead. Variations on this theme are the belief that their organs are rotting away or that they are missing body parts.[18] Auditory hallucinations tend to be transient and are typically insulting or demeaning. It is possible, although less common, that the hallucinations or delusions are not congruent with the patient's mood. A lack of congruency with the patient's mood indicates a poor prognosis.

Studies have shown that up to 15% to 20% of patients with major depressive disorder have psychotic features. This percentage can increase to as high as 45%

in the elderly population. Major depressive disorder with psychotic features is associated with poor short-term outcomes, longer recovery times, greater levels of disability, and higher mortality.[19]

Other variations of a depressive episode include melancholic depression and atypical depression. Melancholic depression (also called endogenous depression) is characterized by severe anhedonia, early-morning wakening, weight loss, and profound feelings of guilt over trivial events.[19,20] Atypical depression is characterized by oversleeping and overeating. These patients typically have a younger age of onset, more severe psychomotor slowing, and higher rates of comorbid anxiety, substance abuse, and somatization disorder. Patients with atypical depression have an increased chance of a longer course of illness, a future diagnosis of bipolar disorder, and a seasonal pattern to their moods.[19,20]

Conversion Disorder

Conversion disorder is a type of somatoform disorder in which a patient experiences medically unexplained neurologic symptoms such as hemianesthesia, blindness, involuntary movements, tics, or nonepileptic seizures. These symptoms are not consciously generated and there is an absence of conscious secondary gain. Conversion disorder typically occurs in a time of psychosocial stress. Van der Kolk and colleagues[21] explain that posttraumatic stress disorder (PTSD), dissociation, somatization, and affect dysregulation represent a spectrum of adaptations to trauma. It is important to gather information about psychosocial stressors and trauma/abuse history when treating patients with conversion disorder. Patients with conversion disorder often present in the context of a stressful situation. Conversion disorder symptoms usually appear abruptly and disappear abruptly and it is rare, but not unheard of, for someone to have chronic conversion disorder.

Two variations of conversion disorders that may present with altered levels of consciousness are discussed: psychogenic nonepileptic seizures and psychogenic coma.

Psychogenic Nonepileptic Seizures

Psychogenic nonepileptic seizures (PNES), often called pseudo seizures, are a common manifestation of conversion disorder. Many would discourage the use of the term pseudo seizure because it implies faking or malingering. A PNES is an episode of altered behavior, motor activity, and perceptions that appear like an epileptic seizure but with an absence of neurologic evidence of seizure activity.[22] Bodde and colleagues[23] offer the following definition: "a psychogenic non-epileptic seizure is an observable abrupt paroxysmal change in behavior or consciousness that resembles an epileptic seizure, but that is not accompanied by the electrophysiologic changes that accompany an epileptic seizure, for which no other evidence is found for other somatic causes for the seizure, whereas there is positive evidence or a strong suspicion for psychogenic factors that may have caused the seizure."

The incidence of PNES in the general population is about 1.5/100,000 persons per year which is about 4% of the incidence of epilepsy; 25% to 30% of patients referred to tertiary epilepsy centers are eventually diagnosed with pseudo seizure.[23] It is important to make the correct diagnosis of PNES to avoid potential iatrogenic hazards of antiepileptic drugs and to decrease the delay in implementing appropriate psychiatric and psychological treatment.[23]

PNES occurs as a result of a complex array of psychosocial and psychological mechanisms. It is believed that certain vulnerable individuals will develop PNES in certain circumstances. First, there is likely an initial psychological cause, such as the experience of abuse or trauma. PNES patients have a high incidence of trauma history and comorbid PTSD.[23] Some people are more predisposed to psychosomatic symptoms. Patients with dependent, avoidant, or borderline personality traits or disorders are more predisposed to psychosomatic symptoms. In addition, those with a combination of high trait anxiety and poor coping mechanisms are at increased risk. Patients with an abuse history and vulnerable personality traits who develop PNES often have a shaping factor, such as a relative with epilepsy, or a previous history of epilepsy themselves, that steer the symptoms in the direction of seizures. There is often a triggering factor in which the maladaptive defense and coping mechanisms are brought into play by a psychosocial stressor. The problem may become chronic given the right prolongation factors, such as secondary gain.[23]

It is important to recognize nonepileptic seizures, as failure to do so may result in iatrogenic injury and death resulting from unnecessary treatments.[24] However, it can be confusing as up to 50% of patients with PNES also have epilepsy and will require antiepileptic treatment.[25]

Patients with PNES often do not show typical seizure activity. They can show motor phenomena uncharacteristic of epileptic seizures such as asynchronous out of phase clonic movements, opisthotonus, side-to-side head movements, atonia, eyes deviating upward, and resistance to eye opening. Patients can also show decreased responsiveness.[26]

One way to understand the presentation of PNES is to compare it with the presentation of a true ictal event, such as a grand mal seizure. A grand mal seizure usually begins with an aura. Following this the patient abruptly loses consciousness and begins a tonic then clonic phase of movement. In a grand mal seizure these are bilaterally symmetric forceful movements. Depending on the position of the patient at the onset of the seizure, injuries can occur. Common injuries occur when the patient falls or bites their tongue. A grand mal seizure typically lasts 30 seconds and rarely more than 2 minutes. Following the seizure there is a 15 to 20 minute postictal period in which the patient is initially nonverbal and disoriented. During this time the patient gradually recovers consciousness and the ability to speak.

Pseudo seizures typically do not follow these expected patterns. A PNES resembling a grand mal seizure may begin gradually instead of abruptly and without a stereotyped progression of seizure activity. Instead of bilaterally symmetric forceful contractions, patients with PNES often have struggling or flailing type movements. Patients with PNES may retain consciousness and attend to their environment during seizure. Patients with PNES rarely bite their tongue, fall, sustain injuries, or lose bladder or bowel continence. It is also uncommon to have postictal symptoms with PNES.

There is a dearth of literature on the efficacy of treatment strategies for patients with PNES, and there are no standardized treatment protocols.[23] However, there are some basic strategies that can be followed.

Treatment begins when the patient is informed of the diagnosis. The way that a patient is informed can have long-term consequences. They should not be abruptly told they do not have seizures and then dismissed. This condition is the unconscious generation of symptoms and patients view it as a significant problem regardless of its cause. Patients with PNES are usually victims of abuse with maladaptive coping mechanisms. The suggestion that there is nothing medically wrong or to suggest they are faking it may traumatize them further. Patients should be informed in a respectful way that acknowledges the problem and steers them toward future treatment.

Effective treatment of PNES is accomplished through a combination of psychotropic medications and psychotherapy. Medications should be considered to address comorbid psychiatric symptoms such as depression and anxiety but do not directly reduce PNES behavior. Patients also need psychotherapy that focuses on abuse issues, emotional modulation, and healthy coping strategies. Some may also benefit from family therapy and case management.

When a diagnosis of PNES is firmly established in the absence of a diagnosis of epilepsy, it is important to withdraw antiepileptic drug treatment. Outpatient treatment is likely more effective. Hospitalization may serve to reinforce somatoform behaviors and should be avoided when it is safe to do so.

Psychogenic Coma

A psychogenic coma is a conversion disorder in which a patient presents in a comatose state with no apparent medical cause. When a patient is unresponsive and no organic cause is found after a thorough and prompt investigation of potentially life-threatening causes, the diagnosis of psychogenic coma may be considered.[27]

First and foremost, investigation into organic and life-threatening causes of unresponsiveness need to be performed. This includes a thorough physical examination, mental status examination, and collection of history from collateral sources. Emphasis should be placed on evaluating CNS pathology. The workup includes a lumbar puncture to culture and examine the CSF, neuroimaging (preferably magnetic resonance imaging for increased resolution and ability to visualize the posterior fossa and brainstem), and an electroencephalogram (EEG). A normal EEG may suggest either a rare localized brainstem abnormality or a psychiatric cause of unresponsiveness.[28]

There are some bedside tests to evaluate for psychogenic coma. However, the response to these maneuvers may be inconsistent and clinical judgment is necessary. Patients may respond to noxious stimuli such as smelling salts, sternal rub, or cotton swabs placed in the nares. Patients with psychogenic coma may hold their eyes tightly shut and resist attempts to open them. Oculovestibular testing, also called caloric testing, can also be used. In a physiologically awake person, irrigation of the ear with warm water produces nystagmus toward the irrigated side and irrigation with cold water produces similar nystagmus away from the irrigated side. Sustained nystagmus may indicate that the patient is unresponsive due to psychogenic causes.[27] The clinician may also try to elicit protective reflexes. An example of this would be to hold the patients hand over their face and drop it. Patients with a psychogenic coma may slightly move their hand to the side as it falls so that it does not hit their face.[27] The physician should catch the hand before it strikes the face to avoid facial injury.

Once the diagnosis of psychogenic coma has been established, conservative management and observation should be practiced. Care should be taken to limit invasive testing and monitoring to avoid iatrogenic medical complications.

The differential diagnosis of psychogenic coma includes the broad differential for all causes of coma. These include CNS events, toxic ingestion, endocrine dysfunction, infectious disease, respiratory abnormalities, cardiovascular events, hepatic dysfunction, renal dysfunction, and Wernike encephalopathy.[28]

There are some neurologic and neuropsychiatric considerations in the differential diagnosis as well. Patients with catatonia may present in an unresponsive state. Maintaining postures for long periods of time, staring, negativism, and mutism are common characteristics of catatonia that may mimic coma. A severe depressive episode may present with profound inanition and abulia to the point of unresponsiveness. Patients in this state may be uninterested in their environment and subsequently may stop talking and eating. A patient with locked-in syndrome resulting from bilateral pontine lesions that affect the pontine motor tracts presents as mute and paralyzed, but appears alert and has preserved intellectual functioning, upward gaze, and eye blinking. Damage to the frontal lobes can result in symptoms of apathy and abulia, as well as impaired executive functioning. Frontal lobe dysfunction from congenital causes or head trauma may not be apparent on brain imaging. Patients with akinetic mutism are unable to move or speak, except for eye tracking and movements to perform certain tasks such as eating. These patients seem to be unconcerned with their lack of ability to communicate, unlike patients with aphasia. This condition is caused by a unilateral or bilateral lesion in the superior mesial region of the frontal lobe. Patients with global aphasia have often incurred a significant ischemic or hemorrhagic event and typically have an array of neurologic impairments. However, there are rare cases where only language has been disrupted and all other cerebral functions remain intact. Patients with isolated global aphasia are unable to communicate or comprehend spoken language. They are unresponsive, but are alert and able to perform meaningful tasks. They may also be able to communicate nonverbally. Malingering is the intentional generation of symptoms for a conscious secondary gain. It is not a neuropsychiatric disorder, merely the intentional manipulation to achieve a goal. It may, at times, be difficult to detect malingering. The clinician may suspect malingering on the observation of inconsistencies in behavior. Circumstantial evidence of malingering may also be obtained through collateral sources. Clinicians have a tendency to over diagnose malingering; malingering does not preclude the presence of an actual physical disorder.[28]

Adverse Drug Reactions to Psychiatric Medications

There are several adverse drug reactions associated with medications that are commonly used to treat psychiatric disorders. Such reactions are not unique to psychiatry, and can occur with many different pharmacologic agents. Information about medications the patient is taking and adherence to the prescribed regime, as well as over-the-counter medications, herbal supplements, and drugs of abuse, is important. How such agents can combine to cause problems must also be considered. Acute dystonic reactions and serotonin syndrome are now discussed (NMS was discussed earlier).

Acute Dystonic Reaction

An acute dystonic reaction (ADR) is a sustained, involuntary, and sometimes painful muscle contraction affecting either a single muscle or a group of muscles caused by a dopamine antagonist medication. Cranial, pharyngeal, cervical, and axial muscles are most commonly affected. This can result in the patient suddenly assuming an abnormal posture or facial expression. Common presentations are oculogyric crisis, grimacing, fixation of the jaw, retrocollis, torticollis, and opisthotonic posturing.[29]

Such reactions are often terrifying to patients and may lead to poor adherence with medications in the future.[30] Laryngeal involvement may lead to respiratory difficulties, and in rare cases may require airway protection.

Any agent with dopamine antagonist activity can cause an ADR, but most are associated with antipsychotic medications. All antipsychotic medications have the potential to cause an ADR, but high-potency antipsychotics such as haloperidol tend to cause more reactions than low-potency antipsychotics such as chlorpromazine. Newer atypical antipsychotics (ie, risperidone, quetiepine) are lower risk.[29]

Young men are at highest risk, especially those with a high muscle mass. African American and Hispanic patients are also at high risk.[30] The risk of an ADR is dose related. Up to 90% of ADRs occur within the first 4 days of neuroleptic exposure. If untreated, such symptoms can last for hours or days or longer with depot preparations.[29]

The pathophysiology of ADRs are unknown. However, dystonia is related to the dopamine pathway and because the symptoms can occur days after the initial blockade of dopamine receptors, it is postulated that secondary dopamine hypersensitivity plays a role.[29]

The cornerstone of treatment is with anticholinergic medications. Prompt intramuscular (IM) or IV administration of anticholinergic medications usually results in rapid resolution of symptoms. Benztropine 1 to 2 mg is usually given either IM or IV. Diphenhydramine 25 mg can also be administered IM or IV. The anticholinergic medication given to reverse an ADR may wear off before the effects of the antipsychotic that caused the condition. Therefore, additional oral dosing of anticholinergic medications should be given for a few days or longer. Amantadine 100 mg by mouth twice a day may be an alternative in those in whom anticholinergic medications are contraindicated.[30]

In high-risk patients, oral anticholinergic medications should be used prophylactically with the initiation of treatment of high-potency antipsychotic medications. The typical regimen is benztropine 1 to 2 mg by mouth twice a day.

Serotonin Syndrome

Serotonin syndrome is a reaction to medication that causes excessive serotonin agonism, centrally and peripherally.[31] Serotonin syndrome is characterized by a triad of symptoms (**Table 3**).[32]

The condition can progress to coma and death, and may require intubation, paralysis, and sedation.

The main treatment of serotonin syndrome is withdrawing the offending agent. This does not usually result in an immediate resolution of symptoms, so supportive measures need to be provided. Benzodiazepines are helpful in decreasing agitation. Diazepam is the best studied, and has been shown in animal models to increase survival by blunting hyperadrenergic symptoms. In mild cases, IV hydration and observation are usually sufficient. In moderate cases 5-hydroxytryptamine 2A antagonists, such as cyproheptadine, can be used. Severe cases with hyperthermia often require intubation, paralysis, and sedation as necessary.[31,33]

Other Adverse Drug Reactions

There are other adverse psychiatric drug reactions that can present to the emergency department with altered levels of consciousness. For example, Kimmel and collegeaus[34] describe a case of encephalopathy caused by increased ammonia levels associated with valproic acid. In addition, cases of lithium toxicity can present with nausea/vomiting, ataxia, and altered mental status including stupor or coma. Patients with psychiatric illness are at increased risk for suicide often times with home medications or street drugs.

Table 3
Symptoms of serotonin syndrome

Neuromuscular hyperactivity	Tremor, clonus, myoclonus, hyperreflexia and, in advanced stages, pyramidal rigidity
Autonomic hyperactivity	Diaphoresis, fever, tachycardia, and tachypnea
Altered mental status	Agitation, excitement and, in advanced stages, confusion

SUMMARY

An overview of several different psychiatric issues that should be considered when confronted with a patient with a decreased level of consciousness is provided. Symptoms commonly regarded as psychiatric may be caused by systemic illness and in turn often what seems to be systemic illness is in fact psychiatric. Although severe cases may present in this fashion, it is uncommon for patients with psychiatric issues to present with a decreased level of consciousness. Medical causes such as systemic illness or adverse drug reactions need to be ruled out first.

REFERENCES

1. Rund DA, Hutzler JC. Emergency psychiatry. St. Louis (MO): C.V. Mosby; 1983.
2. Reeves RR, Pendarvis EJ, Kimble R. Unrecognized medical emergencies admitted to psychiatric units. Am J Emerg Med 2000;18(4):390–3.
3. Sadock BJ, Sadock VA. Kaplan & Sadock's comprehensive textbook of psychiatry. 7th edition. Philadelphia: Lippincott Williams & Wilkins; 2000.
4. Howieson DB. The neuropsychiatric evaluation. In: Yudofsky SC, Hales RE, editors. Essentials of neuropsychiatry and clinical neurosciences. Arlington (VA): American Psychiatric Publishing; 2004. p. 55–80.
5. Lukens TW, Wolf SJ, Edlow JA, et al. Clinical policy: critical issues in the diagnosis and management of the adult psychiatric patient in the emergency department. Ann Emerg Med 2006;47(1):79–99.
6. Taylor MA, Fink M. Catatonia in psychiatric classification: a home of its own. Am J Psychiatry 2003;160(7):1233–41.
7. Caroff SN, Mann SC, Campbell EC, et al. Epdemiology. In: Caroff SN, editor. Catatonia: from psychopathology to neurobiology. 1st edition. Washington, DC: American Psychiatric Pub; 2004. p. 15–31.
8. Fink M, Taylor MA. Catatonia: a clinician's guide to diagnosis and treatment. New York: Cambridge University Press; 2003.
9. Lopez-Canino A, Francis A. Drug induced catatonia. In: Caroff SN, editor. Catatonia: from psychopathology to neurobiology. Washington, DC: American Psychiatric Publishers Inc; 2004. p. 129–39.
10. Carroll B, Thomas C, Jayanti K, et al. Treating persistent catatonia when benzodiazepines fail. Curr Psychiatr 2005;4(3):56–64.
11. Mann SC, Caroff SN, Fricchione GL, et al. Malignant catatonia. In: Caroff SN, Mann SC, Francis A, et al, editors. Catatonia: from psychopathology to neurobiology. Washington, DC: American Psychiatric Publishing Inc; 2004. p. 105–19.
12. Fink M, Taylor MA. The catatonia syndrome: forgotten but not gone. Arch Gen Psychiatry 2009;66(11):1173–7.
13. Carbone JR. The neuroleptic malignant and serotonin syndromes. Emerg Med Clin North Am 2000;18(2):317–25, x.
14. Seitz DP, Gill SS. Neuroleptic malignant syndrome complicating antipsychotic treatment of delirium or agitation in medical and surgical patients: case reports and a review of the literature. Psychosomatics 2009;50(1):8–15.
15. Pelonero AL, Levenson JL, Pandurangi AK. Neuroleptic malignant syndrome: a review. Psychiatr Serv 1998;49(9):1163–72.
16. Lee J. Laboratory findings. In: Caroff SN, Mann SC, Francis A, et al, editors. Catatonia: from psychopathology to neurobiology. Washington, DC: American Psychiatric Publishing Inc; 2004. p. 65–75.
17. Strawn JR, Keck PE Jr, Caroff SN. Neuroleptic malignant syndrome. Am J Psychiatry 2007;164(6):870–6.

18. Pearn J, Gardner-Thorpe C. Jules Cotard (1840–1889): his life and the unique syndrome which bears his name. Neurology 2002;58(9):1400–3.
19. Sadock BJ, Kaplan HI, Sadock VA. Kaplan & Sadock's synopsis of psychiatry: behavioral sciences/clinical psychiatry. 10th edition. Philadelphia: Wolter Kluwer/Lippincott Williams & Wilkins; 2007.
20. American Psychiatric Association Task Force on DSM-IV. Diagnostic and statistical manual of mental disorders: DSM-IV-TR. 4th edition. Washington, DC: American Psychiatric Association; 2000.
21. van der Kolk BA, Pelcovitz D, Roth S, et al. Dissociation, somatization, and affect dysregulation: the complexity of adaptation of trauma. Am J Psychiatry 1996; 153(Suppl 7):83–93.
22. Russell A. The diagnosis and management of pseudoseizures or psychogenic non-epileptic events. Ann Indian Acad Neurol 2006;9:60–71.
23. Bodde NM, Brooks JL, Baker GA, et al. Psychogenic non-epileptic seizures–definition, etiology, treatment and prognostic issues: a critical review. Seizure 2009; 18(8):543–53.
24. Reuber M, Baker GA, Gill R, et al. Failure to recognize psychogenic nonepileptic seizures may cause death. Neurology 2004;62(5):834–5.
25. Benbadis SR, Agrawal V, Tatum WO. How many patients with psychogenic non-epileptic seizures also have epilepsy? Neurology 2001;57(5):915–7.
26. Lesser RP. Psychogenic seizures. Neurology 1996;46(6):1499–507.
27. Downs JW, Young PE, Durning SJ. Psychogenic coma following upper endoscopy: a case report and review of the literature. Mil Med 2008;173(5):509–12.
28. Huffman JC, Stern TA. Assessment of the awake but unresponsive patient. Prim Care Companion J Clin Psychiatry 2003;5(5):227–31.
29. Dressler D, Benecke R. Diagnosis and management of acute movement disorders. J Neurol 2005;252(11):1299–306.
30. Hales RE, Yudofsky SC, Talbott JA. American psychiatric press textbook of psychiatry. 2nd edition. Washington, DC: American Psychiatric Press; 1994.
31. Boyer EW, Shannon M. The serotonin syndrome. N Engl J Med 2005;352(11): 1112–20.
32. Gillman P. Monoamine oxidase inhibitors, opioid analgesics and serotonin toxicity. Br J Anaesth 2005;95:434–41.
33. Dvir Y, Smallwood P. Serotonin syndrome: a complex but easily avoidable condition. Gen Hosp Psychiatry 2008;30(3):284–7.
34. Kimmel RJ, Irwin SA, Meyer JM. Valproic acid-associated hyperammonemic encephalopathy: a case report from the psychiatric setting. Int Clin Psychopharmacol 2005;20(1):57–8.

Delirium in the Older Emergency Department Patient: A Quiet Epidemic

Jin H. Han, MD, MSc[a,*], Amanda Wilson, MD[a,b], E. Wesley Ely, MD, MPH[c]

KEYWORDS

• Delirium • Emergency department • Epidemiology
• Diagnosis • Management

Delirium is an under recognized public health problem that affects 7% to 10% of older patients in the emergency department (ED).[1–3] This form of organ failure has devastating consequences for older patients and poses a significant threat to their quality of life. It has been associated with higher death rates,[4,5] accelerated functional and cognitive decline,[6–8] and longer hospital length of stay.[9,10] Delirium also places a large financial burden on the US health care system, costing more than an estimated $100 billion in direct and indirect charges.[11,12]

Despite its negative consequences, delirium is frequently missed by emergency physicians,[1,3] and this is a serious quality-of-care issue.[13] Currently, 20 million older Americans visit the ED each year,[14–16] and are the fastest growing group of users.[14,17] With the elderly population expected to increase exponentially in the next several decades, the burden of delirium on EDs will intensify.[18] The Society for Academic Emergency Medicine Geriatric Task Force has recommended delirium screening in the ED as one of the key quality indicators for emergency geriatric care.[19] Given this urgency, the purpose of this review is to discuss the definition, risk factors, and

Jin H. Han and Amanda Wilson were supported in part by the Emergency Medicine Foundation Grant Career Development Award. Dr Wes Ely was supported in part by the National Institutes of Health AG01023 and the Veterans Affairs Tennessee Valley Geriatric Research, Education, and Clinical Center (GRECC).

[a] Department of Emergency Medicine, Vanderbilt University Medical Center, 703 Oxford House, 1313 21st Avenue South, Nashville, TN 37232-4700, USA
[b] Department of Psychiatry, Vanderbilt University Medical Center, 1601 23rd Avenue South, Suite 1159, Nashville, TN 37212, USA
[c] Division of Allergy, Pulmonary, and Critical Care, Department of Internal Medicine, Center for Health Services Research, Sixth Floor Medical Center East #6109, Vanderbilt University Medical Center, Nashville, TN 37232-8300, USA
* Corresponding author.
E-mail address: jin.h.han@vanderbilt.edu

Emerg Med Clin N Am 28 (2010) 611–631
doi:10.1016/j.emc.2010.03.005 **emed.theclinics.com**
0733-8627/10/$ – see front matter

consequences of delirium in older ED patients, and its diagnosis and management in the ED setting.

DEFINITION OF DELIRIUM

Delirium is defined as an acute change in cognition that cannot be better accounted for by preexisting or evolving dementia.[20] This change in cognition is rapid, occurring over a period of hours or days, and is classically described as reversible. Patients with delirium typically have inattention, disorganized thinking, altered level of consciousness (somnolent or agitated), and perceptual disturbances.[20]

Delirium is classified into 3 psychomotor subtypes: hypoactive, hyperactive, and mixed.[21] Hypoactive delirium is described as quiet delirium and is characterized by decreased psychomotor activity. These patients can seem depressed, sedated, somnolent, or even lethargic. Conversely, patients with hyperactive delirium have increased psychomotor activity and they seem restless, anxious, agitated, and even combative. Patients with mixed-type delirium exhibit fluctuating levels of psychomotor activity (hypoactive and hyperactive). Several epidemiologic studies have investigated the frequency with which different psychomotor subtypes occur in a variety of settings (**Table 1**); hypoactive delirium and mixed-type delirium seem to be the predominant subtypes in older patients.[22–27] In the ED setting, Han and colleagues[3] observed that 96% of older patients with delirium had the hypoactive or mixed subtype.

Each psychomotor subtype is hypothesized to have a different underlying pathophysiologic mechanism and underlying cause.[21,28] For example, delirium caused by alcohol withdrawal is more likely to be the hyperactive subtype, whereas delirium caused by a metabolic derangement is more likely to be the hypoactive subtype.[29] The various psychomotor subtypes of delirium have a differential effect on clinical course and outcomes,[30,31] and also affect recognition by health care providers. Hyperactive delirium is more easily recognized, whereas hypoactive delirium is often undetected because of its subtle clinical presentation,[32] and is often ascribed to other causes such as depression or fatigue.[33]

Table 1
Studies that have evaluated the psychomotor subtypes of delirium

Author	Age Inclusion (y)	Setting	Psychomotor Subtype (%)		
			Hypoactive	Hyperactive	Mixed
Han et al, 2009[3]	>65	ED	92	4	4
Liptzkin and Levkoff, 1992[22]	>65	Inpatient, medical	19	15	52
O'Keeffe, 1999[23]	Not reported	Inpatient, geriatrics	29	21	43
Marcantonio et al, 2002[24]	>65	Inpatient, hip fracture repair	71	—	29
Kelly et al, 2001[25]	Nursing home	Inpatient, geriatrics	56	3	41
Peterson et al, 2006[26]	None	Inpatient, medical ICU	44	2	55
Pandharipande et al, 2007[27]	None	Inpatient, surgical ICU Trauma ICU	64 60	9 6	0 1

THE DISTINCTION BETWEEN DELIRIUM AND DEMENTIA

Delirium and dementia both cause cognitive impairment, and health care providers often confuse these 2 distinct clinical entities. This confusion is exacerbated by the high frequency in which delirium is superimposed on dementia,[34] which is why delirium is often missed in these patients.[35] However, there are several key distinguishing features between delirium and dementia (**Table 2**), and most delirium assessments capitalize on these differences. Unlike delirium, dementia is characterized by a gradual decline in cognition occurring over months or years, and is usually irreversible. Altered level of consciousness, inattention, perceptual disturbances, and disorganized thinking are not commonly observed in patients with dementia.

However, there are some instances when the clinical features of delirium and dementia overlap, making them difficult to distinguish from each other. This especially the case in patients with severe or end-stage dementia, who can exhibit symptoms of inattention, perceptual disturbance, disorganized thinking, and altered level of consciousness even in the absence of delirium. When these patients develop delirium, an acute change in mental status is usually observed and any preexisting abnormalities with inattention, disorganized thinking, or level of alertness may worsen. For this reason establishing their baseline mental status is crucial to diagnosing delirium in patients with severe dementia.

Although classically thought of as irreversible, there are certain circumstances in which dementia may be reversible. Hypothyroidism, vitamin B_{12} deficiency, normal pressure hydrocephalus, and depression are examples of illnesses that can cause reversible dementia or a dementialike illness (pseudodementia). However, the cognitive decline observed in reversible dementia is usually gradual as opposed to the rapid cognitive decline seen in delirium. Conversely, there is also a proportion of patients whose delirium is not transient; their symptoms can persist for months or even years.[36,37]

Dementia with Lewy bodies (DLB) deserves special mention because it can be difficult to distinguish from delirium. DLB is the second most common subtype of dementia (after Alzheimer's disease) and affects 15% to 25% of elderly patients with dementia.[38] Similar to delirium, DLB is characterized by a rapid decline and fluctuation in cognition, attention, and level of consciousness. Such fluctuations can be observed over several hours or days. Like delirium, perceptual disturbances are frequently observed in patients with DLB. In contrast to delirium, however, patients

Table 2
Differences between delirium and dementia

Characteristic	Delirium	Dementia
Onset	Rapid over a period of hours or days	Gradual over a long period of time
Course	Fluctuating	Stable
Is cognitive decline reversible?	Yes	No
Altered of level of consciousness?	Yes	No[a]
Inattention present?	Yes	No[a]
Disorganized thinking present?	Yes	No[a]
Altered perception present?	Yes	No[a]

[a] May be present in patients with severe dementia.

with DLB have parkinsonian motor symptoms, such as cog wheeling, shuffling gait, stiff movements, and reduced arm swing during walking. Nevertheless, differentiating between DLB and delirium can be difficult in the ED and may require a detailed evaluation by a psychiatrist or neurologist.

CAUSE OF DELIRIUM

Delirium is often the initial manifestation of an underlying acute illness and can be present before fever, tachypnea, tachycardia, or hypoxia.[39] The cause of delirium is multifactorial and involves a complex interrelationship between patient vulnerability and precipitating factors (**Fig. 1**).[40,41] Patients who are highly vulnerable may be older, have severe dementia, and have multiple comorbidities. In these patients, a relatively benign insult, such as a small dose of narcotic medication, can precipitate delirium. Patients who are less vulnerable to developing delirium, like those who are younger and have little comorbidity burden, require higher doses of noxious stimuli (eg, severe sepsis) to develop delirium.[42] Because older patients are more likely to have multiple vulnerability factors, they are disproportionately more susceptible to becoming delirious compared with younger patients. For this reason, patients in nursing homes are especially vulnerable.[43]

Most of what is known about delirium vulnerability factors is from studies performed in hospitalized patients (**Table 3**).[44–46] There are limited data from the ED, but one study identified dementia, premorbid functional impairment, and hearing impairment as independent risk factors for delirium in the ED.[3] Similar observations have been made in the medical and surgical inpatient population.[10,40,47–49] Dementia is probably the most consistently observed independent vulnerability factor for delirium across different clinical settings.[40,48–55] As the severity of dementia worsens, the risk of developing delirium also increases.[56] Other vulnerability factors have also been reported in the hospital literature and include old age,[48,51,54] high comorbidity burden,[55] visual

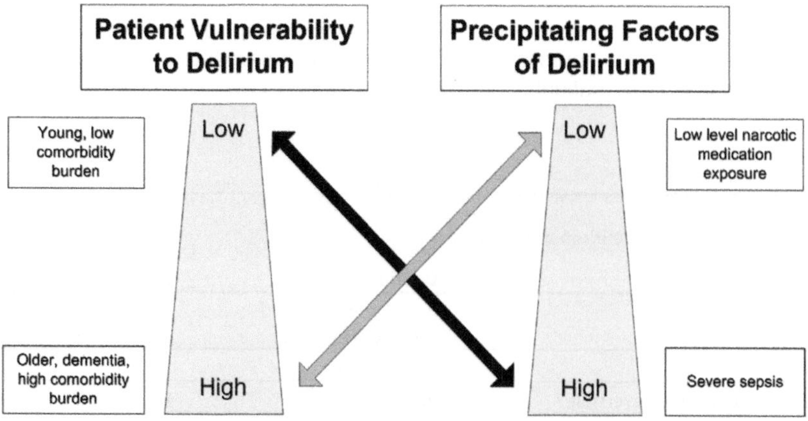

Fig. 1. The interrelationship between patient vulnerability and precipitating factors in the development of delirium. Patients who have little vulnerability require significant noxious stimuli to develop delirium (*black arrow*). Conversely, patients who are highly vulnerable require only minor noxious stimuli to develop delirium (*gray arrow*). (*Data from* Inouye SK, Charpentier PA. Precipitating factors for delirium in hospitalized elderly persons. Predictive model and interrelationship with baseline vulnerability. JAMA 1996;275(11):852–7.)

Table 3
Predisposing and precipitating factors for delirium

Predisposing Factors	Precipitating Factors
Demographics • Advanced age • Male gender Comorbidity • Dementia • Number of comorbid conditions • Severity of comorbid conditions • Chronic kidney disease • End-stage liver disease • Terminal illness Medications and drugs • Polypharmacy • Baseline psychoactive medication use • History of alcohol or other substance abuse Functional status • Functional impairment • Immobility Sensory impairment • Hearing impairment • Visual impairment Decreased oral intake • Dehydration • Malnutrition Psychiatric • Depression	Systemic • Infection • Inadequate pain control • Trauma • Dehydration • Hypo- or hyperthermia Metabolic • Thiamine deficiency (Wernicke encephalopathy) • Hepatic or renal failure • Electrolyte disturbances • Hypoglycemia/hyperglycemia • Thyroid dysfunction Medications and drugs • Medications and medication changes • Recreational drug use or withdrawal Central nervous system • Cerebrovascular accident • Intraparenchymal hemorrhage • Subdural/epidural hematoma • Seizures and postictal state • Meningitis/encephalitis Cardiopulmonary • Acute myocardial infarction • Congestive heart failure • Respiratory failure • Shock Iatrogenic • Procedures or surgeries • Indwelling urinary catheters • Physical restraints

Modified from Refs.[44–46]

impairment,[40] baseline psychoactive drug use such as narcotics, benzodiazepines,[10,48] and medications with anticholinergic properties,[51] history of alcohol abuse,[50,55] and malnutrition.[41,57]

Numerous precipitating factors of delirium have also been reported in the hospital literature (see **Table 3**). Regardless of what the precipitating factors are, patients with higher severities of illness have a higher likelihood of developing delirium.[10,40,47,54] Multiple delirium precipitants can exist concurrently and on occasion, no obvious cause can be found.[58] Infections, such as a urinary tract infection or pneumonia, are one of the most common causes of delirium (34%–43% of cases).[48,52–54,59,60] Dehydration,[40] electrolyte abnormalities,[10,61] organ failure,[10,61] drug withdrawal, central nervous system insults,[52,53,59] and cardiovascular illnesses such as congestive heart failure[54] and acute myocardial infarction[62] have all been implicated as delirium precipitants. Poorly controlled somatic pain may also cause delirium,[48,63,64] and pain control with nonnarcotic or narcotic analgesia may help resolve delirium in this case.[64] Delirium can also be precipitated by iatrogenic events. Inouye and Charpentier[41] observed that the use of physical restraints or bladder catheters, or the addition of more than 3 medications, was associated with delirium development.

PSYCHOACTIVE MEDICATIONS AS RISK FACTORS FOR DELIRIUM

Medications with anticholinergic properties, benzodiazepines, and narcotics are notorious for precipitating and exacerbating delirium. Such medication risk factors are particularly relevant to the older patient population because polypharmacy is highly prevalent.[49] Medications with anticholinergic properties are more frequently associated with delirium than any other drug class.[65–67] More than 600 medications with anticholinergic properties exist, and of these, 11% are commonly prescribed to elderly patients.[68] Some examples of commonly prescribed medications with anticholinergic properties are promethazine, diphenhydramine, hydroxyzine, meclizine, lomotil, and heterocyclic antidepressants (eg, amitriptyline, doxepin).

Benzodiazepines have also been implicated as common delirium precipitants in hospitalized patients.[69–72] However, delirium is heterogeneous and benzodiazepines can have a protective effect in a subgroup of delirious patients. For example, patients who are withdrawing from alcohol have improved mortality and morbidity when given benzodiapezpines.[73] Narcotic medications are also deliriogenic,[48] and meperidine is a consistently observed culprit.[70,72,74–76] Similar to benzodiazepines, there is a subgroup of delirious patients who may benefit from narcotic medications. In patients with poor pain control, narcotic analgesia can reduce delirium severity.[64,65]

To illustrate these points we present a hypothetical case scenario. Mr B is an 83-year-old patient with a past history of dementia, hearing impairment, and depression who presents to an urgent clinic for nausea, vomiting, and diarrhea. He takes amitriptyline for his depression and donezepil for his dementia. The patient has normal vital signs, normal physical examination, and unremarkable laboratory workup. The urgent care clinician diagnoses Mr B with gastroenteritis and prescribes promethazine 25 mg tablets for symptomatic relief. Mr B takes the medication as prescribed and develops an acute change in mental status 24 hours later, which is subsequently diagnosed as delirium at the local ED.

The patient in this scenario was highly susceptible to developing delirium and possessed 2 vulnerability factors (dementia and hearing impairment). In addition, he was already on a medication with anticholinergic properties (amitriptyline) and the addition of promethazine increased the patient's anticholinergic burden, enough to precipitate delirium. This case illustrates how seemingly benign medications can precipitate delirium in a highly vulnerable patient.

THE NEGATIVE CONSEQUENCES OF DELIRIUM

An abundance of hospital-based studies have investigated the deleterious effects of delirium. From these studies, delirium is a powerful prognostic marker and has been associated with in-hospital and long-term mortality.[4,5,77–79] Although some have argued that delirium is simply a surrogate for severity of illness and comorbidity burden,[80] the relationship between delirium and death has been shown to be independent of these factors.[4,5]

Delirium also has a profound effect on the older patient's quality of life. The trajectory of cognitive decline is accelerated in delirious patients compared with nondelirious patients, and this effect is evident in patients with and without preexisting dementia.[6,10,78,81,82] Delirium is also associated with accelerated functional decline,[8,81,83] which can lead to subsequent loss of independent living and future placement in a nursing home.[8,77]

Hospitalized patients with delirium are more prone to developing urinary incontinence, decubitus ulcers, and malnutrition.[11,12,51,84] These conditions can then lead to prolonged hospital stays and increased health care costs.[10,55,84,85] Once discharged from the hospital, delirious patients are more likely to be rehospitalized, further adding to the financial burden.[8,60,77,84] Moreover, there is also a huge emotional cost; many patients are able to recall their experiences with delirium, causing patients and their families significant emotional distress.[86,87]

Only 4 delirium outcome studies have been conducted in the ED setting. In 385 older ED patients, Lewis and colleagues[2] observed that patients with delirium were significantly more likely to die at 3 months (14% vs 8%), but their analysis did not adjust for potential confounders. Kakuma and colleagues[88] studied 107 older patients discharged from the ED and reported that delirium was independently associated with 6-month mortality, but this study excluded patients who were admitted to the hospital. Han and colleagues[89] studied 303 older ED patients who were admitted and discharged. These investigators found that patients who were delirious in the ED were more likely to die at 6 months compared with nondelirious patients (36% vs 10%). This relationship was independent of age, comorbidity burden, and severity of illness.[89] However, they did not incorporate other important confounders such as dementia and functional impairment in the multivariable model. Only one ED study has investigated the relationship between delirium and long-term functional outcomes. Vida and colleagues[90] reported that delirium in the ED was associated with accelerated functional decline at 18 months in patients without preexisting dementia only. However, this association disappeared after adjusting for potential confounders.[90] Even with the small number of ED studies and the limited external validity of hospital studies, delirium in the ED seems to be a marker for adverse patient outcomes.

UNRECOGNIZED DELIRIUM IN THE EMERGENCY DEPARTMENT

Despite the negative consequences of delirium, emergency physicians miss 57% to 83% of cases because of lack of appropriate and routine screening.[1–3,88,91–93] This quality-of-care issue extends beyond the ED as similar miss rates have been observed in the hospital setting.[32,94–97] Delirium is more commonly missed in patients with hypoactive symptomatology, who are aged 80 years and older, have visual impairment, or have dementia.[32,35]

The consequences of missing delirium in the ED are unclear. However, Kakuma and colleagues[88] reported that discharged ED patients in whom delirium was missed by the emergency physician were more likely to die at 6 months compared with patients in whom delirium was recognized (30.8% vs 11.8%). Although the mechanism for this is uncertain, ED patients with undetected delirium may receive inadequate diagnostic workups, and an underlying life-threatening illness may remain undiagnosed. They may also receive inappropriate interventions, such as medications with anticholinergic properties or benzodiazepines. Delirious patients who are discharged from the ED are less likely to understand their discharge instructions,[98] which may potentially lead to noncompliance, recidivism, and potentially increased mortality and morbidity.[99,100]

DIAGNOSING DELIRIUM IN THE ED

Several delirium assessments exist, but the Confusion Assessment Method (CAM) is probably the most widely accepted by clinicians. The CAM was developed for nonpsychiatrists and is based on the *Diagnostic and Statistical Manual of Mental Disorders, Revised 3rd Edition* (DSM-IIIR) criteria.[101] It consists of 4 features: (1) acute onset of mental status changes and a fluctuating course, (2) inattention, (3) disorganized thinking, and (4) altered level consciousness.[101] A patient must have features 1 and 2 and either feature 3 or 4 to meet criteria for delirium (**Fig. 2**). The CAM training manual recommends using a cognitive screening test such as the Mini-Mental State Examination and the Digit Span Test to help determine the features of the CAM.[102]

An acute change in mental status and fluctuating course (feature 1) is a cardinal feature of delirium and must be present for a patient to be CAM positive. In the ED, this feature is determined from interviewing a proxy such as a family member. Feature 1 can be difficult to ascertain if a proxy is not readily available in the ED. If a patient comes from a long-term care facility, contacting the patient's nurse or physician at that facility can often help establish the patient's baseline mental status. Similarly, the patient's primary care provider, if available, is another potential resource. In some patients, an acute change and fluctuation in mental status can be observed first hand during the ED stay.

Features 2, 3, and 4 are assessed during the patient interview and cognitive screen. Similar to feature 1, inattention (feature 2) is considered another cardinal feature of delirium and is described as a patient who is easily distractible and has difficulty maintaining focus. A patient with disorganized thinking (feature 3) may ramble, display tangential thoughts, or have an illogical flow of ideas. Patients with altered level of consciousness (feature 4) may exhibit drowsiness, lethargy (hypoactive), anxiety, hypervigilance, or combativeness (hyperactive).

Inouye and colleagues[101] found the CAM to have excellent sensitivity (94%–100%) and specificity (90%–95%) in hospitalized patients. Subsequent validation studies have shown more variability in diagnostic performances, with sensitivities ranging from 46% to 94% and specificities ranging from 63% to 100%.[103] However, this variability is most likely attributable to the level of training.[104] The CAM has excellent interobserver reliability (κ 0.70–1.00) when performed by trained personnel.[103] The CAM is the only delirium assessment validated for use in the ED. Using lay interviewers to perform the CAM and a geriatrician's assessment as the reference standard, Monette and colleagues[105] observed that the CAM was 86% sensitive and 100% specific in ED patients. They also reported that the CAM had excellent interobserver reliability ($\kappa = 0.91$) in this setting.

However, the CAM takes up to 10 minutes to perform,[102] which can be challenging in a highly demanding ED. The Confusion Assessment Method for the Intensive Care Unit (CAM-ICU) may be more feasible in the ED because it takes less than 2 minutes to perform. The CAM-ICU primarily uses the same the same 4 features as the CAM: (1) acute onset of mental status changes or a fluctuating course, (2) inattention, (3) altered level consciousness, and (4) disorganized thinking. Similar to the CAM, a patient must

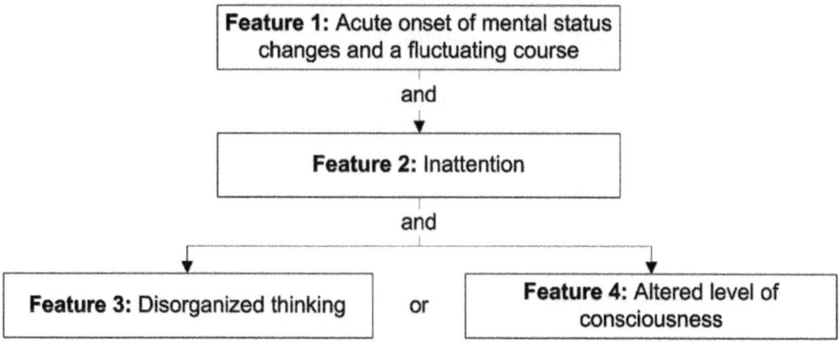

Fig. 2. Features of the CAM. A patient must have features 1 and 2 and either 3 or 4 to meet criteria for delirium. (*Courtesy of* Vanderbilt University, Nashville, TN. Copyright © 2010, Vanderbilt University. Used with permission.)

have features 1 and 2, and either feature 3 or 4 to meet criteria for delirium. However, there are several notable differences between these 2 assessments. The CAM-ICU uses brief neuropsychiatric screening assessments to test for inattention and disorganized thinking. These screening assessments help minimize subjectivity and improve its ease of use. The CAM-ICU also slightly modifies feature 1 of the original CAM, requiring either an acute change in mental status or fluctuating course.[106] In the latest iteration, the CAM-ICU also reorders features 3 and 4 of the CAM: CAM-ICU feature 3 is altered level of consciousness and feature 4 is disorganized thinking. The rationale for this change is detailed in the next paragraph. The CAM-ICU also uses the Richmond Agitation and Sedation Scale to help determine altered level of consciousness.[106]

Testing all 4 features of the CAM-ICU typically takes less than 2 minutes. However, using the algorithm provided in **Fig. 3**, the CAM-ICU can take less than 1 minute to perform. This algorithm provides a stepwise approach to performing the CAM-ICU and allows the rater to stop the assessment early, especially if either feature 1 (acute change in mental status or fluctuating course) or feature 2 (inattention) is negative. Disorganized thinking (CAM-ICU feature 4) is assessed only if features 1 and 2 are both positive, and if there is no evidence of any altered level of consciousness (CAM-ICU feature 3). Because most CAM-ICU–positive patients have altered mental status or a fluctuating course, inattention, and altered level consciousness, disorganized thinking (CAM-ICU feature 4) is usually not assessed in the clinical setting. For this reason, the latest version of the CAM-ICU reverses the order of the original CAM features 3 and 4 as described in the previous paragraph.

The CAM-ICU has been validated in mechanically ventilated and nonmechanically ventilated ICU patients. Ely and colleagues[107,108] reported that the CAM-ICU was highly sensitive (93%–100%) and specific (89%–100%), with excellent interrater reliability ($\kappa = 0.84$–0.96) between nurses and physicians. However, the CAM-ICU has not been validated in ED patients and spectrum bias may exist. A validation study in the ED setting is ongoing.

Several other delirium instruments exist in the literature (**Table 4**). Similar to the CAM, these instruments require subjective assessments and many take up to

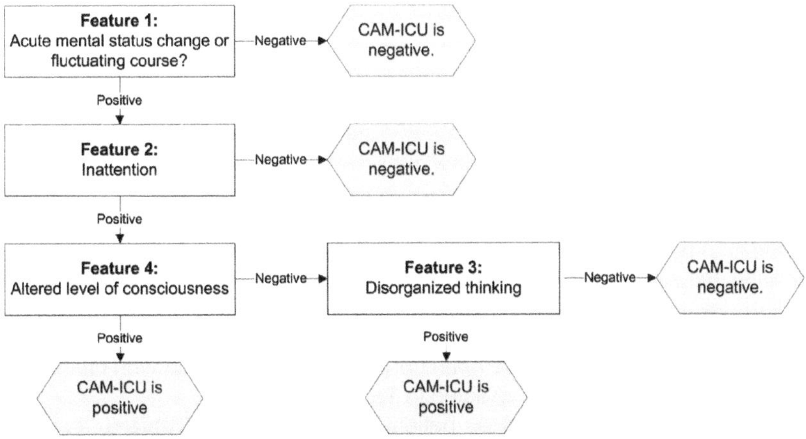

Fig. 3. Algorithm for performing the CAM-ICU in the clinical setting. The shaded hexagons indicate a stopping point for the CAM-ICU. (*Courtesy of* Vanderbilt University, Nashville, TN. Copyright © 2010, Vanderbilt University. Used with permission.)

Table 4
Other delirium assessments

Delirium Instrument	Duration of Items	Interrater Reliability	Reference Standard	Validated in the ED?
Delirium Rating Scale – Revised 98[109]	15–30 min	Excellent	DSM-IV by psychiatrist	No
Delirium Symptom Interview[110]	15 min	Excellent	Psychiatrist or neurologist	No
Memorial Delirium Assessment Scale[111]	10 items	Excellent	DSM-IIIR/IV by psychiatrist	No
Confusional State Examination[112]	22 items	Moderate to excellent	Psychiatrist	No
[a]Confusion Rating Scale[113,114]	2 min	Unknown	CAM, Short Portable Mental Status Questionnaire (SPMSQ)	No
[a]Nursing Delirium Screening Scale[115,116]	2 min	Unknown	CAM, DSM-IV by research assistant	No
[a]NEECHAM Confusion Scale[117–119]	10 min	Excellent	DSM-III by research nurse/CAM	No

[a] These delirium assessments were developed specifically for nurses.

10 minutes to complete, making them difficult to perform in the ED.[109–122] However, the Nursing Delirium Screening Scale (NuDESc) may be potentially useful in the ED because it takes less than 2 minutes to perform. The NuDESc is a checklist that asks nurses about the presence of disorientation, inappropriate behavior, inappropriate communication, hallucinations, and the presence of psychomotor retardation during an 8-hour shift.[116] However, the NuDESc does not assess for an acute change in mental status or fluctuating course and inattention, which are cardinal features of delirium. Despite this, the NuDESc seems to have excellent diagnostic characteristics. Using the CAM as the reference standard, Gaudreau and colleagues[116] reported the NuDESc to be 86% sensitive and 87% specific. Radtke and colleagues[115] observed that the NuDESc was 95% sensitive and 87% specific compared with a research assistant's assessment using the *Diagnostic and Statistical Manual of Mental Disorders, 4th Edition* (DSM-IV) criteria. The interrater or interobserver reliability of the NuDESc are unknown and are important to elucidate given its use of subjective observations. Similar to the CAM-ICU, the NuDESc still requires validation in the ED setting.

DIAGNOSTIC EVALUATION FOR ED PATIENTS WITH DELIRIUM

Once delirium is detected in the ED, the diagnostic evaluation should be focused on uncovering the underlying cause. Although infection is one of the most common causes of delirium in the older ED patient, life-threatening causes should initially be considered and can be recalled using the mnemonic "WHHHHIMPS" (**Box 1**).[123] After these life-threatening causes have been considered, the ED evaluation can focus on ruling out other causes of delirium listed in **Table 3**.

The ED evaluation of the delirious patient is summarized in **Table 5**. If available, obtaining a detailed history from a proxy is crucial. A careful review of the patient's home medication list should also be performed, including eliciting a history of any recent changes or additions to the patient's home medication regimen. Because

Box 1
Life-threatening causes of delirium

Wernicke disease

Hypoxia

Hypoglycemia

Hypertensive encephalopathy

Hyperthermia or hypothermia

Intracerebral hemorrhage

Meningitis/encephalitis

Poisoning (whether exogenous or iatrogenic)

Status epilepticus

Data from Caplan JP, Cassem NH, Murray GB, et al. Delirium. In: Stern TA, ed. Massachusetts General Hospital comprehensive clinical psychiatry. Philadelphia: Mosby/Elsevier; 2008.

alcohol and benzodiazepine abuse can still occur in elderly patients, a careful social history should also be obtained.

The physical examination should look for any vital sign abnormalities, although they will be normal in most cases. A neurologic examination should be performed looking for any focal neurologic findings suggestive of a central nervous system insult. Laboratory and radiologic tests are commonly performed in all patients with delirium (see **Table 5**). A urinalysis should be performed in all patients, because urinary tract

Table 5
Evaluation of the older ED patient with delirium

History	Careful review of home medications Recent changes in home medications History of drug and alcohol abuse
Physical examination	Vital signs Signs of infection Toxidromes Volume status Neurologic examination
Laboratory tests to consider	Urinalysis Blood glucose Electrolytes Blood urea nitrogen and serum creatinine Liver function tests and / or ammonia Thyroid-stimulating hormone Arterial blood gas if hypercarbia is suspected Cardiac biomarkers if acute myocardial infarction is suspected Lumbar puncture if meningitis is suspected Urine drug screen
Radiological tests to consider	Chest radiograph CT of the head
Other tests to consider	12-lead electrocardiogram

infections are common amongst delirious patients. Electrolytes should be obtained to rule out hyper- or hyponatremia, or hypercalcemia. Because organ failure can precipitate delirium, a blood urea nitrogen and serum creatinine test should be obtained to rule out uremia. Liver function tests and ammonia levels can also be considered, especially in patients with physical findings of end-stage liver disease. Because thyroid dysfunction can cause delirium,[124] thyroid-stimulating hormone should also be considered. An arterial or venous blood gas test may be obtained if hypercarbia is suspected, especially in patients with chronic obstructive pulmonary disease. Rarely, patients with acute myocardial infarction can also present with delirium as the sole manifestation[62]; a 12-lead electrocardiogram and cardiac biomarkers can be considered, but their diagnostic yield in ED patients with delirium remains unknown. Lumbar puncture, although not routinely performed, should be considered if there is a clinical suspicion for meningitis/encephalitis and especially if no other causes for delirium are found.

A chest radiograph should also be considered to rule out pneumonia, especially in the setting of hypoxemia, tachypnea, or a history of cough and dyspnea. Performing computed tomography (CT) of the head in all delirious patients is controversial because it may have low diagnostic yield.[125] However, it may be ordered when no other cause for delirium is found. Based on 2 studies, the diagnostic yield of head CT is increased when performed in patients with impaired level of consciousness, a focal neurologic deficit, or a recent history of a fall or head trauma.[125,126] However, these studies were retrospective in nature and have yet to be prospectively validated. Regardless, clinical judgment should be used when deciding if a delirious patient needs a head CT.

DISPOSITION

There is little evidence-based guidance regarding the disposition of older ED patients with delirium. However, admission of delirious patients is likely warranted in most cases. Older delirious patients who are discharged from the ED have higher death rates compared with nondelirious patients, and this effect is magnified when delirium is unrecognized by the emergency physician.[88] In addition, delirious patients may be more likely to return to the ED and be hospitalized.[1] For a small minority, ED discharge can be considered, particularly if close home supervision and follow-up can be arranged. For example, a patient who accidentally overdoses on a narcotic medication can be discharged home if the delirium resolves and if the patient remains delirium free after a period of ED observation. If admitted to the hospital, admission to an inpatient unit that specializes in geriatric care is preferable as it may improve patient outcomes.[127] Regardless of the patient's disposition, if delirium is detected in the ED, this should be communicated to the physician at the next stage of care.

PHARMACOLOGIC MANAGEMENT OF DELIRIUM

The single most effective treatment of delirium is to diagnose and treat the underlying cause. Adjunct pharmacologic treatments have been investigated for delirium, but most studies are limited by their nonblinded trial design, poor randomization, or inadequate power. The American Psychiatry Association recommends avoiding benzodiazepines as monotherapy in delirious patients, except in the setting of alcohol and benzodiazepine withdrawal.[45] As mentioned earlier, benzodiazepines can precipitate and exacerbate delirium in most cases, and they also have high side effect profiles. One randomized trial attempted to compare the efficacy of antipsychotic medications and lorazepam in delirious patients, but was prematurely terminated because the lorazepam arm showed a higher prevalence of treatment-limiting side effects such as oversedation, disinhibition, ataxia, and increased confusion.[128]

Instead, antipsychotic medications should be used, especially in delirious patients with behavioral disturbances, agitation, and overt psychotic manifestations (ie, visual hallucinations and delusions). Haloperidol is a commonly used typical antipsychotic and has been shown to improve delirium severity; Hu and colleagues[129] compared haloperidol with placebo, and reported that 70.4% of patients who received haloperidol showed improvement in their delirium severity at the end of 1 week compared with 29.7% of the placebo group. Intravenous haloperidol should be used cautiously because torsades de pointes have been reported when given in this formulation.[130]

Atypical antipsychotic medications such as olanzapine and risperidone are also frequently used to treat patients with delirium.[131] Compared with typical antipsychotics, this class of medications has a lower incidence of extrapyramidal side effects.[132] Olanzapine has been shown to improve delirium severity compared with placebo in one randomized control trial,[129] but its efficacy may be attenuated in patients aged 70 years and older.[133] Risperdone has also been used to treat delirium, but only one clinical trial has been conducted. Han and Kim[134] compared risperidone with haloperidol and observed that 75% of the haloperidol group versus 42% of the risperidone group showed improvement in their delirium severity. However, this difference was nonsignificant and the trial was underpowered. Some studies have used quetiapine to treat delirium,[131,135,136] but no randomized control trials have been performed.

There are limited data on the effectiveness of typical and atypical antipsychotic medications in patients with different delirium subtypes; their use in patients with hypoactive delirium is controversial. However, a significant proportion of patients with hypoactive delirium have some element of psychosis.[22] For many psychiatrists, when delirium is detected, an antipsychotic is initiated regardless of the subtype.[137]

Similar to benzodiazepines, medications with anticholinergic properties should be avoided. Narcotic medications should not be used to sedate an agitated patient and should only be used to treat acute pain. Although rare, there are reports of histamine-2 blockers, such as famotidine, ranitidine, and cimetidine, causing delirium.[138,139] These blockers should be avoided in delirious patients if at all possible.

NONPHARMACOLOGIC MANAGEMENT OF DELIRIUM

Several nonpharmacologic delirium interventions have been developed for the in-hospital setting and may be tailored for the ED. Most of these nonpharmacologic interventions contain multiple components and involve a multidisciplinary team of physicians, nurses, and social workers or case managers.[140,141] Moreover, geriatricians or geriatric psychiatrists are commonly consulted for these interventions.[140–142]

These interventions usually emphasize decreased use of psychoactive medications, increased mobilization by reducing the use of physical restraints and bladder catheters, and minimized disruptions in normal sleep-wake cycles. Many also encourage reorienting the patient by placing a large white board with the day and date, large clocks, or calendars in the patient's room. Cognitive stimulation, placing familiar objects in the patient's room, and encouraging the presence of family members are also advocated. Although these delirium interventions have shown to be beneficial in the postoperative setting,[141,143] their efficacy in medical patients is equivocal.[140,144] In medical inpatients, Pitkala and colleagues[145] found that their nonpharmacologic intervention improved delirium resolution during hospitalization and cognition at 6 months, but no improvement in nursing home placement or mortality was observed. Additional research is required to determine if nonpharmacologic interventions are feasible and cost-effective in the ED setting.

SUMMARY

Delirium is common in older ED patients and its cause is multifactorial, involving a complex interplay between patient vulnerability and precipitating factors. Based on numerous hospital studies and a limited number of ED studies, delirium has devastating effects on the patient's well-being. As a result, delirium surveillance should be routinely performed in older ED patients, especially those at high risk. The CAM is the only delirium assessment validated for the ED and it has excellent diagnostic characteristics. However, it can take up to 10 minutes to complete and may be difficult to perform in the demanding ED environment. The CAM-ICU and NuDESc take less than 2 minutes to perform and may be more feasible to perform in the ED. However, they still require validation in the ED population. Once delirium is detected in the ED, the primary goal is to find and treat the underlying cause. Other adjunct pharmacologic and nonpharmacologic interventions have been studied in the hospital setting, but their efficacy is equivocal and their usefulness in the ED setting is unknown. Significant knowledge gaps exist in the optimal diagnostic evaluation, disposition, and management of delirious ED patients. Given the impending exponential growth of the elderly patient population, intense research efforts to ameliorate these deficiencies are needed.

REFERENCES

1. Hustey FM, Meldon SW, Smith MD, et al. The effect of mental status screening on the care of elderly emergency department patients. Ann Emerg Med 2003; 41(5):678–84.
2. Lewis LM, Miller DK, Morley JE, et al. Unrecognized delirium in ED geriatric patients. Am J Emerg Med 1995;13(2):142–5.
3. Han JH, Zimmerman EE, Cutler N, et al. Delirium in older emergency department patients: recognition, risk factors, and psychomotor subtypes. Acad Emerg Med 2009;16(3):193–200.
4. Ely EW, Shintani A, Truman B, et al. Delirium as a predictor of mortality in mechanically ventilated patients in the intensive care unit. JAMA 2004;291(14): 1753–62.
5. McCusker J, Cole M, Abrahamowicz M, et al. Delirium predicts 12-month mortality. Arch Intern Med 2002;162(4):457–63.
6. McCusker J, Cole M, Dendukuri N, et al. Delirium in older medical inpatients and subsequent cognitive and functional status: a prospective study. CMAJ 2001; 165(5):575–83.
7. Jackson JC, Gordon SM, Hart RP, et al. The association between delirium and cognitive decline: a review of the empirical literature. Neuropsychol Rev 2004; 14(2):87–98.
8. Inouye SK, Rushing JT, Foreman MD, et al. Does delirium contribute to poor hospital outcomes? A three-site epidemiologic study. J Gen Intern Med 1998; 13(4):234–42.
9. Ely EW, Gautam S, Margolin R, et al. The impact of delirium in the intensive care unit on hospital length of stay. Intensive Care Med 2001;27(12):1892–900.

10. Francis J, Martin D, Kapoor WN. A prospective study of delirium in hospitalized elderly. JAMA 1990;263(8):1097–101.
11. Milbrandt EB, Deppen S, Harrison PL, et al. Costs associated with delirium in mechanically ventilated patients. Crit Care Med 2004;32(4):955–62.
12. Leslie DL, Marcantonio ER, Zhang Y, et al. One-year health care costs associated with delirium in the elderly population. Arch Intern Med 2008;168(1):27–32.
13. Sanders AB. Missed delirium in older emergency department patients: a quality-of-care problem. Ann Emerg Med 2002;39(3):338–41.
14. McCaig LF, Burt CW. National Hospital Ambulatory Medical Care Survey: 2002 emergency department summary. Adv Data 2004;340:1–34.
15. Strange GR, Chen EH, Sanders AB. Use of emergency departments by elderly patients: projections from a multicenter data base. Ann Emerg Med 1992;21(7):819–24.
16. Wofford JL, Schwartz E, Timerding BL, et al. Emergency department utilization by the elderly: analysis of the National Hospital Ambulatory Medical Care Survey. Acad Emerg Med 1996;3(7):694–9.
17. Roskos E, Wilber S. The effect of future demographic changes on emergency medicine [abstract]. Ann Emerg Med 2006;48(Suppl 4):65.
18. He W, Sengupta M, Velkoff VA, et al. Current population reports, P23-209, 65+ in the United States: 2005. Washington, DC: US Government Printing Office; 2005.
19. Terrell KM, Hustey FM, Hwang U, et al. Quality indicators for geriatric emergency care. Acad Emerg Med 2009;16(5):441–9.
20. American Psychiatric Association. American Psychiatric Association. Task Force on DSM-IV. Diagnostic and statistical manual of mental disorders: DSM-IV. 4th edition. Washington, DC: American Psychiatric Association; 1994.
21. Meagher DJ, Trzepacz PT. Motoric subtypes of delirium. Semin Clin Neuropsychiatry 2000;5(2):75–85.
22. Liptzin B, Levkoff SE. An empirical study of delirium subtypes. Br J Psychiatry 1992;161:843–5.
23. O'Keeffe ST. Clinical subtypes of delirium in the elderly. Dement Geriatr Cogn Disord 1999;10(5):380–5.
24. Marcantonio E, Ta T, Duthie E, et al. Delirium severity and psychomotor types: their relationship with outcomes after hip fracture repair. J Am Geriatr Soc 2002;50(5):850–7.
25. Kelly KG, Zisselman M, Cutillo-Schmitter T, et al. Severity and course of delirium in medically hospitalized nursing facility residents. Am J Geriatr Psychiatry 2001;9(1):72–7.
26. Peterson JF, Pun BT, Dittus RS, et al. Delirium and its motoric subtypes: a study of 614 critically ill patients. J Am Geriatr Soc 2006;54(3):479–84.
27. Pandharipande P, Cotton BA, Shintani A, et al. Motoric subtypes of delirium in mechanically ventilated surgical and trauma intensive care unit patients. Intensive Care Med 2007;33(10):1726–31.
28. Ross CA. CNS arousal systems: possible role in delirium. Int Psychogeriatr 1991;3(2):353–71.
29. Ross CA, Peyser CE, Shapiro I, et al. Delirium: phenomenologic and etiologic subtypes. Int Psychogeriatr 1991;3(2):135–47.
30. O'Keeffe ST, Lavan JN. Clinical significance of delirium subtypes in older people. Age Ageing 1999;28(2):115–9.
31. Kiely DK, Jones RN, Bergmann MA, et al. Association between psychomotor activity delirium subtypes and mortality among newly admitted post-acute facility patients. J Gerontol A Biol Sci Med Sci 2007;62(2):174–9.

32. Inouye SK, Foreman MD, Mion LC, et al. Nurses' recognition of delirium and its symptoms: comparison of nurse and researcher ratings. Arch Intern Med 2001; 161(20):2467–73.
33. Nicholas LM, Lindsey BA. Delirium presenting with symptoms of depression. Psychosomatics 1995;36(5):471–9.
34. Fick DM, Agostini JV, Inouye SK. Delirium superimposed on dementia: a systematic review. J Am Geriatr Soc 2002;50(10):1723–32.
35. Fick D, Foreman M. Consequences of not recognizing delirium superimposed on dementia in hospitalized elderly individuals. J Gerontol Nurs 2000;26(1): 30–40.
36. Marcantonio ER, Simon SE, Bergmann MA, et al. Delirium symptoms in postacute care: prevalent, persistent, and associated with poor functional recovery. J Am Geriatr Soc 2003;51(1):4–9.
37. Levkoff SE, Evans DA, Liptzin B, et al. Delirium. The occurrence and persistence of symptoms among elderly hospitalized patients. Arch Intern Med 1992;152(2): 334–40.
38. McKeith IG, Galasko D, Kosaka K, et al. Consensus guidelines for the clinical and pathologic diagnosis of dementia with Lewy bodies (DLB): report of the consortium on DLB international workshop. Neurology 1996;47(5):1113–24.
39. Flaherty JH, Rudolph J, Shay K, et al. Delirium is a serious and under-recognized problem: why assessment of mental status should be the sixth vital sign. J Am Med Dir Assoc 2007;8(5):273–5.
40. Inouye SK, Viscoli CM, Horwitz RI, et al. A predictive model for delirium in hospitalized elderly medical patients based on admission characteristics. Ann Intern Med 1993;119(6):474–81.
41. Inouye SK, Charpentier PA. Precipitating factors for delirium in hospitalized elderly persons. Predictive model and interrelationship with baseline vulnerability. JAMA 1996;275(11):852–7.
42. Inouye SK. Predisposing and precipitating factors for delirium in hospitalized older patients. Dement Geriatr Cogn Disord 1999;10(5):393–400.
43. Han JH, Morandi A, Ely W, et al. Delirium in the nursing home patients seen in the emergency department. J Am Geriatr Soc 2009;57(5):889–94.
44. Pun BT, Ely EW. The importance of diagnosing and managing ICU delirium. Chest 2007;132(2):624–36.
45. Practice guideline for the treatment of patients with delirium. American Psychiatric Association. Am J Psychiatry 1999;156(Suppl 5):1–20.
46. Fearing MA, Inouye SK. Delirium. In: Blazer DG, Steffens DC, editors. The American Psychiatric Publishing textbook of geriatric psychiatry. 4th edition. Washington, DC: American Psychiatric Publishing; 2009. Available at: http://psychiatryonline.com/content.aspx?aid=390561. Accessed May 07, 2010.
47. Hodkinson HM. Mental impairment in the elderly. J R Coll Physicians Lond 1973; 7(4):305–17.
48. Schor JD, Levkoff SE, Lipsitz LA, et al. Risk factors for delirium in hospitalized elderly. JAMA 1992;267(6):827–31.
49. Elie M, Cole MG, Primeau FJ, et al. Delirium risk factors in elderly hospitalized patients. J Gen Intern Med 1998;13(3):204–12.
50. Marcantonio ER, Goldman L, Mangione CM, et al. A clinical prediction rule for delirium after elective noncardiac surgery. JAMA 1994;271(2):134–9.
51. Gustafson Y, Berggren D, Brannstrom B, et al. Acute confusional states in elderly patients treated for femoral neck fracture. J Am Geriatr Soc 1988; 36(6):525–30.

52. Jitapunkul S, Pillay I, Ebrahim S. Delirium in newly admitted elderly patients: a prospective study. Q J Med 1992;83(300):307–14.
53. Kolbeinsson H, Jonsson A. Delirium and dementia in acute medical admissions of elderly patients in Iceland. Acta Psychiatr Scand 1993;87(2):123–7.
54. Rockwood K. Acute confusion in elderly medical patients. J Am Geriatr Soc 1989;37(2):150–4.
55. Pompei P, Foreman M, Rudberg MA, et al. Delirium in hospitalized older persons: outcomes and predictors. J Am Geriatr Soc 1994;42(8):809–15.
56. Voyer P, Cole MG, McCusker J, et al. Prevalence and symptoms of delirium superimposed on dementia. Clin Nurs Res 2006;15(1):46–66.
57. Bourdel-Marchasson I, Vincent S, Germain C, et al. Delirium symptoms and low dietary intake in older inpatients are independent predictors of institutionalization: a 1-year prospective population-based study. J Gerontol A Biol Sci Med Sci 2004;59(4):350–4.
58. Koponen H, Stenback U, Mattila E, et al. Delirium among elderly persons admitted to a psychiatric hospital: clinical course during the acute stage and one-year follow-up. Acta Psychiatr Scand 1989;79(6):579–85.
59. Rahkonen T, Makela H, Paanila S, et al. Delirium in elderly people without severe predisposing disorders: etiology and 1-year prognosis after discharge. Int Psychogeriatr 2000;12(4):473–81.
60. George J, Bleasdale S, Singleton SJ. Causes and prognosis of delirium in elderly patients admitted to a district general hospital. Age Ageing 1997; 26(6):423–7.
61. Foreman MD. Confusion in the hospitalized elderly: incidence, onset, and associated factors. Res Nurs Health 1989;12(1):21–9.
62. Bayer AJ, Chadha JS, Farag RR, et al. Changing presentation of myocardial infarction with increasing old age. J Am Geriatr Soc 1986;34(4):263–6.
63. Lynch EP, Lazor MA, Gellis JE, et al. The impact of postoperative pain on the development of postoperative delirium. Anesth Analg 1998;86(4):781–5.
64. Vaurio LE, Sands LP, Wang Y, et al. Postoperative delirium: the importance of pain and pain management. Anesth Analg 2006;102(4):1267–73.
65. Caeiro L, Ferro JM, Claro MI, et al. Delirium in acute stroke: a preliminary study of the role of anticholinergic medications. Eur J Neurol 2004;11(10):699–704.
66. Tune LE, Egeli S. Acetylcholine and delirium. Dement Geriatr Cogn Disord 1999; 10(5):342–4.
67. Beresin EV. Delirium in the elderly. J Geriatr Psychiatry Neurol 1988;1(3):127–43.
68. Tune LE. Anticholinergic effects of medication in elderly patients. J Clin Psychiatry 2001;62(Suppl 21):11–4.
69. Foy A, O'Connell D, Henry D, et al. Benzodiazepine use as a cause of cognitive impairment in elderly hospital inpatients. J Gerontol A Biol Sci Med Sci 1995; 50(2):M99–106.
70. Marcantonio ER, Juarez G, Goldman L, et al. The relationship of postoperative delirium with psychoactive medications. JAMA 1994;272(19):1518–22.
71. Rogers MP, Liang MH, Daltroy LH, et al. Delirium after elective orthopedic surgery: risk factors and natural history. Int J Psychiatry Med 1989;19(2):109–21.
72. Pandharipande P, Shintani A, Peterson J, et al. Lorazepam is an independent risk factor for transitioning to delirium in intensive care unit patients. Anesthesiology 2006;104(1):21–6.
73. Mayo-Smith MF, Beecher LH, Fischer TL, et al. Management of alcohol withdrawal delirium. An evidence-based practice guideline. Arch Intern Med 2004;164(13):1405–12.

74. Adunsky A, Levy R, Heim M, et al. Meperidine analgesia and delirium in aged hip fracture patients. Arch Gerontol Geriatr 2002;35(3):253–9.
75. Morrison RS, Magaziner J, Gilbert M, et al. Relationship between pain and opioid analgesics on the development of delirium following hip fracture. J Gerontol A Biol Sci Med Sci 2003;58(1):M76–81.
76. Dubois MJ, Bergeron N, Dumont M, et al. Delirium in an intensive care unit: a study of risk factors. Intensive Care Med 2001;27(8):1297–304.
77. Pitkala KH, Laurila JV, Strandberg TE, et al. Prognostic significance of delirium in frail older people. Dement Geriatr Cogn Disord 2005;19(2–3):158–63.
78. Rockwood K, Cosway S, Carver D, et al. The risk of dementia and death after delirium. Age Ageing 1999;28(6):551–6.
79. Pisani MA, Kong SY, Kasl SV, et al. Days of delirium are associated with 1-year mortality in an older intensive care unit population. Am J Respir Crit Care Med 2009;180(11):1092–7.
80. Cole MG, Primeau FJ. Prognosis of delirium in elderly hospital patients. CMAJ 1993;149(1):41–6.
81. Francis J, Kapoor WN. Prognosis after hospital discharge of older medical patients with delirium. J Am Geriatr Soc 1992;40(6):601–6.
82. Fong TG, Jones RN, Shi P, et al. Delirium accelerates cognitive decline in Alzheimer disease. Neurology 2009;72(18):1570–5.
83. Murray AM, Levkoff SE, Wetle TT, et al. Acute delirium and functional decline in the hospitalized elderly patient. J Gerontol 1993;48(5):M181–6.
84. O'Keeffe S, Lavan J. The prognostic significance of delirium in older hospital patients. J Am Geriatr Soc 1997;45(2):174–8.
85. Thomason JW, Shintani A, Peterson JF, et al. Intensive care unit delirium is an independent predictor of longer hospital stay: a prospective analysis of 261 non-ventilated patients. Crit Care 2005;9(4):R375–81.
86. Bruera E, Bush SH, Willey J, et al. Impact of delirium and recall on the level of distress in patients with advanced cancer and their family caregivers. Cancer 2009;115(9):2004–12.
87. Breitbart W, Gibson C, Tremblay A. The delirium experience: delirium recall and delirium-related distress in hospitalized patients with cancer, their spouses/caregivers, and their nurses. Psychosomatics 2002;43(3):183–94.
88. Kakuma R, du Fort GG, Arsenault L, et al. Delirium in older emergency department patients discharged home: effect on survival. J Am Geriatr Soc 2003;51(4):443–50.
89. Han JH, Cutler N, Zimmerman E, et al. Delirium in the emergency department is associated with six month mortality [abstract]. Acad Emerg Med 2009;16(S1):S214.
90. Vida S, Galbaud du Fort G, Kakuma R, et al. An 18-month prospective cohort study of functional outcome of delirium in elderly patients: activities of daily living. Int Psychogeriatr 2006;18(4):681–700.
91. Hustey FM, Meldon SW. The prevalence and documentation of impaired mental status in elderly emergency department patients. Ann Emerg Med 2002;39(3):248–53.
92. Naughton BJ, Moran MB, Kadah H, et al. Delirium and other cognitive impairment in older adults in an emergency department. Ann Emerg Med 1995;25(6):751–5.
93. Elie M, Rousseau F, Cole M, et al. Prevalence and detection of delirium in elderly emergency department patients. CMAJ 2000;163(8):977–81.

94. Rockwood K, Cosway S, Stolee P, et al. Increasing the recognition of delirium in elderly patients. J Am Geriatr Soc 1994;42(3):252–6.
95. van Zyl LT, Davidson PR. Delirium in hospital: an underreported event at discharge. Can J Psychiatry 2003;48(8):555–60.
96. Inouye SK. Delirium in hospitalized older patients: recognition and risk factors. J Geriatr Psychiatry Neurol 1998;11(3):118–25 [discussion: 157–8].
97. Gustafson Y, Brannstrom B, Norberg A, et al. Underdiagnosis and poor documentation of acute confusional states in elderly hip fracture patients. J Am Geriatr Soc 1991;39(8):760–5.
98. Bryce SN, Han JH, Kripilani S, et al. Cognitive impairment and comprehension of emergency department discharge instructions in older patients. Ann Emerg Med 2009;54(3):S80–1.
99. Clarke C, Friedman SM, Shi K, et al. Emergency department discharge instructions comprehension and compliance study. CJEM 2005;7(1):5–11.
100. Hastings SN, Barrett A, Hocker M, et al. Older patients' understanding of emergency department discharge information and its relationship with adverse outcomes [abstract]. J Am Geriatr Soc 2009;57(S1):S71.
101. Inouye SK, van Dyck CH, Alessi CA, et al. Clarifying confusion: the Confusion Assessment Method. A new method for detection of delirium. Ann Intern Med 1990;113(12):941–8.
102. Inouye SK. The Confusion Assessment Method (CAM): training manual and coding guide. New Haven: Yale University School of Medicine; 2003.
103. Wei LA, Fearing MA, Sternberg EJ, et al. The Confusion Assessment Method: a systematic review of current usage. J Am Geriatr Soc 2008; 56(5):823–30.
104. Rolfson DB, McElhaney JE, Jhangri GS, et al. Validity of the Confusion Assessment Method in detecting postoperative delirium in the elderly. Int Psychogeriatr 1999;11(4):431–8.
105. Monette J, Galbaud du Fort G, Fung SH, et al. Evaluation of the Confusion Assessment Method (CAM) as a screening tool for delirium in the emergency room. Gen Hosp Psychiatry 2001;23(1):20–5.
106. Ely EW, Pun BT. The Confusion Assessment Method for the ICU training manual. Nashville: Vanderbilt University; 2002.
107. Ely EW, Margolin R, Francis J, et al. Evaluation of delirium in critically ill patients: validation of the Confusion Assessment Method for the Intensive Care Unit (CAM-ICU). Crit Care Med 2001;29(7):1370–9.
108. Ely EW, Inouye SK, Bernard GR, et al. Delirium in mechanically ventilated patients: validity and reliability of the Confusion Assessment Method for the Intensive Care Unit (CAM-ICU). JAMA 2001;286(21):2703–10.
109. Trzepacz PT, Mittal D, Torres R, et al. Validation of the delirium rating scale-revised-98: comparison with the delirium rating scale and the cognitive test for delirium. J Neuropsychiatry Clin Neurosci 2001;13(2):229–42.
110. Albert MS, Levkoff SE, Reilly C, et al. The delirium symptom interview: an interview for the detection of delirium symptoms in hospitalized patients. J Geriatr Psychiatry Neurol 1992;5(1):14–21.
111. Breitbart W, Rosenfeld B, Roth A, et al. The memorial delirium assessment scale. J Pain Symptom Manage 1997;13(3):128–37.
112. Robertsson B, Karlsson I, Styrud E, et al. Confusional State Evaluation (CSE): an instrument for measuring severity of delirium in the elderly. Br J Psychiatry 1997; 170:565–70.

113. Gagnon P, Allard P, Masse B, et al. Delirium in terminal cancer: a prospective study using daily screening, early diagnosis, and continuous monitoring. J Pain Symptom Manage 2000;19(6):412–26.
114. Williams MA, Ward SE, Campbell EB. Confusion: testing versus observation. J Gerontol Nurs 1988;14(1):25–30.
115. Radtke FM, Franck M, Schneider M, et al. Comparison of three scores to screen for delirium in the recovery room. Br J Anaesth 2008;101(3):338–43.
116. Gaudreau JD, Gagnon P, Harel F, et al. Fast, systematic, and continuous delirium assessment in hospitalized patients: the Nursing Delirium Screening Scale. J Pain Symptom Manage 2005;29(4):368–75.
117. Neelon VJ, Champagne MT, Carlson JR, et al. The NEECHAM confusion scale: construction, validation, and clinical testing. Nurse Res 1996;45(6):324–30.
118. Champagne MT, Neelon VJ, McConnell ES, et al. The NEECHAM confusion scale: assessing acute confusion in the hospitalized and nursing home elderly. [abstract]. Gerontologist 1987;27:4.
119. Milisen K, Foreman MD, Hendrickx A, et al. Psychometric properties of the Flemish translation of the NEECHAM confusion scale. BMC Psychiatry 2005;5:16.
120. Trzepacz PT, Baker RW, Greenhouse J. A symptom rating scale for delirium. Psychiatry Res 1988;23(1):89–97.
121. Trzepacz PT, Dew MA. Further analyses of the Delirium rating scale. Gen Hosp Psychiatry 1995;17(2):75–9.
122. Williams MA. Delirium/acute confusional states: evaluation devices in nursing. Int Psychogeriatr 1991;3(2):301–8.
123. Caplan JP, Cassem NH, Murray GB, et al. Delirium. In: Stern TA, editor. Massachusetts General Hospital comprehensive clinical psychiatry. Philadelphia: Mosby/Elsevier; 2008. Available at: http://www.mdconsult.com/das/book/body/199996226-2/0/1657/167.html?tocnode=57542610&fromURL=165.html#4-u1.0-B978-0-323-04743-2..50020-2_385. Accessed May 7, 2010.
124. El-Kaissi S, Kotowicz MA, Berk M, et al. Acute delirium in the setting of primary hypothyroidism: the role of thyroid hormone replacement therapy. Thyroid 2005;15(9):1099–101.
125. Naughton BJ, Moran M, Ghaly Y, et al. Computed tomography scanning and delirium in elder patients. Acad Emerg Med 1997;4(12):1107–10.
126. Hardy JE, Brennan N. Computerized tomography of the brain for elderly patients presenting to the emergency department with acute confusion. Emerg Med Australas 2008;20(5):420–4.
127. Naughton BJ, Saltzman S, Ramadan F, et al. A multifactorial intervention to reduce prevalence of delirium and shorten hospital length of stay. J Am Geriatr Soc 2005;53(1):18–23.
128. Breitbart W, Marotta R, Platt MM, et al. A double-blind trial of haloperidol, chlorpromazine, and lorazepam in the treatment of delirium in hospitalized AIDS patients. Am J Psychiatry 1996;153(2):231–7.
129. Hu H, Deng W, Yang H. A prospective random control study comparison of olanzapine and haloperidol in senile delirium. Chongging Med J 2004;8:1234–7.
130. Hassaballa HA, Balk RA. Torsade de pointes associated with the administration of intravenous haloperidol: a review of the literature and practical guidelines for use. Expert Opin Drug Saf 2003;2(6):543–7.
131. Lee KU, Won WY, Lee HK, et al. Amisulpride versus quetiapine for the treatment of delirium: a randomized, open prospective study. Int Clin Psychopharmacol 2005;20(6):311–4.

132. Ozbolt LB, Paniagua MA, Kaiser RM. Atypical antipsychotics for the treatment of delirious elders. J Am Med Dir Assoc 2008;9(1):18–28.
133. Breitbart W, Tremblay A, Gibson C. An open trial of olanzapine for the treatment of delirium in hospitalized cancer patients. Psychosomatics 2002;43(3):175–82.
134. Han CS, Kim YK. A double-blind trial of risperidone and haloperidol for the treatment of delirium. Psychosomatics 2004;45(4):297–301.
135. Khouzam HR. Quetiapine in the treatment of postoperative delirium. A report of three cases. Compr Ther 2008;34(3–4):207–17.
136. Kim KY, Bader GM, Kotlyar V, et al. Treatment of delirium in older adults with quetiapine. J Geriatr Psychiatry Neurol 2003;16(1):29–31.
137. Platt MM, Breitbart W, Smith M, et al. Efficacy of neuroleptics for hypoactive delirium. J Neuropsychiatry Clin Neurosci 1994;6(1):66–7.
138. Catalano G, Catalano MC, Alberts VA. Famotidine-associated delirium. A series of six cases. Psychosomatics 1996;37(4):349–55.
139. Picotte-Prillmayer D, DiMaggio JR, Baile WF. H2 blocker delirium. Psychosomatics 1995;36(1):74–7.
140. Cole MG, McCusker J, Bellavance F, et al. Systematic detection and multidisciplinary care of delirium in older medical inpatients: a randomized trial. CMAJ 2002;167(7):753–9.
141. Marcantonio ER, Flacker JM, Wright RJ, et al. Reducing delirium after hip fracture: a randomized trial. J Am Geriatr Soc 2001;49(5):516–22.
142. Cole MG, Primeau FJ, Bailey RF, et al. Systematic intervention for elderly inpatients with delirium: a randomized trial. CMAJ 1994;151(7):965–70.
143. Gustafson Y, Brannstrom B, Berggren D, et al. A geriatric-anesthesiologic program to reduce acute confusional states in elderly patients treated for femoral neck fractures. J Am Geriatr Soc 1991;39(7):655–62.
144. Cole MG, Primeau F, McCusker J. Effectiveness of interventions to prevent delirium in hospitalized patients: a systematic review. CMAJ 1996;155(9):1263–8.
145. Pitkala KH, Laurila JV, Strandberg TE, et al. Multicomponent geriatric intervention for elderly inpatients with delirium: a randomized, controlled trial. J Gerontol A Biol Sci Med Sci 2006;61(2):176–81.

Is Salt, Vitamin, or Endocrinopathy Causing this Encephalopathy? A Review of Endocrine and Metabolic Causes of Altered Level of Consciousness

Jennifer J. Casaletto, MD

KEYWORDS

• Level of consciousness • Mental status • Endocrine
• Metabolic • Seizure • Delirium • Emergency

It's a beautiful Saturday morning, the first one in a while that hasn't started with pulling on a pair of scrubs and heading to the emergency department (ED). While you are sitting out on the porch sipping a steaming cup of latte, the postal carrier arrives bearing a special delivery from the American Board of Emergency Medicine: the ConCert is coming to a testing center near you! You consider early retirement. However, gulping your double-shot latte in the preceding moments of dread has resulted in the awakening of your finely tuned, caffeine-dependent brain and you're off to the races. Fruity breath? Diabetic ketoacidosis (DKA). Buffalo hump? Cushing syndrome. Stones, bones, groans, and moans? Hypercalcemia. Mental status change, ophthalmoplegia, and gait ataxia? Wernicke encephalopathy. Severe abdominal pain and hallucinations after starting oral contraceptives? Umm. Seizures and seborrheic dermatitis in a health care worker? Huh. Nausea, confusion, and agitation in an elderly patient after an outpatient cardiac catheterization? Duh. There's no knowledge gap a little caffeine and light reading can't bridge, so read on...

Altered level of consciousness covers a vast continuum from drowsiness to coma and describes the reason for 3% of critical ED visits.[1] Approximately 85% are found

Department of Emergency Medicine, Virginia Tech-Carilion School of Medicine, CRMH-Admin 1S, 1906 Belleview Avenue, Roanoke, VA 24014, USA
E-mail address: jjcasaletto@carilionclinic.org

Emerg Med Clin N Am 28 (2010) 633–662
doi:10.1016/j.emc.2010.03.013

to have a metabolic or systemic cause, whereas the remaining 15% are caused by structural lesions.[1] Early laboratory studies such as a bedside glucose test, serum electrolytes, or a urine dipstick test often direct the ED provider toward endocrine or metabolic causes. This article examines common endocrine and metabolic causes of altered mentation in the ED via sections dedicated to endocrine-, electrolyte-, metabolic acidosis-, and metabolism-related causes.

ENDOCRINE-RELATED CAUSE

Glucose Metabolism

Hypoglycemia, DKA, and hyperglycemic hyperosmolar state (HHS) make up the triad of glucose metabolism disorders that may result in altered mentation.

Symptoms and signs of hypoglycemia (autonomic [eg, diaphoresis, tremors, weakness, pallor] and neuroglycopenic [eg, disorientation, confusion, lack of coordination, seizures, coma, hypothermia]) are manifest as the serum glucose level decreases to less than 55 mg/dL.[2] Hypoglycemia as a cause of altered mentation is confirmed with a serum glucose measurement and reversed with the administration of glucose or dextrose. Most hypoglycemia is drug induced, with the leading culprits being diabetes mellitus medications, followed by type Ia anti-arrhythmics, dextropropoxyphene, β-blockers, pentamidine, antidepressants, and angiotensin-converting enzyme inhibitors. Factitious hypoglycemia, caused by surreptitious self-administration of sulfonylureas or insulin, must also be considered in nondiabetic patients. With the exception of alcohol-induced hypoglycemias, toxic hypoglycemias (eg, carbon tetrachloride, ethylene glycol, or *Amanita phalloida*) are rare and recognized by their coincident acute liver necrosis. Equally as rare are tumor hypoglycemia, caused by insulinomas and extrapancreatic tumors of mesenchymal origin (eg, rhabdomyosarcoma, leiomyosarcoma, liposarcoma), and autoimmune hypoglycemia, characterized by fasting hypoglycemia, increased serum insulin levels, and autoantibodies to serum insulin. Reactive (postprandial) hypoglycemia occurs after meals as a result of congenital carbohydrate metabolism deficiencies and becomes apparent in infancy. The existence of idiopathic reactive hypoglycemia has been a matter of debate; less than 5% of patients believed to exhibit suggestive symptoms are found to have a serum glucose level less than 55 mg/dL associated with symptomatic episodes.[2]

DKA and HHS occur along the same clinical spectrum, hallmarked by the triad of hyperglycemia, ketonemia, and metabolic acidosis, but differ with regard to severity of each triad component (**Table 1**).[3] DKA occurs more commonly in patients with type 1 diabetes mellitus, accounts for 8% to 29% of hospital admissions with a primary diagnosis of diabetes, and has a mortality that has improved to less than 5%.[3] HHS occurs more commonly in people with type 2 diabetes, makes up less than 1% of diabetes-related hospital admissions, and continues to have a mortality exceeding 40%.[3] Whereas DKA symptoms develop over several hours, HHS symptoms develop in days to weeks and are more likely to include an alteration in mental status. Only 30% of patients with HHS progress to the classic coma; focal neurologic deficits and seizures may also constitute the neurologic findings associated with HHS.[3] Recognizing a history of diabetes, symptoms of hyperglycemia, physical signs of dehydration, and the laboratory triad mentioned earlier are keys to identifying alterations in mental status caused by DKA and HHS. An inverse relationship exists between level of consciousness and serum osmolarity in patients with HHS and in the nearly 30% of patients with DKA with an accompanying hyperosmolar state (**Fig. 1**).[3,4] Mental status changes are rare with a serum osmolarity of less than 320 mOsm/kg, whereas most

Table 1
Admission biochemical data (mean ± standard error of the mean) in patients who have HHS and DKA

Parameters Measured	HHS	DKA
Glucose (mg/dL)	930 ± 83	616 ± 36
Na^+ (mEq/L)	149 ± 3.2	134 ± 1.0
K^+ (mEq/L)	3.9 ± 02	4.5 ± 0.13
SUN (mg/dL)	61 ± 11	32 ± 3
Creatinine (mg/dL)	1.4 ± 0.1	1.1 ± 0.1
pH	7.3 ± 0.03	7.12 ± 0.04
Bicarbonate (mEq/L)	18 ± 1.1	9.4 ± 1.4
BOHB (mmol/L)	1.0 ± 0.2	9.1 ± 0.85
Total osmolality (mosm/kg)	380 ± 5.7	323 ± 2.5
IRI (nmol/L)	0.08 ± 0.01	0.07 ± 0.01
C-peptide (nmol/L)	1.14 ± 0.1	0.21 ± 0.03
FFA (nmol/L)	1.5 ± 0.19	1.6 ± 0.16
Human growth hormone (ng/L)	1.9 ± 0.2	6.1 ± 1.2
Cortisol (ng/L)	570 ± 49	500 ± 61
IRI (nmoL/L)[a]	0.27 ± 0.05	0.09 ± 0.01
C-peptide (umol/L)	1.75 ± 0.23	0.25 ± 0.05
Glucagon (pg/L)	689 ± 215	580 ± 147
Catecholamines (ng/L)	0.28 ± 0.09	1.78 ± 0.4
Anion gap	11	17

Abbreviations: BOHB, β-hydroxybutyrate; FFA, free fatty acid; IRI, immunoreactive insulin.
[a] Values after intravenous tolbutamide.
Data from Kilabehi AE, Umpierrez GE, Murphy MB, et al. Management of hyperglycemic crises in patients with diabetes. Diabetes Care 2001;24:135.

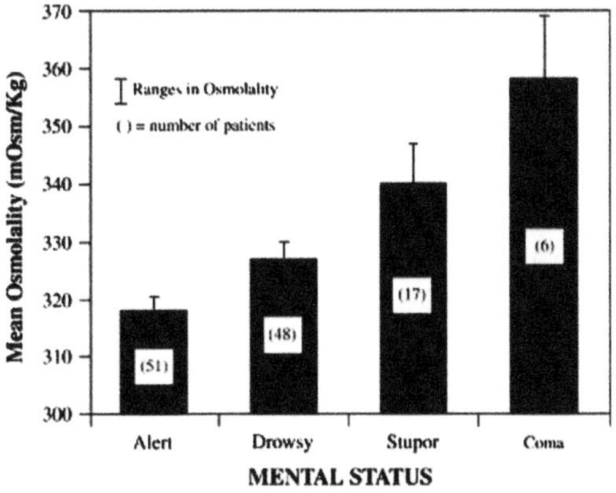

Fig. 1. Relationship between serum osmolality and level of consciousness. (*Adapted from* Kitabchi AE, Wall B. Diabetic ketoacidosis. Med Clin North Am 1995;79(1):10–37; with permission.)

patients with a serum osmolarity greater than 330 mOsm/kg are severely obtunded or comatose.[3,4] Treatment focuses on restoration of intravascular volume and tissue perfusion (approximately 6–9 L deficit), gradual reduction of serum glucose (50–70 mg/dL/h) and plasma osmolarity, correction of electrolyte imbalance, and identification and treatment of the precipitating cause.[3] Inadequate insulin dosing and infection are the most common precipitants; however, pancreatitis, myocardial ischemia, cerebrovascular accident, and drugs that interfere with carbohydrate metabolism (eg, corticosteroids, thiazides, sympathomimetic agents, and second-generation antipsychotic agents) must also be considered in the search for precipitating causes.[3]

Thyroid Disease

As thyroid hormone governs the metabolic state of the body, patients with alterations in mental status stemming from hyperthyroidism or hypothyroidism present with coincident signs of increased or decreased β-adrenergic activity, respectively. Recognition of these signs more often presents a challenge in cases characterized by a shorter duration of illness, lesser magnitude of thyroid hormone excess or shortage, and older patients.

Psychiatric symptoms from hyperthyroidism are numerous and vary widely in rate of onset. A gradual decline in cognitive function (memory loss and decreased attention span), complaints of restlessness, episodic increased emotional lability, and/or anxiety as a result of sleep changes (including insomnia, vivid dreams, and nightmares) prompt less urgent evaluations, which are often performed in the outpatient arena, whereas hyperthyroidism presenting with an acute alteration in mental status prompts urgent or emergent evaluation; acute presentations are most common in elderly patients. Identifying these variable altered mental states as hyperthyroidism is based on recognition of a constellation of multisystem historical and physical examination findings. These findings should prompt confirmation of the diagnosis with a thyroid-stimulating hormone (TSH) and free T4 levels. History can be remarkable for fatigue, nervousness, and anxiety, weight loss, heat intolerance, cardiopulmonary symptoms such as palpitations and dyspnea, nonspecific gastrointestinal (GI) symptoms resulting from decreased pharyngeal muscle effectiveness and rapid bowel transit, menstrual cycle changes in women, gynecomastia in men, and generalized muscle weakness most prominent in the proximal muscle groups. Physical examination findings are also multisystem, including infantlike skin texture, brittle hair, pretibial nonpitting edema, proptosis, enlarged thyroid, tachycardia and tachypnea, proximal muscle weakness or atrophy, and hyperactivity manifest as a rapid resting tremor, rapid speech, or brisk deep tendon reflexes. Suspected hyperthyroidism is confirmed primarily via a free T4 level, which is increased in 95% of hyperthyroid patients; TSH is most often suppressed, except in pituitary-dependent hyperthyroidism.[5] Most treatment is delivered in the outpatient setting and consists of antithyroid medications, radioactive iodine, and/or thyroid surgery. Less frequently, acute or more severe symptoms dictate inpatient management.

Thyroid storm, a severe, life-threatening hyperthyroid state, is differentiated by its more severe clinical presentation. Mental status changes caused by an associated metabolic encephalopathy, characterized by agitation, emotional lability, chorea, delirium, seizures, or coma, aid primarily in correctly identifying this highly lethal form of hyperthyroidism. Profound hyperthermia (reaching as high as 106°F) and tachycardia with rates greater than 140 beats per minute or atrial tachyarrhythmias are trademarks. Dehydration-mediated vascular collapse and severe abdominal pain may also complicate thyroid storm presentations. Despite treatment, mortality ranges from 20% to 50%.[5] Management has 4 tenets:

1. Control the overactive thyroid gland via methimazole or propylthiouracil followed by iodine.
2. Block the peripheral effects of thyroid hormone using β-blockers and/or corticosteroids.
3. Administer supportive care via dextrose-containing intravenous fluids and cooling measures.
4. Identify and treat the precipitating event, most commonly subtherapeutic antithyroid medication or infection. Empiric use of antibiotics is not recommended.[5]

Whereas hypothyroidism may cause mild cognition changes, such as slowing of thought processes and minimal memory changes, the presence of severe hypothyroidism, known as myxedema, is marked by stupor, confusion, or coma. With a mortality approaching 25%, clinical diagnosis and treatment are essential before laboratory confirmation of the diagnosis.[6] Most patients are elderly women with long-standing hypothyroidism whose courses have been complicated by environmental hypothermia, acute cardiovascular events, infection, or drug-induced central nervous system (CNS) depression. Vital sign abnormalities include hypoventilation, bradycardia, hypotension, and/or increased diastolic blood pressure. Physical examination is often notable for dry skin, sparse hair, nonpitting edema, macroglossia, hoarseness, and delayed deep tendon reflexes. The presence of a pericardial effusion or intestinal ileus also points toward myxedema. Laboratory results indicating hyponatremia, caused by reduced renal free water excretion, and anemia are often available before the hallmark findings of increased TSH and low thyroid hormone levels. Patients with myxedema require intensive care management because of frequent need for ventilatory support, rewarming, and management of hypotension. Intravenous administration of glucocorticoids and T4 (alone or in combination with T3) in addition to correction of electrolyte and metabolic disturbances are the mainstays of therapy.

Syndrome of Inappropriate Antidiuretic Hormone

A rapid decrease in serum sodium level can lead to delirium, as seen in patients with syndrome of inappropriate antidiuretic hormone (SIADH). Such a diagnosis must be considered in patients presenting with acute delirium and history of CNS or pulmonary disease, bronchogenic or CNS malignancy, selective serotonin reuptake inhibitor (SSRI) use, or ecstasy (MDMA) abuse.[7] Less common prescription drugs such as amiodarone, carbamazepine, chlorpromazine, and theophylline have also been implicated.[7] SIADH is the most common cause for hypo-osmolar (serum osmolality <275) euvolemic hyponatremia, although hypothyroidism and adrenal insufficiency may result in similar findings. In SIADH, antidiuretic hormone (or vasopressin) decreases free water excretion, resulting in inappropriately concentrated urine recognized by an osmolality greater than 100 mOsm/kg and a sodium concentration less than 20 mEq/L. Normal TSH and serum potassium levels aid in ruling out hypothyroidism and adrenal insufficiency, respectively. In patients with severe, acute neurologic symptoms, the likelihood of cerebral edema outweighs the risk of developing treatment-related osmotic demyelination syndrome. Hypertonic saline is recommended for the first 2 to 4 hours with a maximum rate of sodium correction of 1 to 2 mEq/L/h.[7] Alcoholism and malnutrition place patients at greater risk for osmotic demyelination syndrome.[7] In patients with less severe symptoms, the risks of saline treatment outweigh the benefits.[7] Most cases of SIADH are self-limited and best treated with water restriction.

Cushing Syndrome

Resulting from hypercortisolism, Cushing syndrome, like thyroid disease, most often presents with a constellation of multisystem symptoms that are nonspecific and common in the general population. However, increasing duration and severity of hypercortisolism are hallmarked by new irritability, decreased cognition, and declining short-term memory. Hypertension and glucose intolerance are also common presenting signs. Physical examination is remarkable for abnormal fat distribution in the supraclavicular and temporal fossae, proximal muscle weakness, and wide (>1 cm) purple striae. Although Cushing syndrome may be suspected in the ED setting based on presenting symptoms and physical findings, confirmatory diagnosis and treatment fall to the inpatient team. Diagnosis is confirmed by a 24-hour urine-free cortisol test, dexamethasone suppression test, and/or a midnight plasma cortisol level test.[8] In most cases, Cushing syndrome results from exogenous steroid administration, either prescribed doses or factitious, and resolves as the patient is tapered from steroids.[8] In the remaining cases, treatment is surgical, ideally entailing resection of the adrenocorticotropic hormone (ACTH) or cortisol-producing lesion.

ELECTROLYTE-RELATED CAUSE

Sodium Disorders

In response to changes in sodium concentration, water diffuses between the extracellular and intracellular compartments to maintain osmotic equilibrium. This diffusion is of greatest consequence in the brain. Whereas an increase in cellular volume results in cerebral edema, a decrease in cellular volume results in shrinkage and risks intracerebral hemorrhage.

Decreasing sodium concentration in the extracellular fluid results in a shift of water from the extracellular to the intracellular compartment. The resultant increase in cell volume is of greatest consequence in the brain because of its location in the fixed volume calvarium. The extent of cerebral edema and associated severity of symptoms depend on the rate of development, magnitude, and duration of hyponatremia.[9] Whereas acute onset mild hyponatremia (sodium >125 mEq/L) is often asymptomatic, more severe acute onset hyponatremia presents with nausea, headache, confusion, and agitation.[9] Extreme acute hyponatremia results in seizures, coma, respiratory arrest, and death. Although less severe, alterations in mental status, such as lethargy and confusion, also ensue with chronic hyponatremia. Once hyponatremia has been identified in a patient with a decreased level of consciousness, a search for the cause begins by classifying the hyponatremia as hypo-osmolar (<275), iso-osmolar (275–290), or hyperosmolar (>290) (**Fig. 2**).[7] Osmolality may be determined either by laboratory measurement or by calculation using the following equation:

$$\text{Plasma osmolality} = [2 \times \text{Na}^+ \text{ (mEq/L)}] + \text{glucose (mg/dL)}/18 + \text{blood urea nitrogen (BUN) (mg/dL)}/2.8$$

Patients with hypo-osmolar hyponatremia must be initially subdivided via a clinical assessment of volume status (see **Fig. 2**).[10] Edema, ascites, increased central venous pressure, and crackles indicate hypervolemia, whereas orthostatic hypotension, tachycardia, dry mucous membranes, decreased central venous pressure, and poor skin turgor indicate hypovolemia. Each population should then be further subdivided based on urine osmolarity and/or urine sodium concentration to derive a working

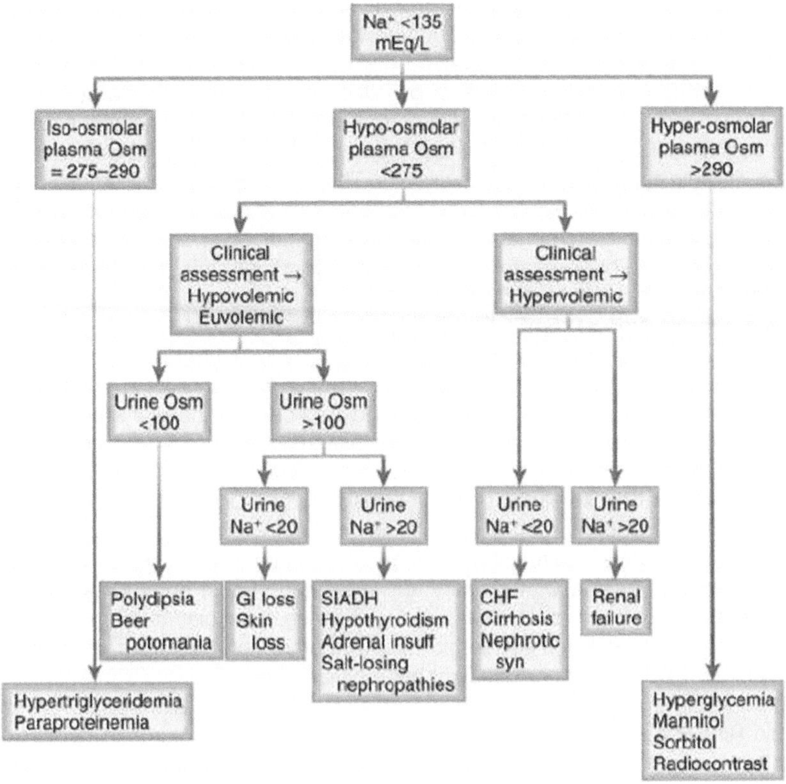

Fig. 2. Diagnostic algorithm for hyponatremia, CHF, congestive heart failure; Osm, osmolality. (*From* Wadman MC. Sodium and water balance. In: Adams J, ed. Emergency Medicine. Philadelphia: Saunders/Elsevier; 2008; with permission.)

diagnosis (see **Fig. 2**).[10] Iso-osmolar hyponatremia is often referred to as pseudohyponatremia, because it results from laboratory artifact caused by the presence of extensive nonaqueous solutes in the plasma (eg, hyperlipidemia, hyperproteinemia). Hyperosmolar hyponatremia occurs secondary to accumulation of an osmotically active nonelectrolyte solute in the extracellular compartment, which shifts water from the intracellular compartment, thereby diluting the sodium concentration. Hence, hyperosmolar hyponatremia requires the clinician to search for a precipitating substance, such as the presence of hyperglycemia or history suggesting mannitol, sorbitol, or radiocontrast administration.

In the past, controversy surrounded the treatment of hypo-osmolar hypovolemic hyponatremia because of the risk of osmotic demyelination syndrome associated with the administration of relatively hyperosmolar intravenous fluids, causing rapid diffusion of intracellular water from CNS cells.[7] However, in patients with severe neurologic symptoms, the risks associated with cerebral edema are now uniformly believed to outweigh the potential risk of treatment-associated osmotic demyelination. Thus, the emergency medicine literature recommends initial treatment with hypertonic (3%) saline; specifically, Wadman[7] recommends infusion of hypertonic saline at 1 to 2 mL/kg/h for the first 2 to 4 hours, with a maximum sodium concentration increase of 1 to 2 mEq/L/h. As soon as neurologic improvement has occurred, the rate of correction should be reduced, ensuring that sodium concentration does not increase greater than 10 to 12 mEq/L in the first 24 hours. In addition, loop diuretics should be used to manage fluid overload as needed. In chronic hypo-osmolar hyponatremic patients or patients with mild symptomatology, the risk of osmotic demyelination syndrome outweighs any benefit of rapid correction, therefore normal saline should be used with a maximum rate of sodium correction of 0.5 mEq/L/h.[7] Water restriction is of critical importance in acute or chronic hypo-osmolar hyponatremia. The treatment of hyperosmolar hyponatremia and hypo-osmolar hypervolemic hyponatremia is more straightforward. Treatment of hyperosmolar hyponatremia requires identification and treatment of the underlying cause. In hypo-osmolar hypervolemic hyponatremia, fluid intake must be restricted to less than 800 to 1000 mL per day.[7]

Hypernatremia (Na^+ >145mEq/L) is less common in the ED, classically presenting in elderly, female residents of nursing homes who have decreased water intake as a result of underlying infection. Hypernatremia usually results from impaired thirst sensation or restricted access to water. Associated cerebral cellular shrinkage leads to restlessness, irritability, lethargy, muscular twitching, hyperreflexia, and spasticity. Determination of the underlying cause again begins with clinical assessment aimed at recognizing the patient's volume status followed by measurement of urine osmolarity and urine sodium concentration (**Fig. 3**).[10] The most common ED presentation is hypovolemic hypernatremia as a result of inadequate fluid intake in the setting of increased free water loss.[7] Patients with primary and metastatic (most commonly breast and lung) hypothalamic tumors, granulomatous disease, vascular malformations, and head trauma are at risk for euvolemic hypernatremia resulting from destruction of hypothalamic thirst centers or deficient hypothalamic vasopression secretion.[9]

The mainstay of hypernatremia treatment is water administration. Use intravenous lactated Ringer solution or normal saline to restore plasma volume in hypovolemic patients, followed by hypotonic fluid via intravenous or oral routes to replace the free water deficit.[7] Beware of dextrose-containing solutions because they can lead to osmotic diuresis, worsening the free water deficit. In those patients with severe symptoms, water deficit can be replaced rapidly, noting the risk for cerebral edema associated with excessively rapid rehydration. In those with less severe presentations, free water deficit should be replaced in 48 hours with a sodium correction of not more than 0.5 to 1.0 mEq/L/h, not exceeding 10 mEq/L over 24 hours.[7] Free water deficit can be estimated using the following equation:

$$\text{Free water deficit (L)} = 0.6 \times \text{body weight (kg)} \times ([\text{plasma sodium}/140] - 1)$$

Substitute a body mass factor of 0.5 for young women and elderly men. A body mass factor of 0.4 for elderly women more accurately reflects their true free water deficit.

Potassium

Moderately to severely hypokalemic patients may have fatigue, proximal muscle weakness, or even ascending paralysis, but usually maintain a clear sensorium.[11] Likewise, hyperkalemia produces fatigue and weakness, although weakness and paralysis are generalized and associated with decreased deep tendon reflexes. Rare changes in mental status associated with disorders of potassium are most often a result of associated acid-base changes.[11]

Calcium

Renal stones, aching bones, abdominal groans, and psychiatric moans make up the rhyming tetrad describing the classic presentation of hypercalcemia. In these

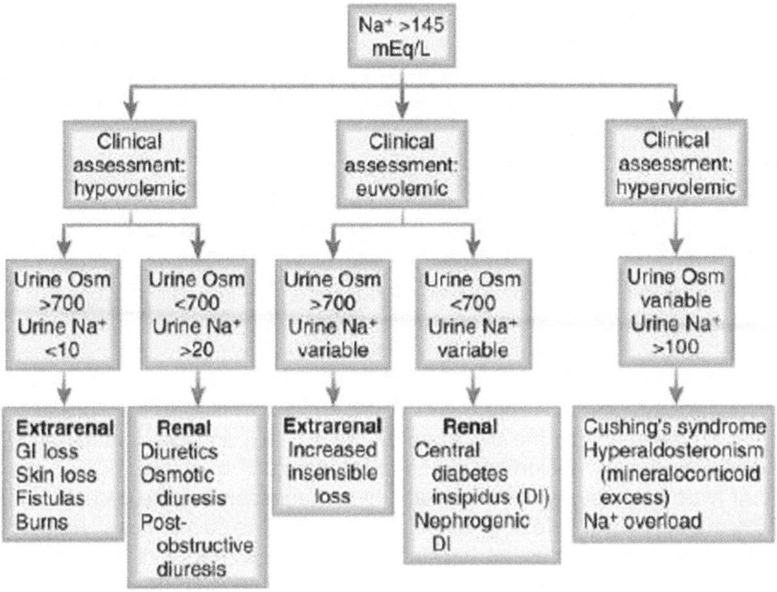

Fig. 3. Diagnostic algorithm for hypernatremia. Osm, osmolality. (*From* Wadman MC. Sodium and water balance. In: Adams J, ed. Emergency Medicine. Philadelphia: Saunders/Elsevier; 2008; with permission.)

instances, psychiatric moans refer to difficulty concentrating, fatigue, and lethargy seen in patients with marked hypercalcemia.[12] In addition, acute hypercalcemia can be complicated by bradycardia, seizures, and coma.[13] Although cardiac arrhythmias are rare, the presence of hypertension, shortening of the QT interval, and first-degree atrioventricular block provide further clues to the diagnosis before laboratory confirmation with an ionized serum calcium level.[13] Malignancy and hyperparathyroidism cause more than 80% of acute hypercalcemia presentations. The remainder are the result of less common causes such as thyrotoxicosis, granulomatous disease, drug-mediated, prolonged immobilization, total parenteral nutrition, and renal disease.[12,14,15] Although the goal is treatment of the underlying cause, patients displaying acute symptoms require urgent reduction of serum calcium levels. Aggressive intravenous normal saline volume expansion at rates of up to 200 to 500 mL/h followed by intravenous loop diuretics blocking the $Na^+K^+2Cl^-$ exchange in the ascending limb of the loop of Henle is used in patients with adequate cardiac and renal function.[13] Expansion of intravascular volume is critical before the administration of the loop diuretic, as the magnitude of urine output is unpredictable.[13] Furthermore, inadvertent use of thiazide diuretics can have disastrous consequences, because these medications decrease urinary calcium excretion. If volume expansion and loop diuretic use are ineffective in reducing acute symptom severity and serum calcium levels, intramuscular calcitonin can be administered. Calcitonin reduces serum calcium rapidly by inhibiting osteoclastic bone resorption, promoting renal excretion of calcium, and by decreasing renal tubular reabsorption; however, its use is often complicated by tachyphylaxis.[13] Additional second-line calcium-lowering therapies must be adapted to fit the underlying cause: intravenous bisphosphonates for malignancy-associated hypercalcemia, glucocorticoids for hypercalcemia associated with granulomatous disorders or lymphoma, and parathyroidectomy in hyperparathyroidism.[12,13] None of these second-line treatments acutely lowers serum calcium.

Although large or abrupt decreases in serum calcium level can result in neurologic symptoms such as carpopedal spasms or even tetany attributable to neuromuscular hyperreactivity, mental status typically remains intact.

Magnesium

Magnesium is not routinely tested in the ED and a normal serum level may be falsely reassuring, as magnesium is primarily an intracellular ion. Therefore, diagnosis of hypomagnesemia requires a high index of suspicion, especially in high-risk patients with malnutrition, alcoholism, or chronic diuretic use.[12,16] In addition, consider hypomagnesemia in the presence of hypokalemia, hyponatremia, hypocalcemia, and hypophosphatemia, because more than half of patients with hypomagnesemia have a coexisting electrolyte abnormality.[16] CNS hyperexcitability (eg, combativeness, disorientation, psychosis, seizures) and neuromuscular irritability are prominent. A prolonged QT segment on the electrocardiogram (ECG) and paroxysmal atrial and ventricular arrhythmias, including torsades de pointes, are hallmarks of clinically significant hypomagnesemia. Symptomatic hypomagnesemia is treated with intravenous 50% magnesium sulfate at a rate of 2 to 4 g over 30 to 60 minutes.[16] Be cautious, as rapid intravenous magnesium infusion can be associated with fluid-responsive hypotension. In life-threatening arrhythmias, the same doses are administered via intravenous push.[16] Benzodiazepines can be used as needed for seizure activity.

Apart from preeclamptic patients treated with magnesium infusion, hypermagnesemia is rare because of the rapid renal response to increased serum levels. Furthermore, preeclamptic patients undergoing magnesium infusion commonly run levels of 4 to 6 mg/dL without showing clinical symptoms, implying that extremely increased serum magnesium concentrations are required before the onset of symptoms.[12] Excessive use of over-the-counter magnesium-containing laxatives or enemas, especially in the setting of renal dysfunction, or lithium-induced impairment of renal magnesium excretion can lead to symptomatic hypermagnesemia. Symptomatic hypermagnesemic patients are confused and lethargic with generalized muscle weakness; ventricular arrhythmias may complicate the course. Ceasing magnesium intake and adequate volume resuscitation reverses symptoms in most patients. Calcium should be used to stabilize the cardiac membrane in patients with arrhythmias.[12] Dialysis may be necessary in symptomatic hypermagnesemic patients with impaired magnesium excretion as a result of renal disease.[12]

Phosphate

Similar to magnesium, phosphate is primarily an intracellular ion; it is essential for energy and transport in all cells. Whereas mild and moderate hypophosphatemia do not result in clinical findings, severe hypophosphatemia (<1 mg/dL) presents with declining CNS, cardiac, respiratory, and muscular function. Common neurologic findings include confusion, seizures, and coma; more rarely, an ascending paralysis can complicate the diagnosis.[17] Rhabdomyolysis and hemolytic anemia arise as phosphate is required to maintain cellular membrane integrity. Intracellular shifts, increased urinary excretion, decreased intestinal absorption, and rarely, dietary deficiencies can all lead to hypophosphatemia. Respiratory alkalosis caused by sepsis, hyperthermia, alcohol withdrawal, DKA, or salicylate toxicity is an important cause of intracellular shift mediated hypophosphatemia seen in the ED. Hypophosphatemia caused by increased urinary excretion (associated with hyperparathyroidism, DKA, and HHS) and decreased intestinal absorption (caused by severe vomiting and/or diarrhea) may also be encountered in the ED. In patients with severe or symptomatic hypophosphatemia, intravenous phosphate replacement is essential. Either sodium phosphate or potassium phosphate may be used, with the initial dose and rate of infusion based on symptom severity.[12,17] Overly aggressive replacement should be avoided, as it may result in hypocalcemia as a result of precipitation and calcium-phosphate tissue deposits.[17]

Hyperphosphatemia does not produce symptoms unless there is precipitation of phosphorus with calcium, leading to hypocalcemia symptoms, which usually do not include alterations in mental status.[12]

METABOLIC ACIDOSIS-RELATED CAUSE

Metabolic Acidoses: MUDPILES and HARDUP

Presence of a metabolic acidosis in the setting of altered mentation must be considered a sign of an underlying disease process, the identification of which is crucial to initiating proper treatment. Lethargy, stupor, and coma occur in severe metabolic acidoses. The most common causes of increased anion gap acidoses can be remembered using the mnemonic MUDPILES: methanol, uremia, diabetic and alcoholic ketoacidosis (AKA), paraldehyde, isoniazid (INH) or iron, lactate, ethylene glycol, and salicylates (**Box 1**). The causes of a hyperchloremic or normal anion gap acidosis can be remembered by the mnemonic HARDUP: hyperalimentation, acetazolamide, renal tubular acidoses and renal insufficiency, diarrhea and diuretics, ureterostomy, and pancreatic fistula (**Box 2**). A subsegment of increased anion gap acidoses referred to as high-anion gap acidoses (defined by the coexistence of an increased anion gap and a decreased serum bicarbonate) are the most common culprits in acidosis-related altered mental status. There are 4 principle causes of high-anion-gap acidosis: lactic acidosis, ketoacidosis, ingested toxins, and renal failure.

Methanol

Methanol is widely available in paints, solvents, antifreeze, and fuel for outdoor stoves and torches. Therefore, a high index of suspicion for exposure plays a large part in diagnosing methanol-induced acidosis. Absorption takes place via GI, dermal, and respiratory routes.[18–20] Signs and symptoms may be delayed for 30 hours or more following exposure.[21] The toxicity of methanol predominantly affects the neurologic, ophthalmologic, and GI systems. The state of inebriation and CNS depression has often elapsed before presentation with neurologic symptoms such as headache and dizziness.[21] However, agitation, acute mania, amnesia, decreased level of consciousness, and seizures can complicate the initial presentation.[18,22–26] In 2 large case series, all

Box 1
Causes of increased anion gap acidoses

*M*ethanol

*U*remia

*D*iabetic, alcoholic, and starvation ketoacidosis

*P*araldehyde

*I*NH and iron

*L*actic acidosis

*E*thylene glycol

*S*alicylates

Box 2
Causes of normal anion gap acidoses

*H*yperalimentation

*A*cetazolamide (carbonic anhydrase inhibitors)

*R*enal tubular acidosis and renal insufficiency

*D*iarrhea and diuretics

*U*reteroenterostomy

*P*ancreatic fistula

patients with acidemia had ophthalmologic complaints.[18,27] The wise clinician should always be on the lookout for visual symptoms associated with wavering mental status. Symptoms include blurred vision, photophobia, visual hallucinations, and varying degrees of visual impairment.[18,26,28–30] Examination findings range from normal to retinal edema associated with unreactive pupils and absent vision.[18,26,28–30] GI effects are frequently limited to nausea and vomiting, but may include severe abdominal pain, GI hemorrhage, diarrhea, liver function abnormalities, and pancreatitis.[18,24–26,30]

In addition to an anion gap acidosis, methanol toxicity also results in a difference between the measured serum and calculated serum osmolalities, referred to as an osmolal gap. Methanol levels can be measured to further confirm diagnostic suspicion of methanol toxicity, however such levels are rarely available in real time and only measure methanol that has not been metabolized. Imaging may reveal cerebral edema or basal ganglia hemorrhages or infarcts in severely ill patients with methanol toxicity.[31–35] Supportive therapy, administration of intravenous bicarbonate and folinic acid (leucovorin), and antidote therapy via intravenous fomepizole (preferred to ethanol because of its ease of administration) are mainstays of treatment. Hemodialysis can be used in the most severe cases.[21]

Uremia

A history of progressive renal dysfunction in conjunction with increased BUN and creatinine levels and an increased gap acidosis are keys to diagnosing uremia-induced mental status change. The normal anion gap metabolic acidosis present with renal insufficiency progresses to an increased gap acidosis as the glomerular filtration rate (GFR) decreases and renal failure ensues.[36]

Physical manifestations of uremia involve multiple systems, with neurologic and cardiovascular signs being most prominent. Neurologically, daytime drowsiness progresses to obtundation, whereas distal dysesthesias result from the effects of uremia on the peripheral neurologic system. Signs of fluid overload and noncardiogenic pulmonary edema predominate among cardiovascular effects. GI manifestations include anorexia, with subsequent nausea and vomiting. Uremic patients commonly complain of diffuse pruritis; dystrophic calcifications and changes in skin pigmentation may be present as well. In addition, anemia as well as platelet dysfunction result from uremia. Hyperglycemia caused by uremia-induced insulin resistance may be encountered in the ED.[37] Definitive treatment requires hemodialysis.

Ketoacidoses: Diabetic, Alcoholic, and Starvation

Without appropriate treatment, patients with any of the ketoacidoses exhibit decreasing levels of consciousness. However, depressed neurologic state is the exception rather than the rule on ED presentation with each of these 3 syndromes.

DKA encompasses a triad of clinical findings: hyperglycemia, ketonemia, and acidemia. It occurs most often in patients with type 1 diabetes; however, there are occurrences in patients with type 2 diabetes. The latter occurs predominantly in obese, African American type 2 diabetic patients.[38,39] Onset of DKA requires the shortage or absence of insulin coupled with increased levels of glucagon. Most often this state is a result of noncompliance with insulin therapy or a period of increased physical stress (eg, infection, surgery).

Patients suffering from DKA often present with nausea, vomiting, and polyuria that may be associated with abdominal pain. Examination reveals Kussmaul respirations and signs of dehydration. Without prompt treatment, DKA progresses, leading to a decreased level of consciousness and rarely, circulatory collapse. Common laboratory abnormalities associated with DKA are listed in **Table 1**. In addition to hyperglycemia, the presence of ketonuria, assessed by the nitroprusside reaction with acetoacetate, helps set the diagnosis of DKA apart from most remaining sources of increased anion gap acidoses. Patients with DKA have a lower β-hydroxybutyrate/acetoacetate ratio, resulting in positive serum ketone testing at dilutions greater than 2:1, setting them apart from patients with alcoholic or starvation ketoacidosis.[40] Treatment is discussed in the glucose metabolism section.

AKA often poses a diagnostic challenge because of a history of chronic alcoholism that is often difficult to elicit, frequently a recent binge followed by abrupt cessation of alcohol use. Similar to DKA, glucagon levels are increased because of insufficient intracellular glucose, leading to ketoacid formation. Clinical presentation is remarkable for vomiting, abdominal pain, and dehydration. In contrast to DKA, serum glucose levels are most often low to normal. Furthermore, the increase in the β-hydroxybutyrate/acetoacetate ratio from 3:1 in DKA to 7:1 in AKA results in a nitroprusside test that is more often negative because of the relative lack of acetoacetate.[36,40] Treatment is supportive, with volume resuscitation and electrolyte replacement.

Starvation ketoacidosis occurs during fasting in the face of physiologic stress, such as illness, exercise, or pregnancy.[41–45] During this time, starvation-induced absence of insulin stimulates the ketogenic pathway discussed earlier, accounting for the acute starvation ketoacidosis.[41] As in AKA, the serum glucose level is low to normal and serum ketones may not be found if the nitroprusside test is used, as a result of a predominance of β-hydroxybutyrate. Treatment is supportive, with volume resuscitation, electrolyte replacement, and measured refeeding.

Paraldehyde

Several decades ago, paraldehyde was used as a pharmacologic treatment of alcohol withdrawal. In overdose, the clinical picture of paraldehyde matches that of a sedative-hypnotic overdose: hypotension, bradypnea, hypothermia, and altered mental status.[46,47] Ingestion leads to formation of acetic and chloracetic acids, which create the increased anion gap in the resultant metabolic acidosis.[48]

INH and Iron

After declining steadily for more than 20 years, the incidence of tuberculosis in the United States rose each year after 1985, peaking in 1992.[49] As the primary antituberculin agent for prophylaxis and initial single-drug and multidrug therapy for tuberculosis, it seems only logical that INH usage has risen. INH toxicity comes in 2 forms: an acute, indirectly mediated toxicity that occurs via depletion of pyridoxine and a chronic, directly mediated, hypersensitivity reaction. The former leads to a relative γ-aminobutyric acid (GABA) deficiency, resulting in refractory generalized, tonic-clonic seizures.[50] The anion gap metabolic acidosis is a product of rapid, excessive accumulation of lactate during these seizures.

Before the onset of seizures and metabolic acidosis, acute INH poisoning presents with vomiting, diaphoresis, tachycardia, and hypertension within 30 minutes of ingestion.[51] Agitation, altered mental status, and hallucinations have all been reported, likely secondary to the decrease in GABA.[50] Associated seizures are classically generalized, prolonged, and refractory to standard antiepileptic therapy.[50] Hemodynamic instability may occur in the patient with seizures and acidosis.[51,52] Supportive care and pyridoxine are the mainstays of treatment; however, sodium bicarbonate and hemodialysis may be necessary in severe cases.[53]

Similar to INH, iron exhibits a direct and indirect toxicity; however, unlike INH, both types occur with acute overdoses in a dose-dependent fashion. Iron mediates direct GI and myocardial toxicity.[54,55] Unbound iron, which remains after transferrin is saturated, uncouples mitochondrial oxidative phosphorylation, thereby devastating adenosine triphosphate (ATP) synthesis. Impaired ATP synthesis has its most damaging effects on GI, cardiovascular, hepatic, and CNS cells because of their high metabolic activity. This damage worsens GI hemorrhage and myocardial dysfunction and adds hepatic failure and CNS dysfunction to the realm of iron toxicity.[56] The increased anion gap is caused by accumulation of lactate produced as a result of hypovolemia, cardiogenic shock, anaerobic metabolism, and unbuffered protons produced as a result of free ferric iron hydration.

When considering iron overdose as part of the differential diagnosis, ideally the history is consistent with iron ingestion or an abdominal radiograph revealing radiopaque tablets. Without these clues, diagnosis is difficult and relies on recognition of the clinical stages of iron poisoning and an increased iron level drawn 3 to 5 hours after ingestion in the presence of an increased anion gap acidosis. Clinically, iron poisoning takes place in 5 stages; altered mentation is prominent only in stages III and IV.[57] The increased anion gap metabolic acidosis is most prominent in stages II to IV, corresponding to several hours up to 5 days after ingestion. Stage I consists of GI symptoms ranging from abdominal pain and vomiting to life-threatening GI hemorrhage. Symptoms begin 1 to 6 hours after an ingestion of greater than 10 to 20 mg/kg of elemental iron and may be delayed with enteric-coated preparations. Stage II represents a period of relative stability in which GI symptoms abate; however, subclinical hypoperfusion and metabolic acidosis persist. This stage may last up to 24 hours. Although some patients may recover from stage II, many who have ingested greater than 40 mg/kg progress to systemic toxicity. The onset of stage III occurs 24 to 48 hours after ingestion and is characterized by reoccurrence of GI symptoms, hypoperfusion, severe metabolic acidosis, altered mental status, and coagulopathy. Although stage III accounts for the highest number of deaths from iron poisoning, iron levels are often normal by this stage. Progression to stage IV is rare; it is marked by acute hepatic failure and encephalopathy. Those patients who recover from an acute iron overdose may present subacutely, 2 to 4 weeks after overdose, in stage IV with a bowel obstruction as a result of GI scarring.[56,58] The treatment of acute iron overdose requires intravascular volume resuscitation and bicarbonate administration; use of decontamination modalities and intravenous chelation therapy with deferoxamine remain controversial and necessitate an estimation of risk and extent of systemic toxicity.[56]

Lactic Acidosis

Similar to ketoacidoses and renal failure, lactic acidoses more commonly result in a high-gap acidosis and marked alterations in mental status. There are 3 general categories of lactic acidosis. Accumulation of the L isomer, measured when obtaining serum lactate levels, is responsible for type A and type B lactic acidoses. These 2 distinctions refer to causes that produce lactic acidosis via tissue hypoxia (type A) and those that are accompanied by normal oxygen delivery (type B). Type A lactic acidosis can be the result of hemodynamic shock, severe hypoxemia or anemia, vigorous exercise (including prolonged seizures or shivering), mesenteric ischemia, or mitochondrial dysfunction. Although most of these causes are familiar to providers, mitochondrial dysfunction may be less so; it may be the consequence of a congenital enzyme deficit or, more commonly, mediated by toxins. Examples of the former include mitochondrial encephalopathy with acidosis and stroke (MELAS) and Pearson syndrome, often diagnosed in childhood after extensive genetic evaluation. Examples of the latter include carbon monoxide, which inhibits delivery of oxygen to the mitochondria via the binding of hemoglobin, and cyanide, which directly binds and inactivates complex IV of the mitochondrion's electron transport chain. In both scenarios, mitochondrial dysfunction results in lactic acid production caused by the anaerobic metabolism of pyruvate.

Type B lactic acidoses result from an overproduction and/or decreased hepatic removal of lactate in the face of maintained oxygen delivery to the tissues. The causes of type B acidoses are as follows: hypoglycemia/glycogen storage disease, diabetes mellitus, ethanol ingestion, hepatic failure, malignancy, and drugs. Most of these underlying causes are familiar; however, further mention of lactic acidosis of malignancy and commonly encountered drugs mediating type B acidoses is worthwhile. Lactic acidosis has been described in patients who have cancer in the absence of tissue hypoperfusion and other known causes of increased lactate production. Known as lactic acidosis of malignancy, it has been reported in patients with Hodgkin disease, acute leukemia, and sarcoma.[59–61] Although many common medications are known to increase lactate levels, some of the most pronounced increased lactate levels are seen in those patients taking biguanides and nucleoside analog reverse transcriptase inhibitors (NRTIs) (eg, zidovudine, didanosine) or those on propofol infusions. Severe, life-threatening lactic acidosis has been associated with biguanides, such as metformin (Glucophage), in 2 clinical settings: renal insufficiency and overdose.[62] The occurrence of mildly symptomatic to severe lactic acidosis in patients positive for the human immunodeficiency virus under treatment with NRTI therapy is believed to be caused by mitochondrial disruption. A recent case review reported female gender to be an independent risk factor for development of lactic acidosis and suggested that duration of NRTI therapy, specific drug use, and genetic predisposition may also be risk factors.[63] Deaths have been reported in children and adults on continuous propofol infusions of greater than 48 hours' duration. The propofol infusion syndrome includes cardiac failure, rhabdomyolysis, severe metabolic acidosis, and renal failure. The metabolic acidosis is thought to be the result of impaired free fatty acid use and mitochondrial activity.[64]

The D isomer is responsible for the third type of lactic acidosis, which occurs in patients with small-bowel resection or jejunoileal bypass. The D lactate is formed by colonic bacteria after ingestion of a large carbohydrate load in the face of carbohydrate malabsorption.[65] It cannot be metabolized by lactate dehydrogenase, leading to accumulation, which presents clinically with an encephalopathy and an increased anion gap acidosis.[66] The treatment of lactic acidosis is specific to the underlying cause and beyond the scope of this article.

Ethylene Glycol

Ethylene glycol lowers the freezing point of water and is therefore most often found in antifreeze, deicing solutions, and brake fluid. As with methanol, a high index of suspicion for exposure plays a large part in the diagnosis of poisoning. Absorption takes place via the GI tract; skin and inhalational exposures are negligible.[21] Signs and symptoms typically occur within 4 to 8 hours of ingestion, but may be prolonged for 12 or more hours if coingested with ethanol.[21] The toxicity of ethylene glycol reveals itself clinically in 4 stages, with predominant effects on the neurologic, cardiopulmonary, and renal systems. Stage I is referred to as the acute neurologic stage in which ethylene glycol results in an inebriated state similar to that of ethanol. Larger ingestions may result in hallucinations, seizures, or coma. Stage II, the cardiopulmonary stage, begins 12 to 24 hours after ingestion and is characterized by hypertension, tachycardia, and tachypnea. Although the tachypnea may occur solely in response to metabolic acidosis, it may also be the harbinger of ensuing pulmonary edema secondary to myocardial depression or direct pulmonary toxicity. In addition, hypocalcemia, secondary to chelation of calcium by oxalic acid, and myositis, heralded by increases in creatine phosphokinase (CPK) levels, may be present. Stage III, the renal stage, occurs 24 to 72 hours after ingestion and is distinguished by flank pain and acute tubular necrosis with or without oliguria. An increased degree of acidosis, a delay in presentation, and increased glycolic acid levels predict progression to renal failure more reliably than ethylene glycol levels.[67–69] Stage IV, the delayed neurologic sequelae stage, presents with cranial nerve palsies approximately 1 week after ingestion.

Similar to methanol toxicity, ethylene glycol toxicity classically results in increased anion and osmolal gaps, but cannot be ruled out by the presence of a normal osmolal gap.[70] In addition, levels greater than 20 mg/dL or those less than 20 mg/dL with an accompanying acidosis, are considered toxic. Unlike methanol, there are many laboratory-based clues that can further the clinician's diagnostic suspicion of ethylene glycol ingestion.[21] Approximately half of patients intoxicated with ethylene glycol exhibit envelope-shaped calcium oxalate dihydrate or needle-shaped calcium oxalate monohydrate crystalluria.[71,72] Freshly voided urine and fresh emesis with a pH greater than 4.5 fluoresce under a Wood lamp if fluorescein-containing antifreeze was ingested.[21] An ECG may show a prolonged QT interval, providing a clue to ethylene glycol-induced hypocalcemia. Cerebral imaging reveals cerebral edema with decreased attenuation in the basal ganglia, thalami, midbrain, and upper pons.[73,74] Supportive therapy, administration of intravenous bicarbonate and folinic acid (leucovorin), and antidote therapy via intravenous ethanol or fomepizole are mainstays of treatment. Hemodialysis may be used in the most severe cases.[21]

Salicylates

Acute and chronic toxicity can result from ingestion of salicylates found in oral medications, either alone or in combination with decongestants, antihistamines, or opioids, as well as from some skin and teething ointments, sunscreens, and antidiarrheals that contain salicylate compounds. Salicylates create a mixed acid-base disturbance via direct stimulation of the medullary respiratory center, leading to a respiratory alkalosis, and uncoupling of oxidative phosphorylation, leading to a metabolic acidosis. Serum salicylate levels peak 2 to 4 hours after an acute ingestion. A level of 30 mg/dL following an acute ingestion is potentially toxic, whereas chronic toxicity may even occur at a therapeutic level of 4 to 6 mg/dL. Clinically, an increased salicylic acid concentration presents with tachypnea and/or hyperpnea, as a result of direct medullary stimulation, and hyperthermia, as a result of the uncoupling of oxidative phosphorylation. CNS manifestations parallel increasing academia. Vasoconstriction of the auditory microvasculature generates tinnitus during the initial presentation of toxicity. Vomiting begins 3 to 8 hours after ingestion as a result of direct stimulation of the medullary chemoreceptors. Severe dehydration may ensue as a consequence of increased ventilation, vomiting, and hyperthermia. Increased capillary permeability in the pulmonary and cerebral tissue may result in edema. Rarely, mucosal bleeding results from platelet inhibition of salicylate and depression of hepatic synthesis of factor VII.

A presentation characterized by hyperthermia, an altered level of consciousness, pulmonary edema, and shock in the face of a mixed acid-base disorder may present a diagnostic dilemma or even point directly toward a septic cause without the available history implicating an acute or chronic salicylate overdose. Although tinnitus may point the clinician in the correct direction early in the course of toxicity, this history is often unavailable. Thus, a high index of suspicion must be maintained in the face of an anion gap acidosis. The urine ferric chloride test provides a timely and simple way to check for the presence of salicylates at the bedside. It is performed by placing a few drops of 10% ferric chloride solution in a patient's urine, which indicates the presence of salicylates by turning purple immediately.[75] Although it does not give a quantitative result and cannot confirm toxicity, a negative results indicates that the metabolic disturbances are unlikely the result of salicylates. An increased serum salicylate level is required to confirm toxicity in an acute overdose, whereas persistent symptoms and associated laboratory abnormalities may indicate the presence of chronic overdose in the face of mildly increased serum salicylate levels. Charcoal decontamination to decrease absorption and enhance elimination, fluid resuscitation, and urinary alkalinization constitute initial therapy. Hemodialysis is required in the face of CNS disturbances as well as in cases of severely increased serum salicylate levels (100 mg/dL in acute ingestions and 60 mg/dL in chronic toxicity), intractable acidosis, renal failure, or pulmonary edema.

Hyperalimentation

Hyperchloremic acidosis results from parenteral hyperalimentation administered without a sufficient amount of bicarbonate or bicarbonate-yielding solutes, such as lactate or acetate.[76] Protons are released from synthetic, positively charged amino acids (eg, arginine, lysine, histidine) in hyperalimentation mixtures as they are metabolized. In the face of a relative bicarbonate deficiency, these protons cannot be buffered, leading to a normal anion gap acidosis. Hyperalimentation hyperchloremic acidosis is a rare cause of CNS depression. Ideal treatment includes discontinuation of the parenteral nutrition and administration of bicarbonate. If parenteral nutrition must be continued, chloride should be reduced and acetate added.

Acetazolamide (and Carbonic Anhydrase Inhibitors)

Acetazolamide may be used in the treatment of high-altitude sickness, glaucoma, hyperuricemia, and hypokalemic periodic paralysis. It should therefore be suspected as a cause of normal gap metabolic acidosis in patients with history of such illnesses and laboratory findings remarkable for an increased serum chloride and decreased serum bicarbonate. Blockade of bicarbonate reabsorption in the proximal tubule by acetazolamide does not cause a severe metabolic acidosis as a result of sustained minimal proximal bicarbonate reabsorption even after inhibition by acetazolamide of carbonic anhydrase, the capability of some bicarbonate to be reabsorbed at more distal nephron sites, and the decreased filtration of bicarbonate as a result of metabolic acidosis.[77] Mild metabolic acidosis resulting from acetazolamide use rarely results in CNS-related effects; however, use in patients with impaired hepatic function, underlying respiratory acidosis, and diabetes mellitus may result in CNS depression and decreased physical coordination believed to be caused by decreased cerebrospinal fluid bicarbonate concentration.[78] Symptoms range from fatigue and drowsiness to ataxia, confusion, seizures, and coma. Stopping acetazolamide and bicarbonate administration are keys to treatment.

Renal Tubular Acidoses and Renal Insufficiency

Early in renal tubular acidosis (RTA), when the GFR is between 20 and 50 mL/min, a hyperchloremic acidosis is present because of the decreased ability of the kidneys to compensate with adequate bicarbonate reabsoprtion.[36] However, the normal anion gap metabolic acidosis present with renal insufficiency progresses to an increased gap uremic acidosis as the GFR decreases and renal failure ensues.[36] This latter stage of RTA is associated with altered levels of consciousness, as described in the section on uremia.

Type 1 RTA (or distal RTA) most often occurs in association with a systemic inflammatory illness such as Sjögren syndrome or multiple myeloma. More rarely, it can be an inherited disorder, a result of chronic renal transplant rejection, or drug induced.[36] Type 1 RTA is a consequence of the failure of one or both of the collecting duct proton pumps (H+-ATPase and H+, K+-ATPase) to excrete hydrogen ions. The failure of these pumps results in the inability to acidify the urine less than a pH of 5.5. The resultant increased urinary pH does not allow adequate trapping of NH4+ in the collecting duct. Hence, the clinical findings of a type 1 or distal RTA include: hypokalemia, hyperchloremic acidosis, low urinary NH4+, and urine pH greater than 5.5. Chronic toluene use as well as lithium, pentamidine, rifampin, and amphotericin use produce a type 1 RTA with similar findings.[36,79–81] Furthermore, chronic toluene abuse produces CNS depression in the face of type 1 RTA. Chronic lithium toxicity is manifest by gradual progression of neurotoxic effects, which begin with CNS depression and progress to hyperreflexia, ataxia, seizures, and coma; coincident type 1 RTA is evident is patients who have been treated with lithium for 10 to 20 years.[82]

Type 2 RTA (or proximal RTA) is also referred to as Fanconi syndrome. Proximal RTA is found most commonly in children. In adults, it is usually associated with multiple myeloma or use of carbonic anhydrase inhibitors. Physiologically, generalized proximal tubular dysfunction leads to bicarbonaturia until steady state is reached and persistent proteinuria, glycosuria, aminoaciduria, and phosphaturia. Unlike type 1 RTA, urinary pH is appropriately acidic. Enhanced chloride reabsorption, stimulated by volume contraction, results in hyperchloremia. In untreated patients, serum bicarbonate is low, reaching a nadir of 15 to 18 mEq/L. The rate of potassium ion excretion is proportional to bicarbonate delivery to the distal nephron, leading to an associated hypokalemia. Diagnosis of type 2 RTA relies on the recognition of a chronic hyperchloremic metabolic acidosis accompanied by acidic urine, hypokalemia, and a low fractional excretion of bicarbonate. With infusion of sodium bicarbonate, bicarbonaturia ensues, and the urine becomes alkaline. An excessive amount of exogenous bicarbonate required to correct plasma bicarbonate is a further diagnostic clue to the diagnosis of type 2 RTA.

Hyperchloremic metabolic acidosis occurs in 50% of patients with hyporeninemic hypoaldosteronism, also known as type 4 RTA.[79] This syndrome occurs in older patients with interstitial renal disease, hypertension, diabetes mellitus, and concurrent congestive heart failure.[76,79] Distal tubular damage produces diminished rates of sodium absorption, hydrogen ion secretion, and potassium secretion. A clinical triad of hyponatremia, hyperkalemia, and hyperchloremic acidosis is the hallmark of this disorder. Diuretics such as triamterene, spironolactone, and amiloride, create a similar syndrome.[76]

Diarrhea and Diuretics

Fatigue, weakness, and lethargy are the most frequent CNS manifestations of profuse diarrhea, the most commonly encountered nongap metabolic acidosis. Stool contains large amounts of bicarbonate in addition to organic ions, which are absorbed and converted to bicarbonate; both are lost with diarrhea. Stool contains a greater amount of sodium relative to chloride, resulting in a diarrhea-induced relative hyperchloremia. Hypokalemia exists in large part because of the large quantities of potassium ions lost in stool but also from a hypovolemia-induced hyperrenin-hyperaldosterone state that enhances renal potassium secretion. Although acidic urine production would be anticipated in the face of such a metabolic acidosis, urine produced in conjunction with diarrheal illness more often has a pH of 6.0 or higher.[83] Increased urine pH occurring in the face of a metabolic acidosis and hypokalemia allows hyperchloremic metabolic acidosis of GI origin to be differentiated from that of RTA.

As mentioned earlier, diuretics such as triamterene, spironolactone, and amiloride interfere with distal tubular Na^+ absorption, H^+ secretion, and K^+ secretion, resulting in a hyperkalemic, hyperchloremic metabolic acidosis resembling that of type 4 RTA.[76]

Ureteroenterostomy and Enterostomy

Although uncommon today, ureteroenterostomy (surgical insertion of the ureters into the bowel) was the first form of diversion to be popularized for patients with exstrophy. This style of diversion results in hyperchloremic metabolic acidosis because the urine reaching the colon is alkalinized by colonic bicarbonate secretion in exchange for chloride.[76] Other types of enterostomies, tube drainage, and fistulae that result in loss of bicarbonate-rich intestinal and biliary fluid also result in normal gap metabolic acidosis. With an appropriate accompanying surgical history in conjunction with an acute illness or renal insufficiency, ureteroenterostomy- or enterostomy-associated acidosis may result in CNS depression.

Pancreatic Fistula

External pancreatic fistulas are a consequence of surgical therapy for chronic pancreatitis or pseudocyst, whereas internal fistulas occur mainly in the setting of chronic pancreatitis after rupture of a pseudocyst.[84] The fluid from an internal fistula may track to the peritoneal cavity or pleural space, a diagnosis that can be established by documenting high levels of amylase within the respective fluid. In either scenario, bicarbonate-rich pancreatic fluid is diverted from the bowel, where normal bicarbonate reabsorption occurs. This loss of bicarbonate results in a normal gap metabolic acidosis and rarely causes CNS depression.

Metabolism-Related Cause

Wernicke encephalopathy

The well-known Wernicke encephalopathy triad of mental status change, ophthalmoplegia, and gait ataxia is present in as few as 10% of cases, perhaps accounting for the fact that 85% of cases are diagnosed postmortem.[85] Furthermore, the myth that Wernicke encephalopathy occurs only in alcoholics may contribute to many diagnostic failures. As a disease process originating from thiamine deficiency, Wernicke encephalopathy is associated with alcoholism, AIDS, malignancy, hyperemesis gravidarum, total parenteral nutrition, and gastric bypass. The most common constant component of the disease is mental status change, which can range from mild confusion to complete coma. Associated Korsakoff syndrome is predominantly an amnestic disorder coupled with confabulation. Following closely behind mental status changes,

96% of patients with Wernicke encephalopathy present with some form of ocular abnormality.[85] Of these patients, 85% have nystagmus, followed by 54% with bilateral sixth nerve palsy, 44% with conjugate gaze palsy, and 19% with pupillary abnormalities.[85] When considering ataxia, this component of the triad may be manifest by a mild gait abnormality to a complete inability to stand. In addition to the triad, hypotension, hypothermia, and lactic acidosis may also occur. Presumptive diagnosis is based on a high level of clinical suspicion in conjunction with 2 of the following 4 findings: nutritional deficiency, mental status change, ocular abnormality, and ataxia. Thiamine levels are unlikely to aid the diagnosis because they not often available in the ED. Furthermore, the sensitivity of computed tomography and magnetic resonance imaging are 13% and 53%, respectively, in active disease.[85] Treatment consists of intravenous dosing of thiamine at a rate of 100 mg per day; however, doses as high as 500 mg per day have been recommended for those with persistent symptoms despite prophylaxis or treatment at the 100 mg per day level.[85]

Pyridoxine deficiency

At risk populations for pyridoxine (vitamin B_6) deficiency include malnourished patients, alcoholics, infants born to deficient mothers, and those being treated with INH or hydralazine, which increase urinary excretion of pyridoxine. Pyridoxine serves as a coenzyme required for dopamine, serotonin, epinephrine, norepinephrine, and GABA synthesis. As such, patients with severe deficiency may present with depression, irritability, confusion, or seizures; seizures are most common in infants and patients with drug-mediated pyridoxine deficiency.[86,87] In addition to CNS effects, pyridoxine deficiency affects the blood and skin, manifesting as microcytic anemia and dermatitis, respectively. The dermatitis is a seborrheic dermatitis most evident in the periorbital, nasal, and perioral regions. Associated peripheral neuropathy, characterized by sensory loss, weakness, and painful paresthesias in the lower extremities, is more common in INH and hydralazine-mediated deficiency states, but can be present regardless of the cause.[87] Seizure cessation following the intravenous injection of a single dose of 100 mg of pyridoxine confirms diagnosis of and treats severe pyridoxine deficiency.[88] Patients with less severe presentations and those with chronic nutritional deficiency require daily oral dosing of pyridoxine.

Pellagra

Pellagra, meaning rough skin, results foremost from niacin deficiency, but may also be the consequence of pyridoxine deficiency, as conversion of tryptophan to niacin is a pyridoxine-dependent process. Worldwide, pellagra occurs in regions in which corn is the dietary staple, but occurs in developed countries in those who are malnourished, suffer from Crohn-associated malabsorption, or are being treated with medications such as INH, sulfonamides, anticonvulsants, antidepressants, and chemotherapeutic regimens containing 6-mercaptopurine and 5-fluorouracil.[89] The CNS alteration hallmarking pellagra is dementia; however, it may be preceded by apathy, weakness, and anorexia. In addition to dementia, the other 3 features making up the 4 Ds of pellagra are: diarrhea, dermatitis, and ultimately, death. The dermatitis, usually beginning after the onset of CNS signs, starts as a symmetric, macular erythema in areas with sun exposure. As it progresses, the rash darkens and may become scaly and crusted or develop vesicles. Dry fissured lips, angular stomatitis, and glossitis accompany the rash in later stages of illness. Oral supplementation with niacin every 6 hours is warranted until the resolution of major acute symptoms occurs; this is followed by oral supplementation twice per day until all skin lesions are healed.[89] Niacin supplementation should be accompanied by a high-protein diet and B-complex vitamin supplementation in most cases.[89]

Acute Intermittent Porphyria

There are 7 forms of porphyria, each resulting from a distinct defect in the heme synthesis pathway, and manifesting with neurovisceral symptoms, photocutaneous symptoms, or both. Acute intermittent porphyria (AIP), an autosomal-dominant inherited defect, is the second most common porphyria and the only form usually associated with psychological manifestations.[90] Psychological signs and symptoms associated with AIP include anxiety, depression, confusion, and psychotic episodes with prominent hallucinations. Furthermore, approximately 15% of patients presenting with an acute exacerbation exhibit generalized seizures; this is more likely in patients who are hyponatremic from AIP-associated vomiting or SIADH.[90]

Although AIP is an inherited defect, drugs, starvation, infection, and hormonal factors precipitate symptoms. Drugs clearly implicated in AIP exacerbations include barbiturates, sulfonamides, griseofulvin, sulfonylureas, phenytoin, and estrogen-containing compounds; however, many others are considered unsafe for use during acute exacerbations and may also be precipitants (**Box 3**).[90] Nearly 90% of patients initially complain of abdominal pain and other GI symptoms believed to be caused by a visceral neuropathy.[90] Low-grade fever, leukocytosis, and rarely, a peritoneal abdominal examination, complicate the diagnosis. In addition to GI symptoms, neurologic and autonomic symptoms occur frequently. Whereas altered mentation and hallucinations are classic, an acute motor neuropathy consisting of proximal muscle weakness, cramping, and wasting may take the place of or coincide with CNS symptoms. Autonomic dysfunction is apparent in 80% of AIP exacerbations and is marked by tachycardia, urinary retention, incontinence, hypertension, or postural hypotension.[90] AIP lacks cutaneous findings common in other porphyrias.

ED diagnosis of AIP is based on clinical suspicion and urine that turns a port-wine color when exposed to sunlight or air. Confirmatory testing requires a 24-hour urine collection and genetic testing. Treatment goals are 3 prong: removing the precipitatant, treating symptoms, and reversing induction of the heme synthesis pathway. Discontinuation of precipitating medications, aggressive resuscitation with glucose-containing solutions, and treatment of underlying infection with a medication safe for use in porphyria (see **Box 3**) comprise initial treatment. Symptomatic treatment must be careful to avoid medications known to exacerbate AIP; phenothiazines, morphine, benzodiazepines other than diazepam, and propranolol are common medications used to relieve symptoms associated with AIP exacerbations. Reversal of the heme synthesis induction is achieved by ensuring glucose intake of at least 400 g per day via a combination of oral and parenteral routes; hematin infusion may be added to further prevent induction of the heme synthesis pathway.[90]

Hyperammonemia

Although ammonia is a normal constituent of all body fluids, serum levels must be maintained less than 35 mg/dL to avoid CNS toxicity.[91] This goal is accomplished by hepatic synthesis of urea, the form in which ammonia is excreted. Congenital deficiencies of urea cycle enzymes, hepatic failure, Reye syndrome, valproate or salicylate toxicity, as well as several other types of congenital metabolic disorders (eg, organic acidemias, congenital lactic acidosis, fatty acid oxidation defects) can result in increased serum concentrations of ammonia. Metabolic disorders are the most common cause of hyperammonemia in pediatric patients, whereas hepatic disease is the most common cause in adults.[91] Pediatric and adult patients present with

Box 3
Safe and unsafe drugs in acute porphyria

Drugs safe in acute porphyria

Acetaminophen

Acetazolamide

Acyclovir

Allopurinol

Amiloride

Aminoglycosides[a]

Aspirin

Atropine

β-blockers

Bromides[a]

Bumetanide

Bupivicaine[a]

Buprenorphine

Chlorpromazine

Codeine

Corticosteroids[a]

Deferoxamine

Demerol

Diazoxide[a]

Digitalis

Epinephrine

Fentanyl

Follicle-stimulating hormone

Fenoprophen[a]

Gabapentin

Gentamicin

Glipizide

Haloperidol

Hepzrin

Ibuprophen[a]

Indomethacin

Insulin

Labetolol

Lithium salts

Metformin

Metoprolol

Morphine

Nadolol
Nitrous oxide
Oxytocin
Pencillin
Procaine
Prochlorperazine[a]
Propofol
Propoxyphene
Quinine
Ranitidine[a]
Salbutamol
Senna
Sulindac
Temazepam
Thyroxine[a]
Warfarin

Drugs unsafe in acute porphyria

Alpha methyldopa[b]
Barbiturates[b]
Captopril
Carbamazepine
Cimetidine
Chloramphenicol[b]
Chlorpropamide
Diazepam
Diliazem
Dimenhydrinate
Doxycycline
Ergot compounds[b]
Erythromycin
Estrogen
Tehanol[b]
Furosemide
Griesofulvin[b]
Hydralazine
Hydrochlorothiazide
Imipramine[b]
Lidocaine
Metoclopramide
Metronidazole

Nifedipine
Oral contraceptives
Orphenadrine[b]
Oxycodone
Pentazocine[b]
Phenobarbital
Phenytoin[b]

[a] Denotes medications that are likely to be safe.
[b] Denotes medications that are known to cause acute attacks.

a depressed level of consciousness ranging from mild lethargy to coma and tachypnea resulting from stimulation of the medullary center by the ammonium ion. Associated findings in infants and children include dehydration as a result of vomiting, hypotonia, and a bulging fontanelle caused by increased intracranial pressure (ICP). Adults more commonly have signs of acute or chronic hepatic failure. Patients with hyperammonemia associated with acute hepatic failure may require intubation for airway protection. Control of increased ICP improves survival and may be achieved initially using mannitol, hypertonic saline, and hyperventilation.[92] Intravenous N-acetylcysteine administration has been shown to improve survival in mild to moderately severe cases of acute hepatic encephalopathy.[92] In patients with hyperammonemia caused by chronic hepatic encephalopathy, treatment is focused on supportive care, reducing colonic bacterial production of ammonia, and enhancing ammonia elimination. Antibiotics including neomycin, metronidazole, vancomycin, and rifaximin can be used to decrease the colonic bacterial population responsible for ammonia production; however, treatment has not been shown to improve outcome.[92] Orally or nasogastrically administered lactulose inhibits production and increases elimination of ammonia in the colon; although its use does improve encephalopathy, it does not provide mortality benefit.[92]

Special Considerations

Pediatrics

Approximately 30 in every 100,000 children present to the hospital each year as a result of a nontraumatic cause of a decreased level of consciousness; the mortality of this group is an alarming 40%.[93] The leading causes of nontraumatic coma are infection, drug intoxication, seizures, and inborn errors of metabolism.[93] In infants and children in whom metabolic diseases are suspected, serum glucose, serum ammonia, and urinary ketone investigations are of paramount importance. Neonatal hypoglycemia may indicate hyperinsulinism, limited or depleted glycogen stores, or decreased glycogenolysis caused by metabolic disorders or adrenal insufficiency. Hypoglycemia in older infants and children calls attention to the possibility of toxicologic or pharmacologic exposures, hepatic disease, organic acidemias, and aminoacidopathies. An increased serum ammonia heralds consideration of urea cycle disorders, organic acidurias, fatty acid oxidation disorders, and other less common inherited metabolic disorders that may present in the neonatal period or later in childhood. Less commonly, serum hyperammonemia may be the result of a urinary tract infection with a urease-producing organism, medications, Reye syndrome, or GI hemorrhage. Ketones in the urine indicate a state of catabolism, which can indicate a period of starvation, or less commonly, a decompensated metabolic disorder. No history of starvation and/or a serum lactate greater than 3.5 mg/dL should prompt examinations for an organic acidemia, aminoacidopathy, fat oxidation defect, or mitochondrial enzyme defect.[93]

Excluding ketoacidosis, the remainder of the metabolic acidoses and electrolyte-related causes in the pediatric population have clinical presentations and courses of treatment similar to those discussed earlier. However, several differences are present in endocrine-related causes, specifically with regard to DKA and thyroid disease. Correction of DKA-related hyperglycemia and acidosis is exacted in a more cautious fashion, with an optimal rate of glucose decline of less than 100 mg/dL/h, no insulin bolus before initiation of the insulin drip, maintenance of serum glucose levels more than 200 mg/dL during the first 4 to 5 hours of treatment, and avoidance of bicarbonate use except in cases of life-threatening acidosis. These changes in treatment are enacted in an attempt to reduce the risk of treatment-associated cerebral edema caused by rapid intracellular fluid shifts.

Neonatal screening for hypothyroidism reveals a 1/4000 prevalence, with the highest rates in Hispanic, Native American, and female infants.[94] As laboratory errors do occur and the consequences of missing this disease result in severe mental and physical growth retardation, knowledge of signs and symptoms must be maintained. Affected infants cry little, sleep excessively, have poor appetites, and exhibit respiratory difficulties, mild hypothermia, and constipation. At the other extreme, neonatal thyrotoxicosis constitutes 1% of childhood thyrotoxicoses and is most commonly associated with low birth weight, premature delivery, accelerated skeletal maturation, microcephaly, poor weight gain, and a history of maternal Graves disease.[5] Diagnosis is confirmed with serum TSH and T4 levels.

Pregnancy

The peak incidence of thyroid disease is in women of childbearing age; furthermore, many of the symptoms of thyroid disease mimic normal pregnancy, making increased clinical suspicion crucial to making the diagnosis. Graves disease complicates 1/500 pregnancies and presents similar to hyperthyroidism in nonpregnant patients, with the exception that weight loss is masked by the normal weight gain associated with pregnancy.[5] Treatment with propylthiouracil is preferred to methimazole; use of β-blockers must be considered on an individual basis because of their association with intrauterine growth retardation, neonatal bradycardia and hypotension, hypoglycemia, and prolonged hyperbilirubinemia.[5,95]

Elderly patients

Mental status changes account for an estimated 30% of emergency evaluations in older patients; delirium is the most common acute change and is associated with a hospital mortality of 25% to 33%.[96,97] Medications and occult infections explain most delirium presentations.[97] However, metabolic disorders, including hypernatremia or hyponatremia, hypercalcemia, acid-base disorders, hypoglycemia and hyperglycemia, and thyroid or adrenal disorders, are also common contributors to delirium in the elderly population. More than 98% of elderly patients presenting with dementia have a primary cause, such as neurodegenerative or cerebrovascular cause; however, 2% may be attributed to secondary causes.[98] Metabolic disorders precipitating a subacute dementia presentation include thyroid disease, B_{12} deficiency, and hypocalcemia or hypercalcemia.[98] Hyperadrenergenic and ocular signs are most often absent in elderly patients with hyperthyroidism.[5] Instead, these signs are replaced by apathetic facies, depression, lethargy, generalized weakness, weight loss, and new onset atrial fibrillation or congestive heart failure: a syndrome referred to as apathetic hyperthyroidism.[5]

SUMMARY

Although the cause of altered mental status in a tachypnic, dehydrated patient with a fruity odor on their breath is obvious, the physician is rarely so fortunate. More often, altered mental status of endocrine or metabolic origin may be considered because of the presence of abnormal serum glucose, abnormal serum electrolytes, a metabolic acidosis, or urine ketones. In nearly every cause discussed in this article, the key to diagnosis can be found with a careful history, most often obtained from family, caretakers, and available medical records. Specific attention to available and prescribed medications, toxic exposures, medical history, recent illnesses, and potential for malnutrition, in addition to a high index of suspicion for toxic or pharmaceutical exposure and a detailed physical examination, are essential to securing diagnosis of an altered mental state that has endocrine or metabolic causes.

REFERENCES

1. Cooke JL, Barsan WG. Altered mental status and coma. In: Adams JG, editor. Emergency medicine. 1st edition. Philadelphia: Saunders Elsevier; 2008. p. 985–92.
2. Virally ML, Guillausseau PJ. Hypoglycemia in adults. Diabete Metab 1999;25: 477–90.
3. Kitabschi AE, Nyenwe EA. Hyperglycemic crises in diabetes mellitus: diabetic ketoacidosis and hyperglycemia hyperosmolar state. Endocrinol Metab Clin North Am 2006;35:725–51.
4. Kitabchi AE, Wall B. Diabetic ketoacidosis. Med Clin North Am 1995;79(1):10–37.
5. McKeown NJ, Tews MC, Gossain VV, et al. Hyperthyroidism. Emerg Med Clin North Am 2005;23:669–85.
6. Devdhar M, Ousman YH, Burman KD. Hypothyroidism. Endocrinol Metab Clin North Am 2007;36:595–615.
7. Wadman MC. Sodium and water balance. In: Adams JG, editor. Emergency medicine. Philadelphia: Saunders Elsevier; 2008. p. 1765–71.
8. Nieman LK. Adrenal cortex. In: Goldman L, Ausiello D, editors. Cecil medicine. 23rd edition. Philadelphia: Saunders Elsevier; 2007. p. 1713–21.
9. Fried LF, Palevsky PM. Hyponatremia and hypernatremia. Med Clin North Am 1997;81(3):585–609.
10. Kumar S, Berl T. Sodium. Lancet 1998;352:220–8.
11. Schaefer TJ, Wolford RW. Disorders of potassium. Emerg Med Clin North Am 2005;23:723–47.
12. Moe SM. Disorders involving calcium, phosphorus, and magnesium. Prim Care 2008;35:215–37.
13. Kacprowicz RF, Lloyd JD. Electrolyte complications of malignancy. Emerg Med Clin North Am 2009;27:257–69.
14. Bilezikian JP, Silverberg SJ. Clinical practice. Asymptomatic primary hyperparathyroidism. N Engl J Med 2004;350:1746–51.
15. Stewart AF. Clinical practice. Hypercalcemia associated with cancer. N Engl J Med 2005;352:373–9.
16. Novello NP, Blumstein HA. Hypomagnesemia. eMedicine. Available at: http://emedicine.medscape.com/article/767546-overview. Accessed November 1, 2009.

17. Moore DJ, Rosh AJ. Hypophosphatemia. eMedicine. Available at: http://emedicine.medscape.com/article/767955-overview. Accessed November 1, 2009.
18. Bennet IL, Cary FH, Mitchell GL, et al. Acute methyl alcohol poisoning: a review based on experiences in an outbreak of 323 cases. Medicine 1953;32(4):431–63.
19. Frenia ML, Schauben JL. Methanol inhalation toxicity. Ann Emerg Med 1993; 22(12):1919–23.
20. Kahn A, Blum D. Methyl alcohol poisoning in an 8-month-old boy: an unusual route of intoxication. J Pediatr 1979;94(5):841–3.
21. Ford MD, McMartin K. Ethylene glycol and methanol. In: Ford MD, Delaney KA, Ling LJ, editors. Clinical toxicology. Philadelphia: WB Saunders; 2001. p. 757–67.
22. Gonda A, Gault H, Churchill D, et al. Hemodialysis for methanol intoxication. Am J Med 1978;64(5):749–58.
23. Keyvan-Larijarni H, Tannenberg AM. Methanol intoxication: comparison of peritoneal dialysis and hemodialysis treatment. Arch Intern Med 1974;134(2):293–6.
24. Naraqi S, Dethlefs RF, Slobodniuk RA, et al. An outbreak of acute methyl alcohol intoxication. Aust N Z J Med 1979;9(1):65–8.
25. Shahangian S, Ash KO. Formic and lactic acidosis in a fatal case of methanol intoxication. Clin Chem 1986;32(2):395–7.
26. Swartz RD, Millman RP, Billi JE, et al. Epidemic methanol poisoning: clinical and biochemical analysis of a recent episode. Medicine 1981;60(5):373–82.
27. Dethlefs R, Naraqi S. Ocular manifestations and complications of acute methyl alcohol intoxication. Med J Aust 1978;2(10):483–5.
28. Greiner JV, Pillai S, Limaye SR, et al. Sterno-induced methanol toxicity and visual recovery after prompt hemodialysis. Arch Ophthalmol 1989;107(5):643.
29. Ingemansson SO. Clinical observations on ten cases of methanol poisoning with particular reference to ocular manifestations. Acta Opthalmol (Copenh) 1984; 62(1):15–24.
30. Jacobsen D, Webb R, Collins TD, et al. Methanol and formate kinetics in late diagnosed methanol intoxication. Med Toxicol 1988;3(5):418–23.
31. Aquilonius SM, Askmark H, Enoksson P, et al. Computerized tomography in severe methanol intoxication. Br Med J 1978;2(6142):929–30.
32. Chen JC, Schneiderman JF, Wortzman G. Methanol poisoning: bilateral putaminal and cerebellar cortical lesions on CT and MR. J Comput Assist Tomogr 1993; 15(3):522–4.
33. Hantson P, Duprez T, Mahieu P. Neurotoxicity to the basal ganglia shown by MRI following poisoning by methanol and other substances. J Toxicol Clin Toxicol 1997;35(2):151–61.
34. Mittal BV, Desai AP, Kahde KR. Methyl alcohol poisoning: an autopsy study of 28 cases. J Postgrad Med 1991;37(1):9–13.
35. Phang PT, Passerini L, Mielke B, et al. Brain hemorrhage associated with methanol poisoning. Crit Care Med 1988;16(2):137–40.
36. DuBose TB Jr. Acidosis and alkalosis. In: Fauci AS, Braunwald E, Isselbacher KJ, et al, editors. Harrison's principles of internal medicine. 14th edition. New York: McGraw-Hill; 1998. p. 277–83.
37. Bailey JL, Mitch WE. Pathophysiology of uremia. In: Brenner BM, editor. The kidney. 7th edition. Philadelphia: Elsevier; 2004. p. 2139–43.
38. Kitabchi A, Wall BM. Management of diabetic ketoacidosis. Am Fam Physician 1999;60(2):455–64.
39. Umpierrez GE, Kelly JP, Navarette JE, et al. Hyperglycemic crises in urban blacks. Arch Intern Med 1997;157:669–75.

40. Umpierrez GE, DiGirolamo M, Tuvlin JA, et al. Differences in metabolic and hormonal milieu in diabetic- and alcohol-induced ketoacidosis. J Crit Care 2000;15(2):52–9.
41. Owen OE, Capiro S, Reichard GA Jr, et al. Ketosis of starvation: a revisit and new perspectives. Clin Endocrinol Metab 1983;12(2):359–79.
42. Toth HL, Greenbaum LA. Severe acidosis caused by starvation and stress. Am J Kidney Dis 2003;42(5):E16–9.
43. Koeslag JH, Noakes TD, Sloan AW. Post-exercise ketosis. J Physiol 1980;301: 79–90.
44. Rudolf MC, Sherwin RS. Maternal ketosis and its effects on the fetus. Clin Endocrinol Metab 1983;12(2):413–28.
45. Mahoney CA. Extreme gestational starvation ketoacidosis: case report and review of pathophysiology. Am J Kidney Dis 1992;20(3):276–80.
46. Delaney KA. Acid-base disturbances in the poisoned patient. In: Ford MD, Delaney KA, Ling LJ, et al, editors. Clinical toxicology. Philadelphia: WB Saunders; 2001. p. 94.
47. Davis CO, Wax PM. Focused physical examination/toxidromes. In: Ford MD, Delaney KA, Ling LJ, et al, editors. Clinical toxicology. Philadelphia: WB Saunders; 2001. p. 32.
48. Disney JD. Acid-base disorders. In: Marx JA, Hockberger RS, Walls RM, editors. Rosen's emergency medicine concepts and clinical practice. 5th edition. St. Louis (MO): Mosby; 2002. p. 1718–9.
49. Center for Disease Control and Prevention. Trends in tuberculosis—United States, 1998–2003. MMWR Morb Mortal Wkly Rep 2004;53(10):209–14.
50. Henry GC, Haynes S. Isoniazid and other antituberculosis drugs. In: Ford MD, Delaney KA, Ling LJ, et al, editors. Clinical toxicology. Philadelphia: WB Saunders; 2001. p. 439–41.
51. Brown A, Mallet M, Fiser D, et al. Acute isoniazid intoxication: reversal of CNS symptoms with large doses of pyridoxime. Pediatr Pharmacol 1984;4(3): 199–202.
52. Hankins DG, Saxena K, Faville RJ Jr, et al. Profound acidosis caused by isoniazid ingestion. Am J Emerg Med 1987;5(2):165–6.
53. Mechem CC. Toxicity, isoniazid: treatment and medication. eMedicine. Available at: http://emedicine.medscape.com/article/815298-overview. Accessed November 1, 2009.
54. Roberts RJ, Nayfield S, Soper R, et al. Acute iron intoxication with intestinal infarction managed in part by small bowel resection. Clin Toxicol 1975;8(1):3–12.
55. Tenenbein M, Kopelow ML, deSa DJ. Myocardial failure and shock in iron poisoning. Hum Toxicol 1988;7(3):281–4.
56. Tenenbein M. Iron. In: Ford MD, Delaney KA, Ling LJ, et al, editors. Clinical toxicology. Philadelphia: WB Saunders; 2001. p. 305–9.
57. Banner W Jr, Tong TG. Iron poisoning. Pediatr Clin North Am 1986;33(2):393–409.
58. Velez LI, Delaney KA. Heavy metals. In: Marx JA, Hockberger RS, Walls RM, editors. Rosen's emergency medicine concepts and clinical practice. 5th edition. St. Louis (MO): Mosby; 2002. p. 2151.
59. Nadiminti Y, Wang JC, Chou SY, et al. Lactic acidosis associated with Hodgkin's disease. N Engl J Med 1980;303(1):15–7.
60. Roth GJ, Porte D Jr. Chronic lactic acidosis and acute leukemia. Arch Intern Med 1970;125(2):317–21.
61. Kachel RG. Metastatic reticulum cell sarcoma and lactic acidosis. Cancer 1975; 36(6):2056–9.

62. Chang CT, Chen YC, Fang JT, et al. Metformin-associated lactic acidosis: case reports and literature review. J Nephrol 2002;15(4):398–402.
63. Arenas-Pinto A, Grant AD, Edwards S, et al. Lactic acidosis in HIV infected patients: a systematic review of published cases. Sex Transm Infect 2003; 79(4):340–3.
64. Vasile B, Rasulo F, Candiani A, et al. The pathophysiology of propofol infusion syndrome: a simple name for a complex syndrome. Intensive Care Med 2003; 29(9):1417–25.
65. Uribiarri J, Oh MS, Carroll HJ. D-lactic acidosis: a review of clinical presentation, biochemical features, and pathophysiologic mechanisms. Medicine 1998;77(2): 73–82.
66. Gauthier PM, Szerlip HM. Metabolic acidosis in the intensive care unit. Crit Care Clin 2002;18(2):289–308.
67. Brent J, McMartin K, Phillips S, et al. Fomepizole for the treatment of ethylene glycol poisoning. Methylpyrazole for Toxic Alcohols Study Group. N Engl J Med 1999;340(11):832–8.
68. Karlson-Stiber C, Persson H. Ethylene glycol poisoning: experiences from an epidemic in Sweden. J Toxicol Clin Toxicol 1992;30(4):565–74.
69. Sabeel AI, Kurkaus J, Lindholm T. Intensified dialysis treatment of ethylene glycol intoxication. Scand J Urol Nephrol 1995;29(2):125–9.
70. White SR, Kosnik J. Toxic alcohols. In: Marx JA, Hockberger RS, Walls RM, editors. Rosen's emergency medicine concepts and clinical practice. 5th edition. St. Louis (MO): Mosby; 2002. p. 2127–33.
71. Jacobsen D, Ovrebo S, Ostborg J, et al. Glycolate causes the acidosis in ethylene glycol poisoning and is effectively removed by hemodialysis. Acta Med Scand 1984;216(4):409–16.
72. Leikin JB, Toerne T, Burda A, et al. Summertime cluster of intentional ethylene glycol ingestions. JAMA 1997;278(17):1406.
73. Zeiss J, Velasco ME, McCann KM, et al. Cerebral CT of lethal ethylene glycol intoxication with pathologic correlation. AJNR Am J Neuroradiol 1989;10(2):440–2.
74. Morgan BW, Ford MD, Follmer R. Ethylene glycol ingestion resulting in brainstem and midbrain dysfunction. J Toxicol Clin Toxicol 2000;38(4):445–51.
75. Donovan JW, Akhtar J. Salicylates. In: Ford MD, Delaney KA, Ling LJ, et al, editors. Clinical toxicology. Philadelphia: WB Saunders; 2001. p. 275–80.
76. Kokko JP. Fluids and electrolytes. In: Goldman L, Bennett JC, editors. Cecil textbook of medicine. 21st edition. St. Louis (MO): WB Saunders; 2000. p. 562.
77. Wilcox CS. Diuretics. In: Brenner BM, editor. The kidney. 7th edition. Philadelphia: Elsevier; 2004. p. 2145–6.
78. Heller I, Halevy J, Cohen S, et al. Significant metabolic acidosis induced by acetazolamide. Arch Intern Med 1985;145(10):1815–7.
79. DuBose TD. Acid-base disorders. In: Brenner BM, editor. The kidney. 7th edition. Philadelphia: Elsevier; 2004. p. 944–61.
80. Colucciello SA, Tomaszewski C. Substance abuse. In: Marx JA, Hockberger RS, Walls RM, editors. Rosen's emergency medicine concepts and clinical practice. 5th edition. St Louis (MO): Mosby; 2002. p. 2537.
81. DuBose TD Jr, Caflisch CR. Validation of the difference in urine and blood CO2 tension during bicarbonate loading as an index of distal nephron acidification in experimental models of distal renal tubular acidosis. J Clin Invest 1985; 75(4):1116–23.
82. Osborn HH, Malkevich D. Lithium. In: Ford MD, Delaney KA, Ling LJ, et al, editors. Clinical toxicology. Philadelphia: WB Saunders; 2001. p. 532–8.

83. Halperin ML, Goldstein MB, Richardson RMA, et al. Distal renal tubular acidosis syndromes: a pathophysiological approach. Am J Nephrol 1985;5(1):1–8.
84. Forsmark CE. Chronic pancreatitis. In: Feldman M, Friedman LS, Sleisenger MH, editors. Sleisenger & Fordtran's gastrointestinal and liver disease. 7th edition. Philadelphia: Elsevier; 2002. p. 965.
85. Donnino MW, Vega J, Miller J, et al. Myths and misconceptions of Wernicke's encephalopathy: what every emergency physician should know. Ann Emerg Med 2007;50(6):715–21.
86. Kinsella LJ, Riley DE. Nutritional deficiencies and syndromes associated with alcoholism. In: Goetz CG, editor. Textbook of clinical neurology. 3rd edition. Philadephia: Saunders Elsevier; 2007. p. 906.
87. Balint JP. Physical findings in nutritional deficiencies. Pediatr Clin North Am 1998; 45(1):245–60.
88. Frye RE, Jabbour SA. Pyridoxine deficiency. eMedicine. Available at:http:// emedicine.medscape.com/article/124947-overview. Accessed November 1, 2009.
89. Rabinowitz SS, ReddyS, Rajakumar K. Pellagra. eMedicine. Available at: http:// emedicine.medscape.com/article/985427-overview. Accessed November 1, 2009.
90. Dombeck TA, Satonik RC. The porphyrias. Emerg Med Clin North Am 2005;23: 885–99.
91. Crisan E, Chawla J. Hyperammonemia. eMedicine. Available at: http://emedicine. medscape.com/article/1174503-overview. Accessed November 1, 2009.
92. Eroglu Y, Byrne WJ. Hepatic encephalopathy. Emerg Med Clin North Am 2009;27: 401–14.
93. Bowker R, Green A, Bonham JR. Guidelines for the investigation and management of a reduced level of consciousness in children: implications for clinical biochemistry laboratories. Ann Clin Biochem 2007;44:506–11.
94. LaFranchi S. Hypothyroidism. In: Kleigman RM, Behrman RE, Jenson HB, et al, editors. Nelson textbook of pediatrics. 18th edition. Philadephia: Saunders Elsevier; 2007. p. 2319–27.
95. Houry DE, Abbott JT. Acute complications of pregnancy. In: Marx JA, Hockberger RS, Walls RM, editors. Rosen's emergency medicine concepts and clinical practice. 6th edition. Philadelphia: Mosby Elsevier; 2006. p. 2739–60.
96. Wilber ST. Altered mental status in older emergency department patients. Emerg Med Clin North Am 2006;24:299–316.
97. Inouye SK. Delirium and other mental status problems in the older patient. In: Goldman L, Ausiello D, editors. Cecil medicine. 23rd edition. Philadelphia: Saunders Elsevier; 2008. p. 131–8.
98. Knopman DS. Alzheimer's disease and other dementias. In: Goldman L, Ausiello D, editors. Cecil medicine. 23rd edition. Philadelphia: Saunders Elsevier; 2008. p. 2667–75.

Drugs of Abuse: The Highs and Lows of Altered Mental States in the Emergency Department

Timothy J. Meehan, MD, MPH[a,b,*], Sean M. Bryant, MD[a,c,d], Steven E. Aks, DO[a,e,f]

KEYWORDS

- Toxidrome • Emergency department
- Malicious intoxication • Seizure

As eloquently stated by Paracelsus in the sixteenth century, "all substances are poisons; there is none which is not a poison. The right dose differentiates a poison from a remedy."[1] Many drugs of abuse encountered by emergency physicians (EP) are also therapeutic agents. However, when these drugs are taken in excess or recreationally to obtain a "high," the inherent toxicity becomes apparent.

Many substances taken in overdose cause an alteration in mental status. Agents as diverse as carbon monoxide, cyanide, and antiepileptic drugs can lead to life-threatening central nervous system (CNS) depression. Pharmaceuticals such as methylxanthines and drugs used for attention-deficit disorder can lead to severe agitation, delirium, and seizures. Some of these drugs may be abused. As Paracelsus articulated, any toxin in an extreme dose can lead to poisoning. Altered mental status commonly plays a part with toxicity. However, discussion in this review is restricted to drugs of abuse (**Table 1**).

[a] Toxikon Consortium, Chicago, IL, USA
[b] Department of Emergency Medicine (MC 724), University of Illinois - Chicago, 808 South Wood Street, 4th Floor, Chicago, IL 60612, USA
[c] Department of Emergency Medicine, Cook County Hospital (Stroger), Chicago, IL, USA
[d] Illinois Poison Center, Chicago, IL, USA
[e] Division of Toxicology, Department of Emergency Medicine, Cook County Hospital (Stroger), Chicago, IL, USA
[f] Department of Emergency Medicine, Rush University, Chicago, IL, USA
* Corresponding author. Department of Emergency Medicine (MC 724), University of Illinois - Chicago, 808 South Wood Street, 4th Floor, Chicago, IL 60612.
E-mail address: tmeeha3@gmail.com

Emerg Med Clin N Am 28 (2010) 663–682
doi:10.1016/j.emc.2010.03.012 emed.theclinics.com
0733-8627/10/$ – see front matter

Table 1
Causes of altered mental status

Toxidrome Category	Agents (Examples)
Anticholinergics	Diphenhydramine Jimson weed Tricyclic antidepressants
Cholinergics	Organophosphates Carbamates
Sympathomimetics	Cocaine Amphetamines Amphetamine derivatives (MDMA, Ecstasy)
Sedative Hypnotics/Alcohols	Benzodiazepines Barbiturates GHB Ethanol Isopropyl alcohol
Opioids	Heroin Morphine Hydromorphone Oxycodone Hydrocodone Methadone Fentanyl Propoxyphene
Hallucinogens	LSD Mescaline Mushrooms (*Amanita muscaria, Psilocybe spp*) Nutmeg
Miscellaneous Agents	Herbals: Kava kava Valerian Salvia
Mixed Agents	MDMA (Ecstasy) Designer amphetamine analogs PCP Ketamine
Malicious Agents	Imidazolines GHB

Abbreviations: GHB, gamma-hydroxybutyrate; LSD, lysergic acid diethylamide; MDMA, 3,4-methylenedioxymethamphetamine; PCP, phencyclidine.

The EP should use all possible means to determine the substance ingested when evaluating the poisoned patient with altered mental status. History obtained from friends, family, or paramedics is extremely important. Any and all information about possible drug use is essential for making the correct diagnosis.

One should not rely on laboratory tests to make the initial diagnosis of a poisoned patient.[2] Qualitative urine toxicology screens have very limited efficacy in the acute setting. Most emergency departments (EDs) use enzyme immunoassay test toxicology screens that are based on the SAMHSA 5 (Substance Abuse and Mental Health Services Administration): opiates, cocaine metabolite (benzoylecgonine), phencyclidine, amphetamines, and marijuana (tetrahydrocannabinol). Other screens may include methadone, oxycodone, hydrocodone, phenobarbital, or tricyclic antidepressants (TCAs) but vary among hospitals. Many of these drugs or their metabolic byproducts may remain in the system for several days, and thus these screens cannot reliably distinguish between acute toxicity and recent exposure.

The most useful data beyond the history are the presenting signs and symptoms. The term toxidrome represents a constellation of signs and symptoms, which, taken together, can point to a specific toxin class. The major toxidromes include anticholinergics, cholinergics, sympathomimetics, sedative hypnotics/alcohol, opioids, and hallucinogenics (**Table 2**). Withdrawal syndromes, which result from the abrupt cessation of chronic intoxicant abuse, should also be considered in the toxicology differential. For example, alcohol and sedative hypnotic withdrawal present with similar signs and symptoms, as chronic use changes the neurobiology of γ-aminobutyric acid (GABA)-mediated transmission in the CNS by downregulating GABA receptors and thus increasing neurologic irritability in the face of GABA agonist removal. In the case of chronic alcohol abuse, withdrawal is a potential threat to life and must be recognized and managed aggressively. As part of this withdrawal syndrome, patients may experience hallucinations, particularly visual in nature. In addition, patients often describe formication, a sensation of bugs crawling on the skin. Opioid withdrawal is not life threatening and should not cause a significantly altered sensorium. If altered mental status is observed in presumed opioid withdrawal, an alternate diagnosis should be considered.

Table 2
Toxidromes

Toxidrome	Mental Status Effect	Signs
Opiate	Decreased	Hypoventilation, decreased depth of respiration, miosis
Anticholinergic	Agitation, delirium, coma	Tachycardia, flushed and dry skin, dry mucous membranes, hyperthermia, decreased bowel sounds, urinary retention, mydriasis
Cholinergic	CNS depression	Muscarinic: SLUGBAM: Salivation, lacrimation, urination, gastrointestinal distress, bronchospasm, bronchorrhea bradycardia, abdominal cramps, miosis Nicotinic: CNS depression, hypertension, tachycardia, fasciculations
Sympathomimetic	Agitation, delirium, seizures, coma	Hypertension, tachycardia, hyperthermia, diaphoresis, hyperpnea, mydriasis
Sedative Hypnotic/Alcohols	CNS depression	Decreased motor tone, hypothermia, hypotension
Hallucinogens	Excitation, agitation, delirium, hallucination, CNS depression	Tachycardia, diaphoresis or dry skin, mydriasis
Withdrawal: Alcohol or Sedative Hypnotic	Excitation, agitation, delirium, hallucination (visual), seizures	Tachycardia, hypertension, mydriasis, diaphoresis, hyperthermia
Withdrawal: Opiate	Clear sensorium, anxiety	Yawning, piloerection, nausea, vomiting, tachycardia, pain

DRUG CLASSES IN DEPTH

Toxidrome recognition is essential for detecting the poisoned patient with altered mental status. The constituent signs and symptoms that define the toxidromes have already been discussed; the underlying pathophysiology, clinical effects, and management strategies have not. By looking at the drugs and substances that can precipitate the signs and symptoms, these latter issues are explored. In most cases, prototypical agents are used as examples that can be generalized; however, wherever a controversy or peculiar finding specific to a certain agent exists, it is discussed separately. Finally, the authors discuss one increasingly common crossroad of drugs, altered mental status, and the ED—drug-facilitated sexual assault (DFSA, "date rape").

Anticholinergics

A 16-year-old male is brought to your ED by his friends. He is uncooperative, agitated, and resists all efforts to "talk him down." He is also hypertensive, tachycardic, and mildly hyperthermic and has dried spittle on his tongue. Although he is quite warm and flushed, his skin is dry. In addition, it takes several doses of intramuscular benzodiazepines to control his agitation. Before his friends disappear from the ED, they tell the triage nurse that they were "drinking a tea we read about on the Internet. It said you could get really high and have an awesome trip." As they are leaving, the nurse calls you back to the patient saying, "he's acting up again and trying to punch me!" What to do next?

"They turned natural fools upon it for several days" illustrates a typical view of the CNS abnormalities experienced by British soldiers stationed in Jamestown, Virginia, in 1676.[3] Their anticholinergic poisoning originated from ingesting salad containing Jamestown weed (better known today as jimson weed or *Datura stramonium*). Today, jimson weed is still abused by ingestion, smoking, brewing of tea, and even mixing with toothpaste to alter sensorium or to hallucinate.[4–6]

Patients poisoned by anticholinergic agents commonly present according to the following mnemonic: "Hot as a Hare, Red as a Beet, Dry as a Bone, Blind as a Bat, and Mad as a Hatter." Interestingly, patients may be initially sleepy with mild-to-moderate CNS depression with therapeutic to supratherapeutic dosing (eg, diphenhydramine). However, CNS excitation and stimulation may follow with higher doses, making patients "Mad as a Hatter" (originally attributed to personality changes secondary to mercury poisoning in hat industry workers in Danbury, Connecticut, during the nineteenth century). Although nicotinic and muscarinic receptors exist peripherally and centrally, it is predominantly blockade of central G-protein–linked muscarinic receptors that is responsible for the central effects of disinhibition and excitation. Commonly noted signs and symptoms limited to the CNS may include agitation (sometimes severe), hallucinations, choreoathetosis, seizures, and coma.[7] In addition, varying degrees of agitation coupled to suppression of sweating from the antimuscarinic effects at the glandular level may result in hyperthermia.

Causes for these central anticholinergic effects stem from pharmacologic and nonpharmacologic agents (**Table 3**). The epileptogenic nature of these poisons has been noted in animal studies in which experimentally administered doses of antihistamines resulted in generalized seizures, whereas histidine (a precursor to histamine) reduced seizure activity.[8–10]

Management of patients poisoned by anticholinergic agents is challenging. Gastric decontamination (gastric lavage or activated charcoal) should be entertained only in patients with early presentations of large overdoses. Decontaminating patients exhibiting CNS hyperstimulation (such as tremor or seizures) or CNS depression is a risky

Table 3
Common anticholinergic agents

Pharmaceutical	Nonpharmaceutical
Over-the-counter agents	*Plants*
Diphenhydramine	Deadly nightshade (*Atropa belladonna*)
Dimenhydrinate	Jimson weed (*Datura stramonium*)
Hydroxyzine	Angel's trumpet (*Cestrum nocturnum*)
Miscellaneous antihistamines	Henbane (*Hyoscyamus niger*) Mandrake (*Mandragora officinarum*)
Prescription drugs	Moonflower seeds (*Ipomoea alba*)
Meclizine	*Mushrooms*
Promethazine	*Amanita muscaria* and *Amanita pantherina* (may appear anticholinergic on presentation; however, manifestations generated by the toxins ibotenic acid and muscimol)
Benztropine	
Ophthalmic agents (homatropine, tropicamide, cyclopentolate, atropine)	
Orphenadrine citrate	
Cyclobenzaprine hydrochloride	
Antipsychotics	
Tricyclic antidepressants	

maneuver, with a greater potential for pulmonary aspiration. Intubated patients whose airways are protected still warrant a risk-benefit approach to decontamination because pulmonary aspiration is possible despite the endotracheal tube and benefit of the procedure is impossible to prove.

Although agitation and hallucinations in the scenario of significant tachycardia and hypertension can be significant, an elevated core temperature is the most vital sign and warrants immediate attention. Treatment measures include aggressive supportive care that includes actively cooling hyperpyrexic patients. Centrally acting antipyretics, such as acetaminophen, have no effect in poisoned patients, as the hyperthermia is not caused by resetting of the hypothalamic thermostat. Rather, the hypermetabolic state is responsible for the elevated core temperatures. Thus, actively cooling by using cooling blankets, large fans (such as those used to dry floors in hospitals) with cool mist, and ice application to maximize evaporative cooling may be life saving. The judicious use of benzodiazepines and intravenous (IV) crystalloids are beneficial in these patients as well. Benzodiazepine therapy reduces agitation and delirium in addition to seizure activity. In contrast, antipsychotic agents from the phenothiazine and butyrophenone classes (eg, haloperidol) may actually worsen the situation—they also have anticholinergic effects and may lower the seizure threshold.[11]

Physostigmine is an acetylcholinesterase inhibitor that blocks the metabolism of acetylcholine within the synaptic cleft. The ideal situation to administer this antidote is when treating a patient with a pure anticholinergic overdose. Despite an indisputable pathophysiologic mechanism, its use is a topic of controversy among practicing EPs and medical toxicologists based upon experience with TCAs. This apprehension largely arose after complications that followed the treatment of two patients with TCA poisoning that ultimately led to bradycardia, asystole, and death.[12] TCAs possess anticholinergic properties and can present with mentation changes, coma, or seizures; but poisoning with these agents is more concerning because of the fast sodium channel blockade that results in QRS widening and alpha-adrenergic blockade, which results in hypotension. More appropriate and accepted therapeutic interventions are necessary in the moderate-to-severe TCA-poisoned patient, such as sodium bicarbonate boluses to overcome QRS lengthening and hypotension and benzodiazepines to treat seizure activity. However, some argue that physostigmine is safe in this population of patients pending a normal QRS while others argue complications may be heart rate dependent.[13] Other groups have reported on the safety and efficacy of physostigmine for therapeutic and diagnostic purposes when compared with conventional benzodiazepines.[14,15] However, it is the opinion of these investigators that physostigmine has no role in treating the TCA-poisoned patient. Patients who are poisoned purely by anticholinergics may benefit from physostigmine, but the provider must be aware of the relatively short duration of action (half-life, 16 minutes and duration of action, approximately 1 hour). Dosing is 1 to 2 mg IV over at least 5 minutes in adults (0.02 mg/kg to maximum of 0.5 mg in pediatric patients), and subsequent doses may be warranted if clinical relapse occurs. Atropine (especially in pediatric patients) should be readily available if cholinergic tone begins to predominate.

Sympathomimetics

A 27-year-old female patient arrives in your ED via the local paramedic service after being found in a drugstore parking lot after a possible seizure. She is agitated, diaphoretic, and uncooperative. Her pupils are large, mucous membranes are moist, heart rate is tachycardic, and pulse is bounding. You suspect a stimulant poisoning, and as you begin your evaluation and management, she becomes unresponsive and begins to seize.

The sympathomimetics are a group of xenobiotics that exert their effects through stimulation of the adrenergic side of the sympathetic nervous system. By activating a combination of α and β receptors (**Table 4**), they result in an excessive "fight-or-flight" reaction. On the whole, intoxicated patients who have used these agents present in a hyperdynamic state as illustrated in **Box 1**.

Cocaine

Many drugs can cause the aforementioned symptoms, with the prototypical agent being cocaine. Cocaine is a naturally derived alkaloid from the plant *Erythroxylum coca*. Cocaine was originally isolated and used in the nineteenth century as a local anesthetic but became a restricted-schedule drug in the early twentieth century. Despite restriction for medical use, cocaine is still a widely abused substance today. According to the most recent National Survey on Drug Use and Health, approximately 34 million Americans aged 12 years or older have used cocaine in some form at least once. Of these, 2.4% are consistent users, with the highest incidence/prevalence in the age range of 18 to 24 years.[16]

Table 4
Adrenergic receptors

Receptor	Where Found	Activation Effects
α_1	Peripheral vasculature	Vasoconstriction
α_2	Presynaptic membranes	Decreased outflow
β_1	Cardiovascular	Dromotropy/inotropy/chronotropy
β_2	Peripheral vasculature/muscle	Vasodilation
β_3	Lipocytes	Lipolysis

Box 1
Signs of hyperdynamic state

Hypertensive	Increased muscular tone
Tachycardic	Diaphoresis
Tachypneic	Cardiac murmur
Hyperthermic	Congestive heart failure/pulmonary edema
Mydriasis	

Cocaine comes in two primary forms—the hydrochloride salt, a powdered form that is insufflated or injected, and a freebase (crack), which is heat-stable and therefore able to be smoked. In either case, delivery of the drug to the thin epithelium of the nose or lung results in rapid absorption. Insufflation results in a slightly slower onset of action but prolonged duration, whereas smoking and IV use causes the opposite. After exposure to cocaine, users exhibit hyperalertness, increased sexual desire, as well as a feeling of euphoria caused by the effect of cocaine on dopaminergic transmission in the reward center of the brain. Modification of these dopaminergic pathways is primarily responsible for addiction and dependence.

After intake, cocaine is rapidly metabolized in the plasma to active and inactive substances. One such active metabolite, cocaethylene, is formed in the presence of ethanol. With a prolonged half-life, as well as the retention of sodium channel activity, this substance can induce neurotoxicity and arrhythmias long after the euphorigenic effects have subsided.[17] The coingestion of cholinesterase inhibitors (organophosphates, carbamates) to prolong the duration of action by slowing degradation of cocaine has been described and discussed earlier.

The mechanism of action of cocaine is two-fold. First, it acts to block reuptake of the biogenic amines, epinephrine, norepinephrine, dopamine, and serotonin. In doing so, it exerts effects on virtually all organ systems, as well as neuropsychiatrically. Second, cocaine possesses membrane-stabilizing activity, resulting in sodium channel dysregulation in the nervous and cardiovascular systems.

Clinically, patients on cocaine rarely present to the ED after ingestion of a small amount, as the effects described earlier are the desired outcomes. However, cocaine poisoning is dose dependent, and the drug has a narrow therapeutic window. Poisoned individuals (corresponding to a serum level of >3 mg/L) can present with evidence of hyperdynamicism (tachycardia, hypertension, diaphoresis) in addition to agitation, delirium, or visual hallucinations. During the initial evaluation it is critical to obtain a rectal temperature, as hyperthermia is an independent predictor of poor outcomes.[18] If the patient is hyperthermic, then active cooling with ice packs and misting fans is emergently indicated. In addition, administration of benzodiazepines benefits poisoned patients by blunting the sympathetic outflow responsible for many of the presenting symptoms.

Cocaine and cerebral injury Cocaine's effects touch virtually every organ system; the most well-known (and feared) effects are the cardiovascular and neurologic complications. The management of cocaine-associated chest pain and its related controversies are not discussed here; for further information, a thorough review is available elsewhere.[19]

The vascular effects implicated in this process, however, have some bearing on the neurologic and psychiatric presentation of cocaine-poisoned individuals. Cocaine has been described extensively as a cause for stroke, both as a direct causal agent and as a risk factor.[20] The type of cerebral injury encountered may vary depending on the form of cocaine abused. One study that compared the alkaloidal (freebase/crack) forms with the hydrochloride salt forms revealed that alkaloidal forms were primarily associated with ischemic insults, whereas individuals using the salt formulation had primarily hemorrhagic (subarachnoid or intraparenchymal) bleeding. Of note, those with intracranial hemorrhage had a high proportion of preexisting vascular malformations, such as aneurysms or arteriovenous malformations.[21] Mechanistically, ischemic and hemorrhagic insults have different causes that are related to cocaine's effects on vascular receptors. Ischemic events result from cerebral vasospasm caused by stimulation of α_1 receptors. Cocaine also directly augments platelet aggregation, supporting thrombus formation.

Rapid elevation of blood pressure and maintenance of high blood pressure by stimulating cardiac β_1 receptors can result in subarachnoid and intraparenchymal hemorrhages (often, but not always, associated with preexisting vascular problems), as well as carotid dissection.[22] This rapid rise in mean arterial pressure is also likely responsible for the hypertensive encephalopathy that is sometimes seen in patients severely poisoned with cocaine. Cocaine has also been implicated in cerebral vasculitis based on angiographic and pathologic findings. However, the cause is not entirely clear; the effects may be because of impurities in the drug, adulteration or contamination, and not specifically a result of cocaine.[23]

Excellent supportive care is paramount. If intubation is necessary, adequate sedation must be ensured to avoid further raising intracranial pressure or systemic blood pressure. First-line therapy again involves benzodiazepines, although there may be some benefit from direct venodilators such as nitroglycerin or nitroprusside. At this time, the use of beta-adrenergic blockade in the setting of cocaine intoxication is controversial.

Cocaine and seizures Cocaine is classified as a type-Ia antiarrhythmic agent. These agents have membrane-stabilizing activity through their blockade of voltage-gated sodium channels. Cocaine's ability to cause QRS-interval prolongation and to predispose to certain arrhythmias is well known and treated similarly to other QRS-widening agents through administration of IV sodium bicarbonate (8.4%, 50 mEq $NaHCO_3$ in 50 mL).

Cocaine-induced seizure activity is not a focal neurologic phenomenon but is rather a global derangement in neurotransmission. Once again, benzodiazepines (IV route preferred) are the recommended first-line treatment agents. If these agents are ineffective, then adding phenobarbital or propofol may be required. Antiepileptics such as phenytoin and valproic acid are not as effective because the seizure activity does not arise from a structural focus within the brain.

Amphetamines

Like cocaine, amphetamines induce a state of adrenergic excess and produce similar sympathomimetic effects. However, compared with cocaine, the amphetamines have significant differences in structure and mechanism of toxicity. As a class, the amphetamines are based on a phenylethylamine core structure, which resembles that of the biogenic amines epinephrine, norepinephrine, and dopamine. Given this similarity, one might expect amphetamines to directly stimulate adrenergic receptors. Instead, they act to increase the amount of adrenergic neurotransmitters that are released for any given stimulus. This results in greater amounts of synaptic excitatory neurotransmission and the subsequent clinical effects. Patients on amphetamines present on a spectrum from mildly "energized" to full-blown adrenergic crisis (see **Box 1**). Presentations can include intracranial hemorrhage, hypertensive crises, and rhabdomyolysis; hyperthermia is again an indicator of severe toxicity and needs to be addressed aggressively with ice packs, misters, and cold-water immersion. These drugs do not possess sodium channel activity, and as such, are much less likely to induce seizures.

The amphetamine core structure is amenable to substitution using some fairly simple chemistry, and "designer" amphetamines such as 3,4-methylenedioxymethamphetamine (MDMA), 3,4-methylenedioxy-N-ethylamphetamine, and "2-bromo-dragonfly" are available. These substances have been synthesized to take advantage of activity at serotonin storage vesicles for the "benefit" of greater hallucinogenicity and enactogen activity. A fairly well-known example is MDMA ("Ecstasy"). Patients intoxicated with MDMA may present as either sympathomimetic, serotonergic, or, more likely, a combination of both. Given that these designer amphetamines have some degree of serotonergic activity, a core temperature is of paramount importance; these substances can directly cause hyperthermia, and interactions with other serotonergic medications (eg, selective serotonin reuptake inhibitors [SSRIs], TCAs) can precipitate serotonin syndrome.[24]

Patients with amphetamine poisoning tend to have a gradual onset of symptoms, so presentation may be delayed. In addition, the effects of amphetamines are longer acting because their metabolism is not as rapid as that of cocaine. Treatment of amphetamine intoxication is similar to that of cocaine intoxication; supportive care and ample benzodiazepines are first line for all manifestations, with intubation as necessary.

Methylxanthines

The final class of sympathomimetics that can cause alterations in mental status is the drug with the greatest use and abuse both domestically and globally—caffeine. Approximately 90% of American adults consume some amount of caffeine daily.[18] It comes in many forms, from beverages (coffee, cola, tea, energy drinks) to tablets, as well as in herbal concoctions (often containing yerba mate or kola extract). Caffeine is a naturally occurring alkaloid of the methylxanthine class, along with theophylline and aminophylline. Methylxanthines act in the CNS as adenosine antagonists as well as inhibitors of phosphodiesterase C, allowing an increased and prolonged response to other stimulatory hormones such as epinephrine and norepinephrine.

Desired clinical effects include hyperalertness, increased focus and concentration, and more energy. The effects of caffeine rapidly induce tolerance, necessitating greater doses to achieve the same effect, and often result in dependency. The danger of this drug is not from withdrawal but from an inadvertent overdose of caffeine to maintain the pleasurable effects of the drug. In overdose, typically greater than 200 mg/kg in a single ingestion, patients can present similarly to those poisoned by other psychostimulants, with delirium, tremor, and flushing (see **Table 2**, **Box 1**). Hypertension, arrhythmias, or rhabdomyolysis can also occur. Seizures in caffeine overdose are particularly worrisome, as they are the result of central adenosine antagonism, and can be very difficult to treat.[25,26] One report describes infusing adenosine (Adenocard) directly into the cerebroventricular system as a therapeutic maneuver.[27] Deaths have been reported from caffeine overdoses, but these cases often involve other substances that interact with caffeine's metabolism, suggesting that drug-drug interactions play a pivotal role in these fatalities.

Sedative Hypnotics

A 44-year-old woman comes to the ED with her son; he states that "mom isn't acting right." Per the son, she has been slurring her words for most of the day and has been sleepier than usual. When he tried to move her into the car so to take her to her regular physician, she could not walk and slumped up against him. Confused and afraid, he brought her to the ED worried she was having a stroke.

Her history is significant for chronic low back pain, depression, and panic disorder, for which she takes naproxen, sertraline, and alprazolam. Her son also states that she has been admitted to psychiatric facilities in the past for suicidal thoughts and that "she really took a hit when the market crashed. I'm worried about her." Her examination reveals the following vital signs: blood pressure, 110/70 mm Hg; heart rate, 65 beats per minute; respiratory rate, 14 breaths per minute; temperature, 96.2°F; and pulse oximetry, 98% on room air. Otherwise, her pupils are midrange and sluggish, the depth of her respirations is somewhat lessened, and her mental status is depressed. She is arousable to touch, but she does not answer questions appropriately. There are no other focal findings on examination, and her urine drug screen is negative.

As a class, the sedative hypnotics are defined by their agonism at $GABA_A$ receptors in the CNS. $GABA_A$ is a chloride channel protein that serves to modulate the resting potential of a neuron; when activated, $GABA_A$ allows greater chloride influx. This influx results in a hyperpolarized neuronal membrane and subsequently slows signal transduction through the CNS. Clinically, this condition manifests as a spectrum of mental status changes from mild anxiolysis to coma. Although many substances have the ability to induce sleep or coma, only those with activity at the $GABA_A$ receptor can be considered true sedative hypnotics. While ethanol is the most available and widely used, there are two major pharmaceutical categories of sedative hypnotics: benzodiazepines and barbiturates.

The benzodiazepines are a diverse class of medications whose specific mechanism aims to increase the frequency of $GABA_A$ opening by sensitizing the receptor to GABA binding, whereas the barbiturates act to increase the duration of opening. Both drugs increase chloride influx, but by virtue of allowing the receptor channel to cycle open and closed, the benzodiazepines are significantly safer in overdose.[28,29] These medications are further defined by their potency and lipid solubility, both of which affect the ability to cross the lipophilic blood-brain barrier and induce GABAergic effects.

Upon presentation, patients invariably have some level of mental status change, ranging from mild confusion to complete obtundation. Additional signs and symptoms include ataxia, dysarthrias, and changes in cerebellar coordination. Patients may also be hypothermic, hypotensive, and bradycardic, as a direct result of the drug (barbiturates) as well as environmental exposure in light of mental status depression. Diagnosis is clinical, as standard ED urine toxicologic assays may be unable to detect the presence of benzodiazepines unless they are metabolized to a 1,4-benzodiazepine, such as oxazepam. Benzodiazepines belonging to the 7-amino family and those with minimal metabolism, such as alprazolam, do not trigger a positive test (**Table 5**). Chloral hydrate, a historical sedative hypnotic that has some importance in regards to drug-related crimes, is radiopaque and therefore may be found on abdominal radiographs.[30]

Appropriate management and therapy for patients poisoned by these agents focuses on aggressive supportive care, especially with respect to the respiratory and ventilatory systems. However, there is no universal antidote for sedative-hypnotic intoxication. Although flumazenil, a benzodiazepine antagonist, does have the ability to reverse the effects of benzodiazepines at the $GABA_A$ receptor, it has no effect on barbiturates. In the case of an unknown ingestion, the use of flumazenil as a "naloxone for benzodiazepines" would be attractive; however, the indiscriminate use of this antidote has resulted in seizures exhibiting resistance to standard therapy.[31–33] Risks for this outcome seem to be either intoxication with a nonbenzodiazepine or chronic use

Table 5
Pharmacokinetics of selected GABAergic agents

Name	Time to Onset (min)	Equipotent Dosage (by mouth) (mg)	Half-life (h)	Active Metabolites	Half-life (h) Metabolite
Diazepam	15–30	10	20–50	Yes	40–120
Lorazepam	30–45	2	10–20	No	—
Alprazolam	30–45	1	6–27	No	—
Midazolam	1–2 (IV)	—	3–8	Yes	Insignificant
Clonazepam	30–45	0.5	18–50	No	—
Phenobarbital	15–30	30	80–120	No	—

of or dependence on benzodiazepines. In both cases, flumazenil administration blocks anticonvulsive effects and allows for potential continued epileptic activity. Perhaps the safest situation in which to use flumazenil would be when the exact dose, timing, and benzodiazepine agent used are known, for example, reversing procedural sedation in the ED.

Provided that supportive care can be initiated in a timely manner, deaths due to isolated benzodiazepine ingestions are rare and often involve the coingestion of ethanol or another GABAergic substance. In combination, they are responsible for a large proportion of drug-related deaths. Because the mechanism of death is frequently cardiorespiratory compromise, rapid and timely supportive airway management is essential and may be lifesaving.

Opioids

A 3-year-old girl is carried into the ED by her frantic mother screaming "my baby isn't breathing! Help me!" Rapid assessment reveals shallow, slow breathing, as well as poor response to stimulation and miosis. While you are preparing to intubate the patient, the mother exclaims "this is the last time I let her stay with her father, that useless dope addict." Astutely, you decide to give 0.1 mg/kg of naloxone in an attempt to avoid intubation; the child arouses and, while still sleepy, has improved respiration and mental status. You leave the child on the monitor, decide not to intubate, and go about your shift. Ninety minutes later when returning to recheck the patient and assess for discharge, you note that she has become obtunded again and call for another round of naloxone while wondering "why was the urine drug screen negative? This child is acting like she is on heroin, but the drug screen says otherwise…"

Extracts of *Papaver somniferum* (the poppy plant) have been used for centuries for recreational and medicinal purposes.[34] The analgesic qualities of this plant are known to many and have been extremely well studied. The plant contains the opiates morphine, codeine, and thebaine. Various laboratory syntheses have given us the semisynthetic and synthetic opioids. Strictly speaking, an opioid is any substance that can have its clinical effects reversed by naloxone. Opiates are naturally occurring alkaloids that share this property. Recreationally, they can be abused through the smoking of opium (approximately 10% morphine by weight) or the abuse of heroin. Heroin, originally marketed by Bayer Pharmaceuticals as an antitussive,[35] is a semisynthetic variation of morphine that exists as a prodrug. After penetrating the CNS because of its increased lipophilicity, it is rapidly deacetylated to monoacetylmorphine, which then binds to various opioid receptors and produces clinical effects.

Clinically, patients present in a typical manner termed the opioid toxidrome. These patients exhibit respiratory depression, mental status changes, and pinpoint pupils. These symptoms are caused by the stimulation of μ receptors (respiratory depression and altered mentation) and κ receptors (miosis). Other symptoms that may accompany this presentation include bradycardia, hypotension, decreased bowel sounds, and any signs of traumatic injury that may have occurred during use. Naloxone, a pure opioid antagonist at the μ receptor, may be therapeutic and diagnostic for patients presenting with this constellation of symptoms. The goal of therapy is partial reversal to ensure airway protection but not full reversal and fulminant opioid withdrawal.[36] Treatment should be begun with doses of 0.2 mg in known or suspected opioid-dependent patients, and titrated to desired effect. In opioid-naive individuals, pediatric patients, or ingestions involving methadone or other high-potency opioids, doses up to 10 mg of naloxone may be required to reach this goal.

Recognition of opioid intoxication is a clinical diagnosis. Standard urine drug screens react with morphine metabolites and thus will be positive for codeine and morphine. Depending on the assay, there may be some cross-reactivity with the semisynthetic opioids (eg, heroin, hydromorphone, oxycodone, and hydrocodone), but the fully synthetic opioids (eg, methadone, tramadol, and fentanyl) will not trigger a positive urine screen.[37]

Certain opioids such as methadone have markedly prolonged elimination half-lives when compared with the 30- to 60-minute half-life of naloxone. As a result, it is likely that the patient will become reintoxicated once the antagonism has worn off. This can be an indication for admission or a continuous naloxone infusion. Similarly, other opioids such as fentanyl are markedly more potent than morphine at the μ receptor and their effects can be much more difficult to reverse. An epidemic of adulterated heroin that had been mixed with fentanyl caused many deaths in Chicago several years ago; at least one hospital ED had to go on "naloxone bypass" as the supply of the opioid antagonist had been exhausted.[38]

Besides mental status depression, many other alterations in CNS function are possible. IV heroin abuse has been associated with embolic stroke, either due to foreign material or through infection (eg, endocarditis). Moreover, meperidine and propoxyphene have been associated with seizures. Meperidine is a synthetic opioid with moderate analgesic efficacy; however, its metabolite, normeperidine, undergoes renal excretion and has a very long half-life. In patients with large doses or renal insufficiency, a buildup of this metabolite occurs and seizures can result.[39] Propoxyphene, on the other hand, has sodium channel stabilizing activity. Similar to TCAs, it can predispose to arrhythmias and seizures. In one case series of propoxyphene overdoses, 20% of individuals had prolonged QRS intervals and approximately 10% suffered at least 1 seizure episode.[40] Because of its purported action on sodium channels, cardiac manifestations should be treated similarly to TCA overdoses, with sodium bicarbonate.

MISCELLANEOUS AGENTS

Hallucinogens

"Turn on, tune in, drop out" was the catchy phrase popularized by Dr Timothy Leary, an advocate and proponent of the therapeutic and emotional benefits of lysergic acid diethylamide (better known as LSD or simply "acid") in the 1960s. Hallucinogen is often a generic term applied to several compounds with similar chemical structures, many of which resemble serotonin. The common and coveted result of using hallucinogens is to escape reality and appreciate heightened sensations that may result in hallucinations—sensory perceptions occurring without any external stimulus. Illusions (altered interpretations of one's surrounding environment) may be commonplace but are usually caused by other agents such as cocaine, phencyclidine (PCP), and marijuana. Pleasantly smelling sounds, hearing bright colors, and tasting words may result in addition to perceived greater introspection or revelation. Patients usually present to the ED only primarily for "bad trips"—severe anxiety after prolonged effects, panic attacks, gastrointestinal upset, or accidental ingestions. Treatment is primarily supportive without specific antidotal therapy. Ensuring a calm and relaxed atmosphere (eg, private room with dim lighting) along with the use of benzodiazepines for anxiety are usually all that is required. Taking an extra minute to talk a patient down from a "bad trip" and providing sympathetic reassurance greatly benefit this patient population.[41]

LSD

LSD could be considered the prototypical hallucinogen or psychoactive agent. Blotter paper (a small square piece of saturated paper often displaying colorful designs or cartoon characters) is a common mode of ingestion. LSD may also be taken as tablets (microdots), impregnated sugar cubes, liquid, and gelatin (window panes). Typical doses range from 25 to 300 μg depending on the patient's tolerance. Massive doses (14,000 μg) can be life threatening or result in uncommon life-threatening sequelae (seizures, coma, hyperthermia, respiratory arrest, and coagulopathy).[42] Onset of symptoms occurs approximately from 15 to 30 minutes, which is relatively short when compared with the duration of action, which may be up to 12 hours. A notorious plant (heavenly blue, pearly gates, flying saucers) commonly abused for the same purpose is morning glory (*Ipomoea violacea*). Because the chemical structure of lysergic acid amide is quite similar to LSD, the psychedelic effects are almost identical. Seeds are commonly ingested, and the number may range from 25 to 400 depending on the tolerance of the user.

Mescaline

The peyote cactus (*Lophophora williamsii*) grows in the southwest United States and Mexico. It is the source of the hallucinogenic alkaloid mescaline (3,4,5-trimethoxyphenylethylamine). The commonly ingested portions of the plant are termed "peyote buttons," the small fleshy tops that are desiccated before consumption either whole or brewed in a tea. Typically, less than a dozen are eaten. It is considered a weaker hallucinogen than LSD, albeit possessing serotonergic agonist properties. The Native American Church may legally use peyote for religious purposes under a special exemption. After consuming the bitter-tasting buttons, profound nausea and vomiting are commonly encountered.[43] Within an hour, hallucinations may occur and last up to 12 hours. Other adverse effects may include lightheadedness, headaches, ataxia, tachycardia, and hypertension.

Mushrooms

"Magic mushrooms" may be grown by budding mycologists or might be ordered over the Internet. The psilocybin-containing mushrooms are the ones associated with the drug culture. Psilocybin and psilocin indoles resemble LSD structurally and produce common CNS effects within an hour of ingestion. In addition to hallucinations, other findings may include headache, vomiting, myalgias, chills, weakness, dyspnea, hyperthermia, renal failure, seizures, and mild methemoglobinemia.[44,45]

Other natural toxins

Naturally occurring tryptamines such as those found in the secretions of *Bufo* toads may be abused as hallucinogens. Bufotenine is found in multiple species and is allegedly the hallucinogenic agent.[46] Since the 1960s, this compound has resurfaced as a psychedelic drug. Although toad licking has been practiced, bufotenine is commonly abused as topical aphrodisiacs made from the dried venom ("stone," "love stone," "black stone," and "rock hard"). One death was reported after IV injection of toad extract.[47] Problematic issues with this toxin are the cardioactive glycosides that may result in significant cardiovascular poisoning, which is similar to digoxin toxicity. Digoxin Fab fragments were successfully used in treating mice poisoned by Chan Su (a traditional Chinese medication derived from dried toad venom).[48]

Myristica fragrans is the evergreen tree from which nutmeg is derived. Myristicin is the toxin found within the glossy brown nut (nutmeg). Significant gastrointestinal distress follows ingestion. Typically, delirium may occur followed by a period of CNS depression. One report of recreational abuse revealed hypothermia with other signs and symptoms consistent with anticholinergic poisoning (ie, tachycardia, mydriasis, dry mouth, and urinary retention).[49]

Salvia divinorum has become a popular hallucinogen in recent years. Common names for the plant include "the Shepherdess" and "the leaf of Mary." Acting as a kappa opioid and serotonergic agonist along with glutamate antagonism, it makes for an ideal hallucinogenic agent.[50] Effects include laughter, feelings of self-consciousness, and the sensation of levitation.[51] It has a quick onset of symptoms with ingestion or smoking, occurring within 1 minute, and subsiding over 30 minutes. Its duration can be likened to that of a trip on dimethyltryptamine which has appropriately been called the "business man's lunch."

Designer Amphetamines

MDMA, alternatively called Ecstasy, X, or E, has become a popular enactogen among partygoers and ravers. The desirable effects include heightened sensations of euphoria, sexuality, physical touch, emotional wellness, and enhanced perception of colors and lights, especially flashing strobes and trails of light. The backbone chemical structure of MDMA is that of amphetamine, which may cause sympathomimetic features albeit to a lesser degree. However, because of its unique chemical alteration and additional side group, it becomes proserotonergic in its ability to enhance serotonin release in the brain.[52] Commonly, 50- to 200-mg tablets with fancy symbols or logos such as bunny ears, smiley faces, stars, peace signs, hearts, cartoon characters, or animals are ingested for effects lasting up to 6 hours. The alterations in mental status from MDMA abuse may be multifactorial. The drug effects are not usually significant enough for presentation to the ED unless brought in by a significant other. Bruxism is a classic finding in abusers; so the patient sucking on a pacifier or a lollipop who presents from a rave club may be a clue to MDMA use. Alterations in sensorium may be the result of hyponatremia. Rehydration stations in rave clubs might be a source of excessive water drinking thus leading to hypervolemic hyponatremia. Alternatively, prolonged dancing in a hot environment can result in patients presenting with hypovolemic hyponatremia. Some patients could be euvolemic with hyponatremia secondary to MDMA's ability to cause syndrome of inappropriate antidiuretic hormone (SIADH).[53] Treatment is primarily supportive: cooling hyperthermic patients, administering benzodiazepines for hyperadrenergic tone, and investigating sodium abnormalities may be warranted. For example, giving normal saline boluses to a patient with SIADH may result in a continued dilutional effect and even lowering of the sodium level, worsening mental status, and/or seizures.

Paramethoxymethamphetamine (PMA) is another amphetamine abused similar to MDMA. PMA has the reputation of being a souped-up version with a notorious slang name "double stack white Mitsubishi (because of the symbol on the tablet)," resulting in a greater likelihood of altered mental status with excessive blood pressure, heart rate, and core body temperature. Patients may present with generalized seizures exacerbating the core temperature elevation. Significant morbidity and mortality may follow PMA ingestion and overdose when compared with that of MDMA.[54]

Because of the inability to grossly tell PMA from MDMA, some communities have established rapid identification centers for users.

Bromo-dragonfly is a common name for another synthetic amphetamine modified from the common phenylethylamine structure. The name is derived from the molecular structure that resembles a dragonfly. Users covet the serotonin agonist inducing hallucinogenic properties that are just less than those of LSD and the longer duration of effect, which may be more than several days. Typical doses are 0.5 to 1 mg and are sold commonly in the form of blotters. Death has been reported from overdose of bromo-dragonfly.[55]

Dissociative Agents

Dissociative agents provide analgesic and anesthetic properties by inducing a dissociation of the patient from the environment. Clinically, they are advantageous in that respiratory or cardiopulmonary compromise is uncommon. Molecularly, they bind to *N*-methyl-D-aspartic acid receptors and noncompetitively antagonize glutamate's excitatory activity.[56]

PCP (angel dust) causes altered mental status unlike the classic hallucinogens and is structurally related to ketamine. PCP may be abused by smoking, injecting, snorting, or ingesting. The dysphoria and CNS stimulation that follow may result in significantly agitated patients who believe that they are invincible; as such, these patients are often violent, and presentations to the ED are usually linked to trauma scenarios, such as leaping from buildings, assaulting other people, or running into traffic. Interestingly, patients can also be comatose and catatonic or mimic a cholinergic or anticholinergic toxidrome. Pupil size is variable, but rotary nystagmus suggests PCP as the cause of a clouded sensorium.[57] Altered episodes generally last up to 6 hours, depending on the dose. Treatment is primarily supportive through creation of a safe environment with adjunctive benzodiazepines as needed. Traumatic injuries are important to address in addition to any other secondary issue that may result from intoxication, such as hyperthermia, seizures, and rhabdomyolysis.

Ketamine (Vitamin K, Special K), commonly used in hospitals for procedural sedation, and as an induction agent during rapid sequence intubation, has become an increasingly popular drug of abuse, especially in clubs and raves. It can be purchased online or obtained illegally from a hospital or veterinary office. Depending on the dose, it is reportedly inexpensive and short acting after intranasal use (15–20 minutes).[58]

Dextromethorphan-containing cough and cold products have been a source of drug misuse and abuse for more than a decade. These drugs share some common pharmacologic and clinical features with PCP and ketamine. Commonly listed as an opioid, it exhibits no analgesic properties. It is abused to provide a dissociative high or an "out of body" experience, but patients instead may experience dysphoria likened to that of PCP or ketamine use. Patients may have an anticholinergic appearance after abuse of these combination products because they often include an antihistamine. Dextromethorphan is proserotonergic, and when abused in the setting of other such medications (eg, monoamine oxidase inhibitors, SSRIs) being used concomitantly, patients could present with serotonin syndrome.[59] Clinicians should also check acetaminophen concentrations because some products also contain this drug for the treatment of cold or flulike illnesses.

MALICIOUS INTOXICATION

A 24-year-old woman arrives in the ED accompanied by 3 friends. She is somnolent and does not respond properly to questioning. The friends state that they were out celebrating her birthday at a local dance club. The friends admit to drinking several alcoholic beverages but state that their friend had only 1 to 2 drinks. They go on to say that she did not feel like dancing and was left alone for a few minutes; upon rejoining their friend at their table there was a very flirtatious man present. Shortly after this, the patient began acting much more inebriated than her amount of alcohol ingested would suggest. Her examination in the ED reveals disorientation, a Glasgow Coma Scale of 10, a blood pressure of 95/65 mm Hg, and a heart rate of 65 beats per minute. Her pupils are small but reactive, her muscular tone is decreased, and her reflexes are 1+ globally. Otherwise, there is no sign of trauma or injury. IV access is obtained, the patient is placed on the cardiac monitor, basic laboratory tests including a serum ethanol level are sent, and IV fluids are begun. Should a urine drug screen be sent? Should blood and urine be set aside for later laboratory analysis?

Drug-facilitated crimes, of which DFSA is a subset, are not infrequently seen in the ED but are often missed. The hallmark of these encounters is ingestion of some substance that facilitates criminal victimization. Occasionally this occurs willingly, but more often is done in a clandestine manner. Most patients present to the ED after being found passed out or confused and upon arrival may not be able to give details leading up to their arrival. As they "look drunk" and oftentimes have a detectable serum ethanol level, the fact that they have been intentionally poisoned by a chemical submissive agent (CSA) may be overlooked and thus undercounted. Although the true prevalence is unknown, it is frequently underreported.[60] In today's age of pharmaceutical excesses, it stands to reason that it occurs with some regularity.

Agents that are used for this purpose tend to have very similar characteristics that make them favorable for facilitating sexual assault. These drugs tend to be rapidly absorbed, as to produce a "knockdown" effect. They are rapidly metabolized and often chosen because they do not trigger a positive test on most standard urine toxicology screens. This property ensures that by the time the victim is aware of what has transpired, the likelihood of detecting the intoxicant is low. Finally, the desired pharmacodynamic properties include sedation/hypnosis, proamnesia, and muscle relaxation. Ingestion of a substance with these properties has been reported to have the effect of lowering inhibitions, impairing judgment, feeling uncoordinated/unsteady, feeling "out of control," being unable to recall events, and losing consciousness. Patients may present to the ED exhibiting signs of trauma or sexual assault, thus enhancing the likelihood of drug detection. Alternatively, patients may present exhibiting the effects of the CSA and appear simply intoxicated, which likely decreases detection.

The most frequently used CSA is ethanol, and the US Department of Justice estimates that approximately 40% of DFSA cases involve ethanol.[61] It is a fairly ubiquitous substance on the social scene and can oftentimes mask the taste of another CSA that has been slipped into the drink. Ethanol also acts synergistically to enhance the effects of most pharmaceutical CSAs, as it also works on the GABA receptor to cause a generalized decrease in neuronal firing.

Gamma-hydroxybutyrate (GHB) and its precursors γ-butyrolactone and 1,4-butanediol are also frequently used for this purpose. GHB has potent sedative/hypnotic effects, induces anterograde and retrograde amnesia, and is rapidly metabolized to substances normally found in blood, thus giving it an "ideal" CSA profile for DFSA. Originally investigated in the 1960s as an adjunct to general anesthesia, GHB was found to have an unpredictable dose-response profile, and its use for this purpose was discontinued. It later gained traction in the bodybuilding community as a growth hormone stimulator, likely because of its sleep-inducing quality. It is currently prescribable as a schedule II drug as sodium oxybate (Xyrem), which is used to treat narcolepsy. GHB is also readily obtainable on the street, and its precursor substances can be purchased online. GHB has a relatively rapid onset of action (within 15 minutes) and a short duration of action and rapid half-life resulting in near undetectability within 6 hours. Its precursors can be given unadulterated, and they undergo metabolism in vivo to GHB. Alternatively, simple chemical processes can be used in the home environment to produce GHB. Patients often present with a waxing/waning mental status. In fact, the hallmark of intoxication is a patient markedly obtunded that requires intubation, only to self-extubate within 4 to 6 hours without any knowledge of events or adverse effects.

Another easily obtained CSA is tetrahydrozoline, the active ingredient in Visine. This belongs to the imidazoline family of drugs, which include clonidine, naphazoline (Naphcon), and oxymetazoline (Afrin). The mechanism of action involves the stimulation of α_2 presynaptic receptors. α_2 Receptors modulate synaptic transmission, and stimulation results in decreased neurotransmitter release. In addition, there are intracellular effects similar to μ receptor stimulation. As such, these medications produce a rapid and profound depressed mental state, and patients often present similar to opioid overdoses—bradypneic, comatose, and with pinpoint pupils.[62] A 30-mL dose of 0.05% tetrahydrozoline (500 μg/mL; total, 15 mg) has been reported to produce bradycardia and obtundation in an adult; as little as 2 to 5 mL (1–2.5 mg) has been reported to induce coma in children.[62,63] Clonidine overdoses have been reported to be variably reversible with moderate-to-high–dose naloxone. These medications may also be amenable to this therapy, although no studies have been published illustrating this effect.

Other medications that can be used for DFSA include the benzodiazepines and barbiturates, as well as any medication with anticholinergic properties.

SUMMARY

The management of altered mental status in the ED encompasses a broad differential and almost limitless possibilities for causation. Within the domain of toxicologic causes, there are several central tenets to patient care. Excellent and meticulous supportive care is the mainstay of management, and attention to the details will help ensure the likelihood of good outcomes. Recognition of possible poisoning based on objective physical findings and vital signs, for example, toxidrome recognition, can assist the clinician in directing care without the need for a cooperative, awake, or nondelirious patient.

The sympathomimetic and anticholinergic toxidromes present in a very similar manner; distinction can often be difficult. However, compared with patients poisoned by a sympathomimetic, patients poisoned by anticholinergics will often have dry mucous membranes and axillae/groins as a result of sweat gland inhibition. In either case, if the patient is hyperthermic, they need to be actively cooled and receive benzodiazepines as first-line pharmacotherapy. Opioid-poisoned patients present clinically with pinpoint pupils, decreased respiration, and depressed mental status. Naloxone can be diagnostic and therapeutic; however, it can sometimes wear off before the offending drug has been metabolized, and reintoxication can occur. Also, a negative urine drug screen for opiates does not prove the absence of opioid and should not be used to deny diagnosis. Sedative hypnotics act similarly on urine drug screens, as not all of these substances are metabolized to the byproduct that reacts with the screen. Flumazenil reverses the effects of benzodiazepines but not other sedative hypnotics and can be dangerous if used indiscriminately. The authors recommend limiting its use to the patient with a known (both amount and timing) exposure, such as with postprocedural sedation in the ED. Otherwise, support of ventilatory function is often all that is required for these patients.

One should be wary of any patient brought in from "a party" or "a club," as there is always the possibility of an attempted drug-facilitated assault and not simply "alcohol on board, metabolize to freedom." Regional poison center consultation may be helpful with intoxication from novel or trendy substances; in the United States, the phone number is 800-222-1222.

REFERENCES

1. Langman LJ, Kapur BM. Toxicology: then and now. Clin Biochem 2006;39: 498–510.
2. Hammett-Stabler CA, Pesce AJ, Cannon DJ. Urine drug screening in the medical setting. Clin Chim Acta 2002;315:125–35.
3. Beverly R. History and present state of Virginia. Richmond (VA): JW Randolph; 1855.
4. Sopchak CA, Stork CM, Cantor RM. Central anticholinergic syndrome due to Jimson weed: physostigmine therapy revisited. Clin Toxicol 1998;36:43–5.
5. Klein-Schwartz W, Oderda GM. Jimsonweed intoxication in adolescents and young adults. Am J Dis Child 1984;138:737–9.
6. Pereira CA, Nishioka SA. Poisoning by the use of Datura leaves in a homemade toothpaste. Clin Toxicol 1994;32:329–31.
7. Jones J, Dougherty J, Cannon L. Diphenhydramine-induced toxic psychosis. Am J Emerg Med 1982;4:369.
8. Yokoyama H, Sato M, Linuma K, et al. Centrally acting histamine H1 antagonists promote the development of amygdala kindling in rats. Neurosci Lett 1996; 217(2–3):194–6.
9. Kamei C, Ohuchi M, Sugimoto Y, et al. Mechanism responsible for epileptogenic activity by first generation H1 antagonists in rats. Brain Res 2000;887(1):183–6.
10. Wills B, Erickson T. Drug and toxin associated seizures. Med Clin North Am 2005; 89:1297–321.
11. Dubin WR, Feld JA. Rapid tranquilization of the violent patient. Am J Emerg Med 1989;7:313.
12. Pentel P, Peterson CD. Asystole complicating physostigmine treatment of tricyclic antidepressant overdose. Ann Emerg Med 1980;9:588.
13. Suchard JR. Assessing physostigmine's contraindication in cyclic antidepressant ingestions. J Emerg Med 2003;25:185–91.
14. Schneir AB, Offerman SR, Ly BT, et al. Complications of diagnostic physostigmine administration to emergency department patients. Ann Emerg Med 2003;42:14–9.
15. Burns MJ, Linden CH, Graudins A, et al. A comparison of physostigmine and benzodiazepines for the treatment of anticholinergic poisoning. Ann Emerg Med 1999;35:374–81.
16. The National Institutes for Drug Abuse. Cocaine: abuse and addiction. Available at: http://www.nida.nih.gov/researchreports/cocaine/cocaine.html. Accessed October 8, 2009.
17. Bourland JA, Martin DK, Mayersohn M. In vitro transesterification of cocaethylene (ethylcocaine) in the presence of ethanol. esterase-mediated ethyl ester exchange esterase-mediated ethyl ester exchange. Drug Metab Dispos 1998; 26:203–6.
18. Callaway CW, Clark RF. Hyperthermia in psychostimulant overdose. Ann Emerg Med 1994;24(1):68–76.

19. McCord J, Jneid H, Hollander JE, et al. American Heart Association Acute Cardiac Care Committee of the Council on Clinical Cardiology, Management of cocaine-associated chest pain and myocardial infarction: a scientific statement from the American Heart Association Acute Cardiac Care Committee of the Council on Clinical Cardiology. Circulation 2008;117(14):1897–907.
20. Petitti DB, Sidney S, Quesenberry C, et al. Stroke and cocaine or amphetamine use. Epidemiology 1998;9(6):596–600.
21. Levine SR, Brust JC, Futrell N, et al. A comparative study of the cerebrovascular complications of cocaine: alkaloidal versus hydrochloride – a review. Neurology 1991;41(8):1173–7.
22. Farooq MU, Bhatt A, Patel M. Neurotoxic and cardiotoxic effects of cocaine and ethanol. J Med Toxicol 2009;5(3):134–8.
23. Merkel PA, Koroshetz WJ, Irizarry MC, et al. Cocaine-associated cerebral vasculitis. Semin Arthritis Rheum 1995;25(3):172–83.
24. Boyer EW, Shannon M. The serotonin syndrome. N Engl J Med 2005;352(11): 1112–20.
25. Eldridge FL, Paydarfar D, Scott SC, et al. Role of endogenous adenosine in recurrent generalized seizures. Exp Neurol 1989;103:179–85.
26. Young D, Dragunow M. Status epilepticus may be caused by loss of adenosine anticonvulsant mechanisms. Neuroscience 1994;58:245–61.
27. Shannon M, Maher T. Anticonvulsant effects of intracerebroventricular Adenocard in theophylline-induced seizures. Ann Emerg Med 1995;26:65–8.
28. Finkle BS, McCloskey KL, Goodman LS. Diazepam and drug-associated deaths. A survey in the United States and Canada. JAMA 1979;242:429–34.
29. Greenblatt DJ, Allen MD, Noel BJ, et al. Acute overdosage with benzodiazepine derivatives. Clin Pharmacol Ther 1977;21:497–514.
30. Savitt D, Hawkins H, Roberts J. The radiopacity of ingested medications. Ann Emerg Med 1987;16(3):331–9.
31. Spivey WH. Flumazenil and seizures: analysis of 43 cases. Clin Ther 1992;14(2): 292–305.
32. Marchant B, Wray R, Leach A, et al. Flumazenil causing convulsions and ventricular tachycardia. BMJ 1989;299(6703):860.
33. Hoffman RS, Goldfrank LR. The poisoned patient with altered consciousness. Controversies in the use of a 'coma cocktail'. JAMA 1995;274(7):562–9.
34. Mann J. Murder, magic and medicine. Oxford, England: Oxford University Press; 1995.
35. Sneader W. The discovery of heroin. Lancet 1998;352:1697–9.
36. Buajordet I, Naess AC, Jacobsen D, et al. Adverse events after naloxone treatment of episodes of suspected acute opioid overdose. Eur J Emerg Med 2004; 11:19–23.
37. Moeller KE, Lee KC, Kissack JC. Urine drug screening: practical guide for physicians. Mayo Clin Proc 2008;83(1):66–76.
38. Schumann H, Erickson T, Thompson T, et al. Fentanyl epidemic in Chicago, Illinois, and surrounding Cook County. Clin Toxicol (Phila) 2008;46(6):501–6.
39. Armstrong PJ, Bersten A. Normeperidine toxicity. Anesth Analg 1986;65(5): 536–8.
40. Sloth Madsen P, Strom J, Reiz S, et al. Acute propoxyphene self-poisoning in 222 consecutive patients. Acta Anaesthesiol Scand 1984;28(6):661–5.
41. Miller PL, Gay GR, Ferris KC, et al. Treatment of acute, adverse psychedelic reactions: "I've tripped and I can't get down". J Psychoactive Drugs 1992;24(3): 277–9.

42. Klock JC, Boerner U, Becker CE. Coma, hyperthermia, and bleeding associated with massive LSD overdose. Clin Toxicol 1975;8:191.
43. Nolte KB, Zumwalt RE. Fatal peyote ingestion associated with Mallory-Weiss lacerations. West J Med 1999;170:328.
44. Curry SC, Rose MC. Intravenous mushroom poisoning. Ann Emerg Med 1985;14: 900–2.
45. Franz M, Regele H, Kirchmair M, et al. Magic mushrooms: hope for a cheap high resulting in end-stage renal failure. Nephrol Dial Transplant 1996;11: 2324–7.
46. Lyttle T, Goldstein D, Gartz J. Bufo toads and bufotenine: fact and fiction surrounding an alleged psychedelic. J Psychoactive Drugs 1996;28:267–90.
47. Kostakis C, Byard RW. Sudden death associated with intravenous injections of toad extract. Forensic Sci Int 2009;188:e1–5.
48. Brubacher JR, Lachmanen D, Ravikumar, et al. Efficacy of digoxin specific Fab fragments (Digibind) in the treatment of toad venom poisoning. Toxicon 1999; 37:931–42.
49. McKenna A, Nordt SP, Ryan J. Acute nutmeg poisoning. Eur J Emerg Med 2004; 11:240–1.
50. Roth BL, Baner K, Westkaemper R, et al. Salvinorin A: a potent naturally occurring nonnitrogenous kappa opioid selective agonist. Proc Natl Acad Sci U S A 2002; 99:11934–9.
51. Singh S. Adolescent salvia substance abuse. Addiction 2007;102:823–4.
52. Callaway CW, Johnson MP, Gold LH, et al. Amphetamine derivatives induce locomotor hyperactivity by acting as indirect serotonin agonists. Psychopharmacology 1991;104:293–301.
53. Ajaelo I, Koenig K, Snoey E. Severe hyponatremia and inappropriate antidiuretic hormone secretion following ecstasy use. Acad Emerg Med 1998;5:839–40.
54. Caldicott DG, Edwards NA, Kruys A, et al. Dancing with "death": p-methoxyamphetamine overdose and its acute management. J Toxicol Clin Toxicol 2003;41: 143–54.
55. Andreasen MF, Telving R, Birkler R, et al. A fatal poisoning involving bromo-dragonfly. Forensic Sci Int 2009;183:91–6.
56. Wong EH, Kemp JA. Sites for antagonism of N-methyl-D-aspartate receptor channel complex. Annu Rev Pharmacol Toxicol 1991;31:401–24.
57. McCarron MM, Schulze BW, Thompson GA, et al. Acute phencyclidine intoxications: incidence of clinical findings in 1,000 cases. Ann Emerg Med 1981;10:237.
58. Jansen KL. Non-medicinal use of ketamine. BMJ 1993;306:601–2.
59. Bryant SM, Kolodchak J. Serotonin syndrome resulting from an herbal detox cocktail. Am J Emerg Med 2004;22:625–6.
60. Kilpatrick DG, Edmonds CN, Seymour A. Rape in America: a report to the nation. Arlington (VA): National Center for Victims of Crime and Crime Victims Research and Treatment Center; 1992.
61. Negrusz A, Juhascik M, Gaensslen RE. Estimate of the incidence of drug facilitated sexual assault in the U.S. Report no. NCJ 212000. Washington, DC: U.S. Department of Justice; 2005.
62. Lev R, Clark RF. Visine overdose: case report of an adult with hemodynamic compromise. J Emerg Med 1995;13:649–52.
63. Jensen P, Edgren B, Hall L, et al. Hemodynamic effects following ingestion of an imidazoline-containing product. Pediatr Emerg Med 1989;5:110–2.

Twenty per Hour: Altered Mental State Due to Ethanol Abuse and Withdrawal

Henry Z. Pitzele, MD[a,b,*], Vaishal M. Tolia, MD, MPH[c]

KEYWORDS

- Ethanol intoxication • Ethanol withdrawal
- Central nervous system • Altered mental state

Among drugs of abuse, ethanol is by far the most pervasive with nearly ubiquitous penetrance within Western civilization. Although ethanol retains a place in religious and traditional ceremonies, its properties as a social lubricant have led to its overuse, abuse, and often, toxicity and addiction. The prevalence of alcohol abuse and dependence in the United States was 8.5% in 2001, representing 17 million people.[1] In 1998, the overall economic cost in the United States, mostly secondary to lost productivity, was estimated to be 185 billion dollars.[2] The medical system represents a significant fraction of this cost, with alcohol-related complaints comprising 14.3% of health care expenditure; the total estimated cost in 1998 was $26.3 billion.[3]

No demographic group of patients is unaffected by ethanol. Although pediatric exposure and toxicity remain rare, alcohol is still the cause of appreciable numbers of calls to poison centers (>10,000/y[4,5]), as well as pediatric intensive care unit (ICU) admissions, and consultations to local municipal departments of Family and Children's Services. In addition to its constant presence in its beverage and nonbeverage forms, the blossoming popularity of alcohol (ethanol)-based hand sanitizers provides another significant source of exposure, especially for children, whose propensity for the tasting experience is high.[6]

Elderly patients are affected by ethanol similar to young adults[7] but are more likely to present to emergency departments (EDs) for treatment of the sequelae of chronic ethanol abuse, mostly gastrointestinal (GI) complaints.[8] The group most likely to

[a] Section of Emergency Medicine, Jesse Brown Veterans Affairs Medical Center, 820 South Damen Avenue, Chicago, IL 60607, USA
[b] Department of Emergency Medicine, University of Illinois at Chicago, 808 South Wood Street, Room 471, Chicago, IL 60612, USA
[c] Department of Emergency Medicine, University of California San Diego, 200 West Arbor Drive, #8676, Room 3-340, San Diego, CA 92103, USA
* Corresponding author. Section of Emergency Medicine, Jesse Brown Veterans Affairs Medical Center, 820 South Damen Avenue, Chicago, IL 60607.
E-mail address: Henry.Pitzele@va.gov

Emerg Med Clin N Am 28 (2010) 683–705
doi:10.1016/j.emc.2010.03.006
0733-8627/10/$ – see front matter. Published by Elsevier Inc.

present for acute ethanol intoxication (as well as toxicity) are adolescents and young adults.[9] This group is most likely to present for evaluation of various forms of acute trauma. The 2 are related with a disturbing coefficient of variance; up to 50% of consecutive patients suffering from trauma at a level I trauma center met the legal definition of intoxication.[10]

EDs are affected disproportionately within the health care system for the evaluation and treatment of acute ethanol intoxication.[11] In addition to alcohol-associated injuries and major trauma, patients with a primary complaint of intoxication represent a significant proportion of ED volumes and usage of resources. In a broad cross-sectional study, alcohol-related complaints accounted for approximately 2.7% of all patient visits[12] (approximately 7% of visits were between 2 AM and 4 AM).[9]

PATHOPHYSIOLOGY

Ethanol is readily absorbed through the proximal GI tract and rapidly achieves equilibrium between intra- and extracellular compartments.[13] Although up to 10% of serum ethanol can be directly excreted in the lungs, urine, and sweat,[14] the main portion of the metabolism (>90%) occurs in the liver, where alcohol dehydrogenase reduces it to acetaldehyde.[15] Although ethanol has some direct actions on the cardiovascular system, its main clinical action in acute intoxication is that of a central nervous system (CNS) depressant. These effects are mediated through 2 pathways: an increase in CNS inhibition and a decrease in CNS excitation.

The main neurotransmitter responsible for CNS inhibition is γ-aminobutyric acid (GABA). Endogenous GABA binds to $GABA_A$ receptors, allowing negatively charged chloride ions to enter the cell, thereby decreasing cellular excitability. Ethanol has a high affinity for binding to the $GABA_A$ receptor, thereby activating this inhibitory cascade, resulting clinically in sedation, motor incoordination, and cognitive dysfunction.[16] Moreover, with the chronic use of ethanol, the number of GABA receptors is upregulated, necessitating larger and larger doses to create the same level of CNS inhibition. This GABA upregulation partially explains the awakeness of some chronic ethanol users at blood alcohol concentrations (BAC) that would routinely induce coma[17] or death[18] in nontolerized individuals. Benzodiazepines work at the $GABA_A$ receptor, which explains their primary role in the treatment of alcohol withdrawal.

Excitation in the CNS is largely mediated through the neurotransmitter glutamate, which is also inhibited by ethanol. Ethanol executes this inhibition by preferentially binding to a common glutamate receptor in the CNS, the *N*-methyl-D-aspartate (NMDA) receptor.[19] To maintain wakefulness in the face of the chronic presence of alcohol, alcoholics express increased numbers of NMDA receptors as well as increased sensitivity of NMDA receptors to glutamate. Alcoholics reach a new basal level of excitatory tone, which also helps to explain the over excitation of the CNS (seizures, hallucinations) when alcohol is withdrawn.[20]

CLINICAL FEATURES OF INTOXICATION

The Diagnostic and Statistical Manual of Mental Disorders defines 4 criteria for alcohol intoxication: (1) recent ingestion of alcohol; (2) clinically significant maladaptive behavioral or psychological changes developing during or shortly after alcohol ingestion, including inappropriate sexual or aggressive behavior, mood lability, impaired judgment, and impaired social or occupational functioning; (3) clinical signs developing during or shortly after alcohol ingestion, including slurred speech, incoordination, unsteady gait, nystagmus, impairment of attention or memory, or stupor/coma; and

(4) lack of a general medical condition or other mental disorder that better accounts for the signs and symptoms.[21]

The type of signs and symptoms manifested during alcohol intoxication varies with BAC (**Table 1**).[22,23] The extent of these symptoms is influenced by the rapidity of increase and decrease of the BAC. Because 80% of ethanol is absorbed in the duodenum and terminal ileum,[24] the largest determinant of the speed of alcohol absorption is the speed of gastric emptying, and therefore dependent on the presence of coingested food. Therefore, BAC increases faster with the ingestion of ethanol on an empty stomach than after a meal.[24,25] Lesser adjuvants speeding up the absorption of alcohol are female sex, lack of concurrent smoking of cigarettes,[22] the use of ranitidine, the use of carbonated alcoholic beverages, and drinks containing approximately 20% ethanol; higher and lower concentrations slow the absorption.[26]

However, in addition to the significant intraindividual differences in the rate of alcohol absorption, there are even larger interindividual differences in symptoms at a given BAC. These interindividual differences are mainly dictated by existing tolerance to ethanol; as previously mentioned, a significant ethanol history can allow a patient to be conscious, alert, cohesive, and relatively free of gross motor effects, even at BACs that would create stupor, coma, or death in nontolerized individuals. One group whose symptoms are not dose-dependent is the approximately 50% of Asians who have a deficiency in mitochondrial aldehyde dehydrogenase. Although the decreased activity of this enzyme does not clearly alter the rate of ethanol metabolism, the build up of acetaldehyde causes facial flushing and tachycardia after ingestion of trivial doses of ethanol.[27]

DIFFERENTIAL DIAGNOSIS

Unfortunately, the differential diagnosis for acute alcohol intoxication spans the entire clinical spectrum of altered mental status. Commonly, concurrent or masquerading causes of alterations in level of consciousness include trauma (especially cranial trauma), sepsis/CNS infection, metabolic derangement (including carbon dioxide narcosis and hepatic encephalopathy), seizure, and nonalcoholic toxicologic ingestion. Maintaining a broad differential, even in the face of historical data (ie, many previous visits for ethanol intoxication, emergency medical services report) or physical data (such as a perceived smell of alcohol on the patient), can obviate the need to scramble at the end of a shift, when an intoxicated patient fails the test of timely metabolism. Specifically, a low threshold for diagnostic laboratory workup and

Table 1
Effects of varying BACs

BAC (mg/dL)	Clinical Manifestations
0–50	Diminished fine motor control, relaxation, increased talkativeness
50–100	Impaired judgment and coordination
100–200	Ataxia/gait instability; slurred speech; mood, personality, and behavioral changes
200–400	Amnesia, diplopia/nystagmus, dysarthria, hypothermia, nausea/vomiting
>400	Respiratory depression, coma, death

Data from Kleinschmidt K. Ethanol. In: Shannon MW, Borron SW, Burns MJ, editors. Haddad and Winchester's clinical management of poisoning and drug overdose. 4th edition. Philadelphia: Saunders; 2007. Chapter 31, p. 591; and Charness ME, Simon RP, Greenberg DA. Ethanol and the nervous system. N Engl J Med 1989;321(7):442–54.

computed tomography (CT) of the head is useful when treating the apparently intoxicated patient with an altered mental state.

The physical finding of the scent of alcohol coming from a patient can be particularly deceptive. Fundamentally, the smell commonly attributed to ethanol is not actually the smell of ethanol but that of nonalcoholic adulterants and botanicals in the alcoholic beverage.[28] Therefore, a small amount of ingested beer causes a much more potent smell than a lethal amount of ingested grain alcohol. The smell emitted by an intoxicated patient is by no means dose-dependent[29]; the patient with an initial BAC of 400 mg/dL may have a stronger smell of alcohol after the concentration decreases to 100 mg/dL than he or she did upon presentation. This fact stands in stark contrast to the dose-dependent manner in which the actual ethanol concentration in human breath makes it reliably reflective of the BAC.[30]

A further complication in the arena of volatile components of alcohol intoxication is intoxication with nonbeverage ethanol (NBE). In addition to the accidental alcohol abusers (mostly pediatric ingestion of mouthwash, cologne, and cough medicine), there is a subsegment of chronic alcohol abusers who repeatedly present after ingestion of NBE (ie, mouthwash, cologne, cough syrup, and isopropanol). The reason that this group of patients repeatedly chooses NBE despite the broad availability of low-cost beverage ethanol is unclear. Considerations for choosing NBE are its low price and availability during times of limited beverage availability (Sundays, during hospitalization, incarceration), which can explain the 15% to 20% of patients in Veterans Affairs alcohol treatment programs who have ingested NBE.[31] The smell of the nonbeverage intoxicant can sometimes be a clue in discovering the identity of the agent (for eg, mouthwash intoxication produces a strong and pervasive minty smell within the examination room).

The danger of the nonbeverage alcohol ingestion varies with the intoxicant. Mouthwash, while predominantly containing ethanol (often approaching 30% by volume), can also contain toxic volatiles such as phenol, which have additional toxicologic concerns. Cough syrup, also heavily ethanol-based, presents with an anticholinergic toxidrome because of antihistamines, which are active therapeutic agents. Isopropanol, the most commonly abused of the toxic alcohols, has many of the same clinical features as ethanol; the predominant features are dose-dependent CNS and respiratory depression. However, isopropanol (especially in large-volume ingestions) can also cause metabolic acidosis and renal damage, occasionally necessitating emergent hemodialysis.

Methanol and ethylene glycol must also be considered in the setting of altered mental status after alcohol ingestion. Ethylene glycol, a sweet-tasting alcohol, is most often ingested in the form of antifreeze and causes some inebriation, severe metabolic acidosis, oxalate crystalluria causing renal failure, and at higher doses, hypocalcemia and death.[32] Methanol, often an ingredient in paint removers and a byproduct of homemade ethanol production, also causes metabolic acidosis, multisystem organ failure, and death, but visual deficits and blindness can be added to its manifestations.[32] The toxicity of ethylene glycol and methanol are due to their metabolites, oxalic acid and formic acid, respectively. Both these metabolites are formed when the alcohol is metabolized by hepatic alcohol dehydrogenase.[33] Therefore, the mainstay of clinical therapy has been the prevention of metabolism by alcohol dehydrogenase by competitive inhibition of the enzyme, in the past using intravenous (IV) ethanol and more recently using fomepizole (4-methylpyrazole).[32]

Once ethanol use has been confirmed in an alcoholic patient with altered mental status, the patient must be considered for a concurrent secondary cause of CNS depression caused by the sequelae of drinking, specifically Wernicke encephalopathy

(WE) and hepatic encephalopathy (HE). WE is an initially reversible neuropsychiatric condition caused by low intracellular stores of vitamin B_1 (thiamine). Because thiamine is a necessary cofactor in several neuronal pathways, the lack of thiamine in brain neurons can cause the typical clinical effects of WE: oculomotor abnormalities, ataxia, and global confusion.[34] Because these symptoms overlap with the symptoms of acute intoxication, WE is often missed and many hospital protocols involve the repletion of thiamine in all intoxicated patients[35] to prevent the 15% to 20% mortality[36] in untreated patients.

HE is another potentially confounding factor in the evaluation of an acutely intoxicated chronic alcoholic patient. The prevalence of HE in patients with cirrhosis is estimated at 30% to 45%,[37] which makes it commonplace among patients in the ED. A decompensation of chronic HE can be caused by acute ethanol intoxication, as well as infection, GI bleeding, or increased dietary protein load,[38] as well as many other metabolic derangements and insults. Clinical diagnostic criteria for overt HE are (1) slow, monotonous speech pattern, (2) loss of fine motor skills, (3) extrapyramidal type movement disorders, (4) hyperreflexia, (5) asterixis, (6) hyperventilation, (7) seizures, (8) confusion/coma, and (9) decerebrate/decorticate posturing.[37] Although the venous level of ammonia does not appear in the diagnostic criteria of HE, it has been shown to correlate with the severity of HE[39] and should therefore be assayed. However, a single ammonia level is not sensitive or specific enough to establish (or rule out) the diagnosis of HE,[39] therefore the testing of serum ammonia in the ED remains an area of controversy.[40]

TREATMENT

The treatment of acute alcohol intoxication is largely supportive. The main goals of ED treatment are airway protection (which can include intubation), the diagnosis of concurrent disease processes, and the provision of a safe location in which the patient may regain their normal level of consciousness. Aspiration precautions should be taken in all such patients until a normal level of consciousness is regained. Life-threatening alcohol poisoning can be treated with hemodialysis, but active treatments for the patient acutely intoxicated with ethanol are usually constrained to intravenous fluids (IVFs), multivitamins, thiamine, and glucose.

Although IVFs are given almost ubiquitously to patients presenting with acute alcohol intoxication, the reasoning behind this treatment decision varies a great deal. A common reason for IVF administration is the treatment of perceived hypovolemia secondary to acute dehydration. The diuretic properties of ethanol in the acute state are well characterized, with one study showing the elimination of 600 to 1000 mL of urine after ingestion of 50 g of ethanol in 250 mL of water (approximately 4 drinks).[41] This diuresis is effected by the suppression of endogenous antidiuretic hormone secretion,[42] a suppression which only functions as the BAC increases,[43] as in acute intoxication. The acute loss of fluid through diuresis is compounded by losses through vomiting, diarrhea, and increased sweating. Therefore, the treatment of the nonalcoholic patient with acute intoxication, who presents with evidence of hypovolemia, remains an indication for IVF.

Chronic alcoholics, however, will not always benefit from administration of IVF. The chronic abuser may suffer the same dehydrating effects of vomiting and overall poor fluid intake as the occasional binge drinker. However, when the BAC remains steady, as it does in many alcoholics, alcohol acts as an antidiuretic, causing the retention of water and electrolytes.[44] Therefore, the chronic alcoholic patient usually presents to the ED in a state of overall isotonic over hydration.[44,45] Thus, experts recommend that administration of IVF not be routine but rather carefully considered on a case-by-case basis, particularly in chronic alcohol abusers or those who have or are at risk for alcohol-induced cardiomyopathy.[45–47]

Multivitamins are commonly administered intravenously to intoxicated patients in the ED.[13] These vitamins are often combined in the form of a "banana bag", containing dextrose, thiamine, folate, and sometimes magnesium sulfate but always including the multivitamin solution that gives it the characteristic yellow color. Although many authors advocate the routine administration of vitamins to alcoholic patients,[48] citing studies that show alcoholics in the ambulatory setting to have multiple vitamin deficiencies,[15] the few studies that have been performed on intoxicated ED populations fail to show significant deficiencies in serum vitamins.[35,49] The conclusion of these studies is that the routine use of IV multivitamins in patients with acute intoxication is not warranted and once again should be carefully considered on an individualized basis.

The routine administration of thiamine is recommended for alcoholic patients, especially those presenting with altered mental status. The difficulty in detecting occult thiamine deficiency and early WE, combined with the significant prevalence of WE (approximately 12%[50]) and relatively high mortality, has made the cost/benefit analysis fall in favor of administering the drug; it is the timing and method of administration that are controversial. Traditionally, thiamine has been administered intravenously, usually at a dose of 100 mg.[50] Traditional literature stresses that the IV administration of thiamine should always precede the administration of dextrose, else the dextrose might precipitate an acute onset of WE in the thiamine-depleted individual. As the data suggesting this possibility are extremely limited (a single article summarizing 4 case studies, only 1 of whom was alcoholic),[51] the timing of the recommended thiamine administration to patients receiving glucose has become more relaxed. It is now recommended to be given at approximately the same time[34,52] rather than the previous insistence on before the administration of glucose.

As mentioned previously, the route of thiamine administration has also come into question. There is an increasing amount of data suggesting that oral repletion of thiamine is sufficient for routine administration,[34] decreasing the cost and risk of anaphylaxis associated with IV administration. The proponents of IV administration counter with evidence that absorption through the oral route is decreased in the intoxicated alcoholic and that sufficient blood levels are rarely achieved by single-dose administration.[53] The recommended route of administration of thiamine remains controversial, but it is clear that alcoholic patients with suspected WE should receive IV therapy, whereas most routine alcoholic patients can safely be given thiamine by mouth.[34,54]

The routine administration of glucose to the intoxicated patient presenting with altered mental status has been tempered by the usual ease of obtaining an immediate bedside fingerstick glucose level. If rapid testing is impossible, IV dextrose administration is recommended. This recommendation is even more important in cases of pediatric ethanol ingestion, who present with hypoglycemia more often than adults, even with BACs of 20 to 30 ng/dL.[55] Dextrose 5% with 0.45% sodium chloride is also the most common IV crystalloid chosen to resuscitate alcoholics because they often present with depleted glycogen stores and occasionally present with alcoholic ketoacidosis (AKA).[13]

Several drugs have been proposed for use in the management of acute alcohol intoxication, almost none of which have shown any benefit in decreasing symptom intensity or duration. The failure of caffeine,[56] naloxone,[57,58] and flumazenil[59] have been documented. IV saline, in addition to its previously mentioned indications for dehydration, is also commonly given in an attempt to hasten the drop in BAC.[46] This myth, too, has been debunked.[46,60] There is growing experimental literature suggesting that metadoxine (an ion-pair between pyridoxine and pyrrolidone carboxylate) actually increases the speed of elimination and clinical improvement in ethanol intoxication.[61,62] The mechanism of action is unknown but is thought to enhance the metabolism of ethanol to acetaldehyde by alcohol dehydrogenase and renal clearance rates through direct action of the CNS. With a small amount of data and limited availability, this therapy (available for sale in Mexico and Asia, under the brand names Alco-liv and Viboliv, respectively[63]) requires more rigorous study before widespread use is recommended.

MEDICOLEGAL SEQUELAE: DISPOSITION OF THE INTOXICATED PATIENT

Discharging an acutely intoxicated patient in the ED is predicated on the patient's return to a nonintoxicated state. Discharge while the patient is still intoxicated opens the practitioner and the discharging hospital to theoretical liability if the patient comes to subsequent harm, whether by exposing himself to traumatic injury, later manifesting an occult life threat masked by the intoxication, or causing harm to a third party while in an intoxicated state.[64] Therefore, the most common practice is to observe the intoxicated patient in the ED until the practitioner is confident that the BAC is less than the threshold for intoxication.

One of the more difficult challenges facing emergency physicians (EP) is whether or not to obtain a BAC in an intoxicated patient. Clear indications to order a BAC assessment exist in patients who present in coma or with significant alterations in consciousness; it is unlikely for an adult patient to present in a coma as a result of ethanol alone at a blood concentration less than 300 mg/dL. However, if there is no clinical evidence of concurrent occult traumatic or metabolic/infectious cause for the patient's altered mental state and the patient does not deny imbibing ethanol, it is acceptable to observe the patient without obtaining a BAC.[65,66]

Sparse definitive literature exists on the decision to obtain a BAC. Simel and Feussner[65] published several surveys attempting to quantify consensus on standard of care and liability by examining the role of BAC assays in the context of counseling alcohol-impaired patients to avoid driving after discharge. These investigators found that 88% of the EPs surveyed preferred to avoid documentation of BAC in moderately intoxicated patients, with more than half of those opting to draw a level, doing so for legal concerns. In a subsequent study, Simel and Feussner[66] surveyed attorneys to see which physician behavior was perceived as most risky for lawsuit generation. The responding attorneys judged that the greatest risk for suit was present when a BAC was documented but no instructions against driving were given (43%). This judgment was followed in riskiness by the lack of a documented BAC in combination with proper discharge instructions forbidding driving (17%), with the least risk perceived with a documented BAC and documented instructions against driving (3.5%).[66] It is therefore wise to expend the additional effort to ensure careful documentation of the patient's fitness for discharge.

Although it is preferable to discharge an intoxicated patient to the care of a responsible, nonintoxicated adult, it is also acceptable (if a responsible adult is not available) to discharge the patient directly if they show marked clinical improvement and are clearly no longer intoxicated. Although there is no legal consensus for an acceptable BAC suitable for discharge, the threshold commonly used in practice is approximately 100 mg/dL, in accordance with many state laws prohibiting driving above this level. Some investigators advocate a repeat BAC to document that a patient's BAC is less than 100 mg/dL before discharge; many others feel that the calculation of predicted decline in BAC is sufficient.

The rapidity of alcohol metabolism varies among individuals but has been shown in patients in the ED to be approximately 20 mg/dL/h.[67,68] In these ED studies, the speed of metabolism in individuals varied little, even across differences in sex, age, and drinking history. These ED-based studies agree with previous research, mostly performed on healthy volunteers[30] rather than on patients in the ED, that shows that at most commonly encountered BACs, the elimination of alcohol occurs according to zero-order kinetics or a fixed rate of elimination per hour, with each patient having their own rate of decrease.[30] Therefore, with 2 samples, we can calculate a patient's rate of elimination and quite accurately predict the time to elimination. However, at extremely high BACs, these kinetics seem to be much more complex.[69]

Serial examinations to document improvement in neurologic status should be performed according to an ED protocol, especially in cases when a BAC is not obtained. Failure of a patient's mental status to improve in a timely manner should provoke a more complete workup, usually including CT of the head. The length of time expected before clinical improvement depends largely on a patient's tolerance and alcohol intake. In one study involving 105 acutely intoxicated patients, the average time for normalization of mental status was 3.2 hours.[70] However, within that study population, 25% of patients failed to normalize within 7 hours, and 1 patient took 11 hours to normalize. The study concluded that any patient who does not show clinical improvement within 3 hours should be carefully evaluated for other causes of mental status depression.

One frightening theoretical scenario is of an alcohol-impaired patient walking out of an ED and into or under an automobile. Searches of US case law through the Lexis and Loislaw legal databases reveal a wealth of cases involving patients whose intoxication in the ED masked a life-threatening illness that exhibited itself after ED discharge,[71–74] but nearly none dealing with the discharge of intoxicated patients who bring traumatic harm to themselves (although such cases certainly exist[75]). There is now some precedent to support the liability of physicians to unrelated third parties who might be injured by discharged intoxicated patients.[76] The plaintiff in a seminal case of third-party liability was in an auto accident with a woman who had just received Compazine for a headache in an ED. The plaintiff sued the hospital that gave the woman the Compazine. The case was appealed to the Missouri Supreme Court and was ultimately dismissed on the grounds of statute of limitations.

Restraints are necessary for intoxicated patients who attempt to leave and for unruly patients who are endangering themselves and others in the ED. Chemical restraints are usually preferred over physical restraints,[77] but both methods are fraught with risk, clinical and medicolegal. The mainstays of chemical therapy are haloperidol and lorazepam,[78] either alone or acting synergistically together. The danger of adding further chemically induced respiratory depression to that already caused by ethanol intoxication is inherent in the use of these medications and must be weighed against the behavioral benefit achieved. The use of physical restraints has been shown to be safe and efficacious in patients in the ED[79] but is still recommended as a temporizing measure until chemical restraint takes effect. The longer-term use of physical restraints is not only dissuaded by the Centers for Medicare and Medicaid Services[80] and the Joint Commission on the Accreditation of Healthcare Organizations,[81] but has also prompted significant numbers of lawsuits for injuries sustained by restrained patients.[82]

MORBIDITY AND MORTALITY

The primary morbidity and mortality caused by alcohol intoxication is from resulting accidental and intentional trauma. Second most common are the effects of chronic alcohol abuse, such as liver failure/upper GI bleeding, alcoholic cardiomyopathy, and electrolyte derangements. However, acute intoxication can itself prompt life-threatening sequelae, especially in the nonalcoholic individual.

Respiratory depression is a significant cause of death in lethal ethanol overdose in children and adults.[28] Several mechanisms exist by which ethanol leads to respiratory depression. The largest effect is seen from depression of the central chemoreceptors' response to hypercapnia, thereby decreasing minute ventilation.[83] At higher doses, ethanol can increase upper airway pressures, presumably through decreases in the muscular tone, which maintains airway patency.[83] In addition to direct respiratory drive depression, ethanol intoxication can often be complicated by aspiration. Moreover, chronic alcoholics are more likely to develop acute respiratory distress syndrome given a concurrent metabolic insult, such as aspiration, hypertransfusion (after a GI hemorrhage), and acute pancreatitis.[84]

AKA is a potentially life-threatening metabolic derangement that is often overlooked in the evaluation of the acutely intoxicated patient.[85] Patients with AKA are usually chronic alcoholics who present after a large ethanol binge that was terminated by nausea, vomiting, and epigastric abdominal pain.[86] This volume depletion, in combination with the alcoholic patient's low caloric intake, low glycogen stores, and relative hypoglycemia, decreases insulin levels and promotes the formation of ketone bodies, especially β-hydroxybutyrate.[86] This acidosis can become profound, and AKA has been implicated as a possible cause of sudden death in alcoholics.[87]

On presentation, patients commonly have tachycardia, hypotension, and tachypnea, with epigastric tenderness and minimal alteration in their level of consciousness.[87] Laboratory findings include an anion gap metabolic acidosis, normal or low serum glucose level, and a low or undetectable BAC because vomiting forces the cessation of intake.[87] Urine ketone levels may be low or undetectable because the ketones are predominantly β-hydroxybutyrate, and urine ketone test strips test only for acetone and acetoacetate.[88] The fundamental treatment of AKA is volume repletion with 5% dextrose solution because volume repletion with normal saline has been shown to worsen the acidosis,[89] presumably because of a chloride overload. Similar to diabetic ketoacidosis, potassium, magnesium, and phosphorus levels must be monitored and the ions repleted as necessary.

ETHANOL WITHDRAWAL

Beyond ethanol toxicity is the complex syndrome of ethanol withdrawal. Many of the symptoms and complications of ethanol withdrawal are directly related to changes in the CNS neurotransmitters and receptor binding, leading to absence of inhibitory stimuli and the surge of excitatory pathways. This condition is caused by the response of the body to chronic ethanol exposure in an attempt to maintain a homeostatic balance. Over a half-million episodes of withdrawal from ethanol that require medication intervention for management occur each year.[90] Of the 1.2 million admissions for alcohol-related conditions, up to 5% go on to develop the most dreaded complication: delirium tremens (DTs). This complication historically had a high mortality, close to 40% in the early 20th century, with a dramatic reduction to near 5% today, presumably because of improvements in supportive and pharmacologic therapy.[91] Predicting the severity of withdrawal is not an easy task. In the mid-1950s, experiments on healthy volunteers demonstrated that prolonged use of alcohol followed by abrupt cessation led to the highest vulnerability for more severe withdrawal symptoms.[92] It is important to understand the neurochemical effects of alcohol consumption to explain the effects of withdrawal.

Pathophysiology

As mentioned previously, ethanol toxicity relies heavily on its binding to the $GABA_A$ receptor complex postsynaptically and $GABA_B$ presynaptically, with an overall effect leading to decrease in neuronal firing and increased sedation.[93] Ethanol also inhibits glutamate-modulated excitation at the NMDA receptor with a resultant upregulation of NMDA binding sites, which may be responsible for withdrawal seizures because it is a response to increase excitatory tone in chronic ethanol exposure, again to maintain a baseline arousal state.[94] This finding was demonstrated in animal models in which the hippocampus of ethanol-fed rats was analyzed and the alterations to the GABA and NMDA receptor complexes were confirmed.[95] Ethanol also has an interesting effect on opioid receptors. In vitro studies demonstrate inhibition of opioid binding to opiate receptors with chronic exposure leading to receptor upregulation and increased responsiveness. Ethanol-induced dopamine release is modulated and thus contributes to ethanol craving.[96] One of the adjunctive treatments for alcohol dependence is naltrexone, which showed efficacy in the multicenter COMBINE study of 1383 patients and showed that treatment over 16 weeks resulted in improved clinical outcomes and longer periods of abstinence.[97]

Symptoms of Ethanol Withdrawal

There is a wide range of ethanol withdrawal symptoms and most are related to the elapsed time since the last drink. Other key historical items include the duration of abuse, comorbid conditions (such as chronic liver disease from hepatitis B/C), the reason for stoppage of consumption, previous withdrawal and degree of severity, and co-ingestions. Much of the data was elucidated from early studies performed by Victor and Adams[98] who also described the 3 main features of mild, moderate, and severe ethanol withdrawal: tremulousness, convulsions, and DT, respectively. This was the first time that the time spent consuming alcohol before the cessation was correlated with the development of withdrawal symptoms and its severity.

Mild Withdrawal

Early CNS hyperactivity can lead to tremulousness, which begins only a few hours after cessation or decrease in ethanol consumption. The study by Isabell and colleagues[92] confirmed dose dependency in the development of withdrawal symptoms previously discovered by Victor and Adams.[98] The tremors can be accompanied by insomnia, anxiety, nausea, vomiting, anorexia, headache, diaphoresis, and palpitations. Some patients, who can still be managed on an outpatient basis, may also progress to have hypertension and fever. If there is no progression of symptoms, resolution usually begins within 24 to 48 hours. As symptoms progress, however, there is increased adrenergic stimulation leading to hyperthermia, hyperreflexia, tachycardia, and agitation.

Moderate Withdrawal

After 12 hours of abstinence, hallucinations in the form of altered perceptions can develop. This symptom is significantly different from DTs in that there is generally maintained sensorium. The patient usually has visual disturbances but may also have auditory and tactile hallucinations.[92] Vitals signs are usually normal in this phase of withdrawal but patient agitation and paranoia can lead them to cause harm to self and others. Thus, patients in this stage typically require hospitalization and close monitoring. The symptoms of alcoholic hallucinosis can last from 24 hours to 6 days and occur in approximately 25% of those with a history of extended ethanol abuse.[99]

Another manifestation of acute ethanol reduction or cessation in the chronic abuser is that of generalized tonic-clonic convulsions, once called rum fits. They occur in approximately 10% of alcoholic patients and can occur in patients with no previous history of seizures.[100] On further epileptic workup, patients are usually found to have a normal electroencephalogram. Recurrence or evidence of status epilepticus is rare because approximately 40% are singular and short events.[101] If status epilepticus occurs, it should lead to a more detailed workup, such as CT of the head, lumbar puncture, and analysis of cerebrospinal fluid, to exclude structural, traumatic, or infectious causes. Withdrawal seizures can occur any time from 7 to 48 hours after cessation or significant reduction in ethanol consumption but incidence peaks at 12 to 24 hours. Acute intervention usually consists of benzodiazepines and, if necessary, phenobarbital. Chronic anticonvulsant therapy is rarely required or recommended. A third of these patients will go on to develop serious withdrawal symptoms of DT.[102]

Severe Withdrawal

Approximately 5% of ethanol abusers who undergo withdrawal develop DT and incur its 5% mortality.[91] DTs typically begin 48 to 96 hours after the last drink and can last up to 2 weeks. The symptoms are caused by a hyperactive autonomic nervous system initiated by the prolonged glutamate-induced stimulation and an increase in the available binding sites on the NMDA receptor complex. Moreover, DT is defined by disorientation, hallucinations, tachycardia, hypertension, agitation, fever, and tremulousness in the setting of profound confusion.[103] Care has to be taken to assess every patient in the ED individually because not all symptoms may be present (eg, patient is on β-blockers). Risk factors for the development of DTs include[104]

- Age above 30 years
- History of previous episodes of DTs
- Chronic heavy alcohol abuse
- Concurrent illness
- Withdrawal symptoms with a still measurable alcohol level
- Presenting to health care provider after a longer period of abstinence.

Blood flow parameters in DT reveal abnormal cardiac indices and rebound hyperventilatory respiratory alkalosis leading to a decrease in cerebral blood flow.[105] The most clinically emergent effect is on the fluid and electrolyte status. Furthermore, hyperthermia was found in more than half of the patients who died from DT in a study by Tavel and colleagues.[106] In response to the findings in this study, early recognition, adequate fluid replacement, and electrolyte repletion have helped to reduce the once significant mortality. In addition to hyperthermia, chronic alcoholics may also have hypoglycemia, hypokalemia, hypomagnesemia, and hypophosphatemia. A combination of these are responsible for the malignant arrhythmias often implicated as the cause of death in those with DT.

Hypovolemia is common, secondary to vomiting and insensible losses from diaphoresis, hyperventilation, and an increased metabolic rate. Hypoglycemia is common as a result of ethanol inhibition of gluconeogenesis (as discussed in AKA), which was first observed in animal models and could contribute to the overall state of confusion in DT. Almost all patients in the withdrawal stage, particularly those in DT, need IV glucose replacement as well as its cofactor in metabolism, thiamine. Hypokalemia results from an increase in aldosterone levels in response to hypovolemia, extrarenal losses, as well as changes in intracellular distribution of potassium through membrane effects.[107] Hypomagnesemia must be corrected along with hypokalemia because the combination could lead to malignant ventricular arrhythmias and sudden cardiac death. Hypophosphatemia is usually a result of the malnourished state in which alcoholics present and can contribute to cardiovascular collapse, muscle breakdown, and rhabdomyolysis.[108]

Prompt recognition and treatment of ethanol withdrawal states, particularly DT, and concurrent or confounding illnesses are essential for the EP to reduce mortality and maximize chances for a good outcome.

MANAGEMENT AND DISPOSITION OF ETHANOL WITHDRAWAL STATES

The goal of management in ethanol withdrawal states is to minimize symptoms, prevent progression to entities such as seizure and DTs, and make an appropriate disposition of the patient. The importance of supportive care such as fluid replacement and electrolyte correction has already been emphasized. Thiamine and glucose are often the first interventions in the withdrawal state and can be initiated even in the prehospital setting, particularly with the ubiquitous availability of rapid blood glucose measuring tools. The mainstay of pharmacologic therapy has been benzodiazepines, which were first used in the 1950s.[109] Benzodiazepines have a favorable safety profile compared with ethanol as well as other drugs previously used, such as phenothiazines, antihistamines, and paraldehyde.[110] This drug acts at the GABA receptor complex and increases the affinity of GABA for its binding sites. Benzodiazepines have similar sedating effects as ethanol and also work as anticonvulsants without the adverse reactions of ethanol abuse.

The most commonly used benzodiazepines to treat the psychomotor agitation of mild withdrawal are diazepam, lorazepam, and chlordiazepoxide.[111] Minor withdrawal symptoms can be controlled with oral and outpatient therapy, although discharge from the ED with prescriptions for oral benzodiazepines is a controversial practice that is not supported by the literature. There is an advantage of lorazepam and oxazepam in cirrhotic patients because of their shorter half-life and prevention of over sedation. If oral medication is not sufficient and parenteral therapy is required, the IV route is superior to intramuscular because of more predictable bioavailability.

The dosing regimens for benzodiazepines are variable. chlordiazepoxide, because of its extended half-life, is a common oral agent used to manage patients on an outpatient basis. No agent in this class has been shown to be superior to another and several meta-analyses have determined that benzodiazepines reduce the risk of seizures and delirium.[110] Determining the type of therapy is often based on the planned disposition for the patient. The main quantitative instrument that is used to assist in this determination is the Clinical Institute Withdrawal Assessment for Alcohol Scale (CIWA-Ar) (**Table 2**).[112] This scale is based on the following symptoms, each of which has an assigned score and the total is the cumulative sum: nausea and vomiting, paroxysmal sweats, anxiety, agitation, tremor, headache, auditory disturbance, visual disturbance, tactile disturbance, and orientation or clouding of sensorium. Although the CIWA-Ar has been validated in the literature, its use in the ED has not[113]; this is thought to be because of the length and level of detail required to complete it.

On the CIWA-Ar, outpatient treatment may be appropriate for scores between 8 and 15, but inpatient treatment and monitoring should be considered for scores greater than 15. Outpatient therapy generally uses either chlordiazepoxide or diazepam. In addition to having a CIWA score between 8 and 15 (those <8 only need symptom-based treatment), the following represent the criteria for outpatient therapy[114]

- Able to take oral medications
- Have a reliable person to assist and monitor the patient for deterioration

- Compliance with medical regimen and appropriate follow-up
- No unstable psychiatric or medical condition or concurrent ingestions
- Not pregnant
- No history of DT or alcohol withdrawal seizures.

Benzodiazepines are usually given according to a fixed schedule and tapered over a period of 3 to 7 days. Less severe withdrawal therapy can be given as symptoms arise.

For inpatient treatment of more moderate or severe ethanol withdrawal, symptom-driven therapy, although more cumbersome for the treating practitioner and staff, has been shown to require less overall medication and decrease the length of stay. In a 1994 study by Saitz and colleagues,[115] 101 patients were assigned to either a fixed schedule of chlordiazepoxide or a schedule based on symptom triggers. For the same outcome, approximately one-quarter (100 mg vs 425 mg) of the medication and one-eighth of the length of stay (9 hours vs 68 hours) was required in the symptom-triggered group. All end points were clinically superior, but it does force frequent reassessment by the provider, especially in the early phases of treatment. There is also some evidence for the benefit of front loading therapy in which higher doses are given initially to more quickly achieve sedation and decrease withdrawal symptoms. Some studies have shown that a significant reduction in overall medication is required compared with conventional regimens without reaching toxic levels because the initial loading dosages are titrated to the response of the individual patient.[116]

Patients with more severe withdrawal symptoms are best cared for in the ICU so that close attention can be paid to vital signs, neurologic status, fluids and electrolytes, and cardiac monitoring. Multiple comorbidities, hemodynamic/electrolyte/respiratory insufficiency, and need for high doses of sedatives or continuous infusion are some of the criteria for ICU admission.[117]

Barbiturates are another set of medications that have been used successfully to treat severe ethanol withdrawal. They also work at the GABA receptor complex by increasing the duration of chloride channel opening, as opposed to benzodiazepines, which affect the frequency. Barbiturates are especially useful when high doses of benzodiazepines are not showing reduction in autonomic symptoms.[118] Propofol can also affect the chloride channel even in the absence of GABA. Generally, because of the respiratory depression that is seen with propofol and barbiturates, airway protection by means of endotracheal intubation and mechanical ventilation is often required. Besides respiratory depression, barbiturates (and propofol) can cause hypotension, which is usually fluid responsive.[119]

Other agents such as β-blockers and clonidine are generally not recommended in acute withdrawal states because of their inability to decrease hyperactivity of the CNS, particularly seizures and DT.[120] Some patients with alcoholic hallucinosis are wrongly diagnosed with a primary psychiatric disorder and given phenothiazines or butyrophenones, which are known to lower the seizure threshold and, in rare cases, have been documented to cause malignant hyperthermia and ventricular arrythmias.[121] Anticonvulsants such as phenytoin also have no role in ethanol withdrawal states (even withdrawal-related seizures), unless the patient has an underlying seizure disorder. This situation is sometimes seen when chronic ethanol abusers suffer head trauma and have epileptogenic foci, in which case anticonvulsants may be adjunct therapy to benzodiazepines in the emergency setting.[122] There has been some evidence derived from ambulatory patients in Europe that carbamazepine is equal in efficacy to phenobarbital and oxazepam (the benzodiazepine used for comparison). There was also evidence of no significant toxicity, reduction of emotional distress, and

Table 2
Clinical Institute Withdrawal Assessment for Alcohol Scale (CIWAS-Ar)

Nausea and vomiting: ask "Do you feel sick to your stomach? Have you vomited?" Observation	0 No nausea and no vomiting 1 Mild nausea with no vomiting 2 3 4 Intermittent nausea with dry heaves 5 6 7 Constant nausea, frequent dry heaving, and vomiting
Tactile disturbances: ask "Have you any itching, pins and needles sensations, any burning, any numbness, or do you feel bugs crawling on or under your skin?" Observation	0 None 1 Very mild itching, pins and needles, burning, or numbness 2 Mild itching, pins and needles, burning, or numbness 3 Moderate itching, pins and needles, burning, or numbness 4 Moderately severe hallucinations 5 Severe hallucinations 6 Extremely severe hallucinations 7 Continuous hallucinations
Tremor: arms extended and fingers spread apart. Observation	0 No tremor 1 Not visible but can be felt fingertip to fingertip 2 3 4 Moderate, with patient's arms extended 5 6 7 Severe, even with arms not extended
Auditory disturbances: ask "Are you more aware of sounds around you? Are they harsh? Do they frighten you? Are you hearing anything that is disturbing to you? Are you hearing things you know are not there?" Observation	0 Not present 1 Very mild harshness or ability to frighten 2 Mild harshness or ability to frighten 3 Moderate harshness or ability to frighten 4 Moderately severe hallucinations 5 Severe hallucinations 6 Extremely severe hallucinations 7 Continuous hallucinations

Paroxysmal sweats. Observation	0 No sweat visible 1 Barely perceptible sweating 2 3 4 Beads of sweat obvious 5 6 7 Drenching sweat
Visual disturbances: ask "Does the light appear to be too bright? Is its color different? Does it hurt your eyes? Are you seeing anything that is disturbing to you? Are you seeing things you know are not there?" Observation	0 Not present 1 Very mild sensitivity 2 Mild sensitivity 3 Moderate sensitivity 4 Moderately severe hallucinations 5 Severe hallucinations 6 Extremely severe hallucinations 7 Continuous hallucinations
Anxiety: ask "Do you feel nervous?" Observation	0 No anxiety, at ease 1 Mild anxious 2 3 4 Moderately anxious or guarded, so anxiety is inferred 5 6 7 Equivalent to acute panic states as seen in severe delirium or acute schizophrenic reactions
Headache, fullness in head: ask "Does your head feel different? Does it feel like there is a band around your head?" Do not rate for dizziness or lightheadedness. Otherwise, rate severity	0 Not present 1 Very mild 2 Mild 3 Moderate 4 Moderately severe 5 Severe 6 Very severe 7 Extremely severe

(continued on next page)

Table 2
(continued)

Agitation. Observation	0 Normal activity 1 Somewhat more than normal activity 2 3 4 Moderately fidgety and restless 5 6 7 Paces back and forth during most of the interview or constantly thrashes about
Orientation and clouding of sensorium: ask "What day is this? Where are you? Who am I?"	0 Oriented and can do serial additions 1 Cannot do serial additions or is uncertain about date 2 Disoriented for date by no more than 2 calendar days 3 Disoriented for date by more than 2 calendar days 4 Disoriented for place or person
Total score (maximum of 67)	

From Sullivan JT, Sykora K, Schneiderman J, et al. Assessment of alcohol withdrawal: the revised Clinical Institute Withdrawal Assessment for Alcohol scale (CIWA-Ar). Br J Addict 1989;84:1353.

a faster return to work. Common side effects, however, are dizziness, nausea, and vomiting. Data from human trials are limited and it has not been evaluated for moderate or severe withdrawal states.[123]

SUMMARY

Ethanol is a common causative agent in the presentations of patients in the ED with altered mental status. The maintenance of a broad differential, especially the consideration of a concurrent brain injury, is important in the evaluation of acute alcohol intoxication. Supportive therapy is called for in the care of the acutely intoxicated individual, with the judicious use of IV fluids, thiamine repletion in the alcoholic patient, and close observation for clinical deterioration. Special consideration should be given to the sequelae of chronic alcoholic disease, especially hypoglycemia, WE, HE, and AKA. Alcoholic patients presenting after cessation or decrease of ethanol consumption should be carefully evaluated for signs of impending withdrawal, with a goal of preventing progression to life-threatening severe withdrawal and DT. The patients with the highest risk for these symptoms include those with previous episodes of life-threatening withdrawal, concurrent serious illness, and large quantities of daily alcohol intake. The patients undergoing withdrawal can be risk stratified using several systems, including the CIWA-Ar. The mainstay of prevention and treatment of these withdrawal symptoms are benzodiazepines, most often administered in the inpatient or detoxification unit settings. Patients with severe withdrawal symptoms may need monitoring in the ICU for the acute phase of their withdrawal.

ACKNOWLEDGMENTS

Dr Pitzele appreciates the expert help of Drs Monika Pitzele, Barnett Pitzele, and Sarah Unterman with manuscript review, and that of Dr Jennifer Cheng with legal research. Dr Vaishal Tolia would like to acknowledge the expert help of Dr Payal Parikh with manuscript review, and both would like to thank Dr Chad Kessler for granting us this opportunity.

REFERENCES

1. Grant BF, Dawson DA, Stinson FS, et al. The 12-month prevalence and trends in DSM-IV alcohol abuse and dependence: United States, 1991-1992 and 2001-2002. Drug Alcohol Depend 2004;74(3):223–34.
2. Harwood H. Updating estimates of the economic costs of alcohol abuse in the United States: estimates, update methods, and data. Online report prepared for the National Institute on Alcohol Abuse and Alcoholism; 2000.
3. Secretary of Health and Human Services. Tenth special report to the U.S. Congress on Alcohol and Health. Available at: http://pubs.niaaa.nih.gov/publications/10report/intro.pdf; 2000. Accessed November 4, 2009.
4. Watson WA, Litovitz TL, Klein-Schwartz W, et al. 2003 annual report of the American Association of Poison Control Centers Toxic Exposure Surveillance System. Am J Emerg Med 2004;22(5):335–404.
5. Watson WA, Litovitz TL, Rodgers GC, et al. 2004 Annual report of the American Association of Poison Control Centers Toxic Exposure Surveillance System. Am J Emerg Med 2005;23(5):589–666.
6. Miller M, Borys D, Morgan D. Alcohol-based hand sanitizers and unintended pediatric exposures: a retrospective review. Clin Pediatr (Phila) 2009;48(4):429–31.

7. Adams WL, Magruder-Habib K, Trued S, et al. Alcohol abuse in elderly emergency department patients. J Am Geriatr Soc 1992;40(12):1236–40.
8. Onen S, Onen F, Mangeon J, et al. Alcohol abuse and dependence in elderly emergency department patients. Arch Gerontol Geriatr 2005;41(2):191–200.
9. Li G, Keyl PM, Rothman R, et al. Epidemiology of alcohol-related emergency department visits. Acad Emerg Med 1998;5(8):788–95.
10. Fantus RJ, Zautcke JL, Hickey PA, et al. Driving under the influence–a level-I trauma center's experience. J Trauma 1991;31(11):1517–20.
11. Whiteman PJ, Hoffman RS, Goldfrank LR. Alcoholism in the emergency department: an epidemiologic study. Acad Emerg Med 2000;7(1):14–20.
12. Nelson CR, Stussman BJ. Alcohol- and drug-related visits to hospital emergency departments: 1992 National Hospital Ambulatory Medical Care Survey. Adv Data 1994;251:1–16.
13. Marco CA, Kelen GD. Acute intoxication. Emerg Med Clin North Am 1990;8(4):731–48.
14. Barry RE, Williams AJ. Metabolism of ethanol and its consequences for the liver and gastrointestinal tract. Dig Dis 1988;6(4):194–202.
15. Lieber CS. Hepatic, metabolic and toxic effects of ethanol: 1991 update. Alcohol Clin Exp Res 1991;15(4):573–92.
16. Mihic SJ, Harris RA. GABA and the GABAA receptor. Alcohol Health Res World 1997;21(2):127–31.
17. Jones AW. The drunkest drinking driver in Sweden: blood alcohol concentration 0.545% w/v. J Stud Alcohol 1999;60(3):400–6.
18. Johnson RA, Noll EC, Rodney WM. Survival after a serum ethanol concentration of 1 1/2%. Lancet 1982;2(8312):1394.
19. Nagy J. Alcohol related changes in regulation of NMDA receptor functions. Curr Neuropharmacol 2008;6(1):39–54.
20. Fadda F, Rossetti ZL. Chronic ethanol consumption: from neuroadaptation to neurodegeneration. Prog Neurobiol 1998;56(4):385–431.
21. American Psychiatric Association. Diagnostic and statistical manual of mental disorders, fourth edition, text revision (DSM-IV-TR). 4th edition. Arlington (VA): American Psychiatric Association; 2000.
22. Kleinschmidt K. Ethanol. In: Shannon MW, Borron SW, Burns MJ, editors. Haddad and Winchester's clinical management of poisoning and drug overdose. 4th edition. Philadelphia: Saunders; 2007. Chapter 31, p. 591.
23. Charness ME, Simon RP, Greenberg DA. Ethanol and the nervous system. N Engl J Med 1989;321(7):442–54.
24. Norberg A, Jones AW, Hahn RG, et al. Role of variability in explaining ethanol pharmacokinetics: research and forensic applications. Clin Pharmacokinet 2003;42(1):1–31.
25. Fraser AG, Rosalki SB, Gamble GD, et al. Inter-individual and intra-individual variability of ethanol concentration-time profiles: comparison of ethanol ingestion before or after an evening meal. Br J Clin Pharmacol 1995;40(4):387–92.
26. Paton A. Alcohol in the body. BMJ 2005;330(7482):85–7.
27. Wall TL, Peterson CM, Peterson KP, et al. Alcohol metabolism in Asian-American men with genetic polymorphisms of aldehyde dehdydrogenase. Ann Intern Med 1997;127(5):401–3.
28. Fleming M, Mihic SJ, Harris RA, et al. Ethanol. In: Brunton LL, editor. Goodman & Gilman's the pharmacological basis of therapeutics. 11th edition. New York: McGraw-Hill; 2006. Chapter 22, p. 591–606.

29. Patel Y, Garmel G. Management of intoxicated/violent patients. In: Mattu A, Goyal D, editors. Emergency medicine: avoiding the pitfalls and improving the outcomes. Malden (MA): Wiley-Blackwell; 2007. Chapter 13, p. 99.
30. Winek CL, Murphy KL. The rate and kinetic order of ethanol elimination. Forensic Sci Int 1984;25(3):159–66.
31. Hoo GWS, Hinds RL, Dinovo E, et al. Fatal large-volume mouthwash ingestion in an adult: a review and the possible role of phenolic compound toxicity. J Intensive Care Med 2003;18(3):150–5.
32. Brent J. Fomepizole for ethylene glycol and methanol poisoning. N Engl J Med 2009;360(21):2216–23.
33. Kraut JA, Kurtz I. Toxic alcohol ingestions: clinical features, diagnosis, and management. Clin J Am Soc Nephrol 2008;3(1):208–25.
34. Thomson AD, Cook CCH, Touquet R, et al. The Royal College of Physicians report on alcohol: guidelines for managing Wernicke's encephalopathy in the accident and Emergency Department. Alcohol Alcohol 2002;37(6):513–21.
35. Li SF, Jacob J, Feng J, et al. Vitamin deficiencies in acutely intoxicated patients in the ED. Am J Emerg Med 2008;26(7):792–5.
36. Al-Sanouri I, Dikin M, Soubani AO. Critical care aspects of alcohol abuse. South Med J 2005;98(3):372–81.
37. Eroglu Y, Byrne WJ. Hepatic encephalopathy. Emerg Med Clin North Am 2009; 27(3):401–14.
38. Lock BG, Pandit K. Evidence-based emergency medicine/systematic review abstract. Is flumazenil an effective treatment for hepatic encephalopathy? Ann Emerg Med 2006;47(3):286–8.
39. Ong JP, Aggarwal A, Krieger D, et al. Correlation between ammonia levels and the severity of hepatic encephalopathy. Am J Med 2003;114(3):188–93.
40. Arora S, Martin CL, Herbert M. Myth: interpretation of a single ammonia level in patients with chronic liver disease can confirm or rule out hepatic encephalopathy. CJEM 2006;8(6):433–5.
41. Baïsset A, Montastruc P. [The effect of alcohol on thirst]. Nouv Presse Med 1976; 5(9 Oct 76):2171–3 [in French].
42. Roberts KE. Mechanism of dehydration following alcohol ingestion. Arch Intern Med 1963;112(2):154–7.
43. Eggleton MG. The diuretic action of alcohol in man. J Physiol 1942;101(2): 172–91.
44. Beard JD, Knott DH. Fluid and electrolyte balance during acute withdrawal in chronic alcoholic patients. JAMA 1968;204(2):135–9.
45. Schuckit M. Alcohol and alcoholism. In: Fauci AS, Braunwald E, Kasper DL, et al, editors. Harrison's principles of internal medicine. 17th edition. New York: McGraw-Hill; 1998. Chapter 387, p. 2724.
46. Li J, Mills T, Erato R. Intravenous saline has no effect on blood ethanol clearance. J Emerg Med 1999;17(1):1–5.
47. Ragland G. Electrolyte abnormalities in the alcoholic patient. Emerg Med Clin North Am 1990;8(4):761–73.
48. Vonghia L, Leggio L, Ferrulli A, et al. Acute alcohol intoxication. Eur J Intern Med 2008;19(8):561–7.
49. Schwab RA, Powers RD. Prevalence of folate deficiency in emergency department patients with alcohol-related illness or injury. Am J Emerg Med 1992;10(3): 203–7.
50. Reuler JB, Girard DE, Cooney TG. Current concepts. Wernicke's encephalopathy. N Engl J Med 1985;312(16):1035–9.

51. Watson AJ, Walker JF, Tomkin GH, et al. Acute Wernickes encephalopathy precipitated by glucose loading. Ir J Med Sci 1981;150(10):301–3.
52. Gussow L. Myths of toxicology: thiamine before dextrose. Emergency Medicine News 2007;29(4):3,11.
53. Thomson AD. Mechanisms of vitamin deficiency in chronic alcohol misusers and the development of the Wernicke-Korsakoff syndrome. Alcohol Alcohol Suppl 2000;35(1):2–7.
54. Krishel S, SaFranek D, Clark RF. Intravenous vitamins for alcoholics in the emergency department: a review. J Emerg Med 1998;16(3):419–24.
55. Vogel C, Caraccio T, Mofenson H, et al. Alcohol intoxication in young children. Clin Toxicol 1995;33(1):25–33.
56. Nuotto E, Mattila MJ, Seppälä T, et al. Coffee and caffeine and alcohol effects on psychomotor function. Clin Pharmacol Ther 1982;31(1):68–76.
57. Jefferys DB, Flanagan RJ, Volans GN. Reversal of ethanol-induced coma with naloxone. Lancet 1980;1(8163):308–9.
58. Nuotto E, Palva ES, Lahdenranta U. Naloxone fails to counteract heavy alcohol intoxication. Lancet 1983;2(8342):167.
59. Flückiger A, Hartmann D, Leishman B, et al. Lack of effect of the benzodiazepine antagonist flumazenil (Ro 15-1788) on the performance of healthy subjects during experimentally induced ethanol intoxication. Eur J Clin Pharmacol 1988;34(3):273–6.
60. Toups VJ, Pollack CV, Carlton FB, et al. Blood ethanol clearance rates. J Emerg Med 1992;10(4):491–2.
61. Díaz Martínez MCLR, Díaz Martínez A, Villamil Salcedo V, et al. Efficacy of metadoxine in the management of acute alcohol intoxication. J Int Med Res 2002; 30(1):44–51.
62. Shpilenya LS, Muzychenko AP, Gasbarrini G, et al. Metadoxine in acute alcohol intoxication: a double-blind, randomized, placebo-controlled study. Alcohol Clin Exp Res 2002;26(3):340–6.
63. Online pharmacy. Available at: http://www.generics.ws/Generic_Viboliv_Metadoxine_500_mg_Pills-p-758.html. Accessed January 5, 2010.
64. Mayer D. Refusal of care and discharging 'difficult' patients from the emergency department. Ann Emerg Med 1990;19(12):1436–46.
65. Simel DL, Feussner JR. Blood alcohol measurements in the emergency department: who needs them? Am J Public Health 1988;78(11):1478–9.
66. Simel DL, Feussner JR. Does determining serum alcohol concentrations in emergency department patients influence physicians' civil suit liability? Arch Intern Med 1989;149(5):1016–8.
67. Brennan DF, Betzelos S, Reed R, et al. Ethanol elimination rates in an ED population. Am J Emerg Med 1995;13(3):276–80.
68. Gershman H, Steeper J. Rate of clearance of ethanol from the blood of intoxicated patients in the emergency department. J Emerg Med 1991;9(5):307–11.
69. Lands WE. A review of alcohol clearance in humans. Alcohol 1998;15(2):147–60.
70. Todd K, Berk WA, Welch RD, et al. Prospective analysis of mental status progression in ethanol-intoxicated patients. Am J Emerg Med 1992;10(4):271–3.
71. Haney v. Mizell Memorial Hospital. 1984: 744 F.2d 1467.
72. Randall Lee Sledge v. Colbert County Northwest Alabama Healthcare Authority. 1995: 669 So. 2d 182.
73. Gunn v. Saint Elizabeth Medical Ctr. 1993 Ohio App.
74. Dagner v. Anderson. 2007: 651 S.E.2d 640.
75. Nguyen DA, Nguyen AVT. Learning from medical errors: legal issues. Abingdon (UK): Radcliffe; 2005.

76. Robinson v. Health Midwest Development. 2001: 58 S.W.3d 519.
77. ACEP Board of Directors. ACEP Policy Statement: use of patient restraints. Available at: http://www.acep.org/practres.aspx?id=29836. Accessed January 5, 2010.
78. Nobay F, Simon BC, Levitt MA, et al. A prospective, double-blind, randomized trial of midazolam versus haloperidol versus lorazepam in the chemical restraint of violent and severely agitated patients. Acad Emerg Med 2004;11(7):744–9.
79. Zun LS. A prospective study of the complication rate of use of patient restraint in the emergency department. J Emerg Med 2003;24(2):119–24.
80. Centers for Medicare and Medicaid Services. Medicare and Medicaid programs; hospital conditions of participation: patients' rights. Fed Regist 2006;71(236):71378–428.
81. Joint Commission for Accreditation of Healthcare Organizations. Revised 2009 Accreditation Requirements as of March 26, 2009-Hospital Accreditation Program. Available at: http://www.jointcommission.org/AccreditationPrograms/Hospitals/Standards/. Accessed December 10, 2010.
82. Heastie v. Roberts. 2007: 226 Ill 2d 515.
83. Dawson A, Lehr P, Bigby BG, et al. Effect of bedtime ethanol on total inspiratory resistance and respiratory drive in normal nonsnoring men. Alcohol Clin Exp Res 1993;17(2):256–62.
84. Moss M, Bucher B, Moore FA, et al. The role of chronic alcohol abuse in the development of acute respiratory distress syndrome in adults. JAMA 1996; 275(1):50–4.
85. Thompson CJ, Johnston DG, Baylis PH, et al. Alcoholic ketoacidosis: an under-diagnosed condition? Br Med J (Clin Res Ed) 1986;292(6518):463–5.
86. Adams SL. Alcoholic ketoacidosis. Emerg Med Clin North Am 1990;8(4):749–60.
87. McGuire LC, Cruickshank AM, Munro PT. Alcoholic ketoacidosis. Emerg Med J 2006;23(6):417–20.
88. Alberti KG, Hockaday TD. Rapid blood ketone body estimation in the diagnosis of diabetic ketoacidosis. Br Med J 1972;2(5813):565–8.
89. Miller PD, Heinig RE, Waterhouse C. Treatment of alcoholic acidosis: the role of dextrose and phosphorus. Arch Intern Med 1978;138(1):67–72.
90. Kosten TR, O'Connor PG. Management of drug and alcohol withdrawal. N Engl J Med 2003;348:1786.
91. Saitz R, O'Malley SS. Pharmacotherapies for alcohol abuse. Withdrawal and treatment. Med Clin North Am 1997;81:881.
92. Isbell H, Fraser HF, Wikler A, et al. An experimental study of the etiology of rum fits and delirium tremens. Q J Stud Alcohol 1955;16:1.
93. Macdonald R. Benzodiazepines: mechanisms of action. In: Levy RH, Mattson RH, Meldrum BS, editors. Antiepileptic drugs. 4th edition. New York: Raven Press; 1995. p. 695–703.
94. Davidson M, Shanley B, Wilce P. Increased NMDA-induced excitability during ethanol withdrawal: a behavioral and histological study. Brain Res 1995;674:91–6.
95. Snell LD, Tabakoff B, Hoffman PL. Radioligand binding to the N-methyl-D-aspartate receptor/ionophore complex: alterations by ethanol in vitro and by chronic in vivo ethanol ingestion. Brain Res 1993;602:91–8.
96. Diamond I, Gordon AS. Cellular and molecular neuroscience of alcoholism. Physiol Rev 1997;77:1–20.
97. Anton RF. Naltrexone for the management of alcohol dependence. N Engl J Med 2008;359(7):715–21.

98. Victor M, Adams RD. The effects of alcohol on the nervous system. Res Publ Assoc Res Nerv Ment Dis 1953;32:526–73.
99. Turner RC, Lichstein PR, Peden JG. Alcohol withdrawal syndromes: a review of pathophysiology, clinical presentation, and treatment. J Gen Intern Med 1989;4: 432–8.
100. Johnson R. Alcohol and fits. Br J Addict 1985;80:227–32.
101. Thompson WL. Management of alcohol withdrawal syndromes. Arch Intern Med 1978;138:278–83.
102. Earnest MP, Feldman H, Marx JA, et al. Intracranial lesions shown by CT scans in 259 cases of first alcohol-related seizures. Neurology 1988;38:1561–5.
103. Debellis R, Smith BS, Choi S, et al. Management of delirium tremens. J Intensive Care Med 2005;20:164.
104. Ferguson JA, Suelzer CJ, Eckert GJ, et al. Risk factors for delirium tremens development. J Gen Intern Med 1996;11:410.
105. Berglund M, Risberg J. Regional cerebral blood flow during alcohol withdrawal related to consumption and clinical symptomatology. Acta Neurol Scand Suppl 1977;64:480.
106. Tavel ME, Davidson W, Batterton TD. A critical analysis of mortality associated with delirium tremens: review of 39 fatalities in a 9-year period. Am J Med Sci 1961;242:58–69.
107. Elisaf M, Liberopoulos E, Bairaktari E, et al. Hypokalaemia in alcoholic patients. Drug Alcohol Rev 2002;21:73.
108. Victor M. The role of hypomagnesemia and respiratory alkalosis in the genesis of alcohol-withdrawal symptoms. Ann N Y Acad Sci 1973;215:235.
109. Mooney HB, Ditman KS, Cohen S. Chlordiazepoxide in the treatment of alcoholics. Dis Nerv Syst 1961;22(Suppl):44–51.
110. Kaim SC, Klett CJ, Rothfeld B. Treatment of the acute alcohol withdrawal state: a comparison of four drugs. Am J Psychiatry 1969;125:1640–6.
111. Bird RD, Makela EH. Alcohol withdrawal: what is the benzodiazepine of choice? Ann Pharmacother 1994;28:67.
112. Sullivan JT, Sykora K, Schneiderman J, et al. Assessment of alcohol withdrawal: the revised Clinical Institute Withdrawal Assessment for Alcohol scale (CIWA-Ar). Br J Addict 1989;84:1353.
113. Kahan M, Borgundvaag B, Midmer D, et al. Treatment variability and outcome differences in the emergency department management of alcohol withdrawal. CJEM 2005;7(2):87–92.
114. Blondell RD. Ambulatory detoxification of patients with alcohol dependence. Am Fam Physician 2005;71:495.
115. Saitz R, Mayo-Smith MF, Roberts MS, et al. Individualized treatment for alcohol withdrawal. A randomized double-blind controlled trial. JAMA 1994; 272:519.
116. Manikant S, Tripathi BM, Chavan BS. Loading dose diazepam therapy for alcohol withdrawal state. Indian J Med Res 1993;98:170–3.
117. Carlson RW, Keske B, Cortez D. Suggested criteria for intensive care unit admission of patients with alcohol withdrawal. J Crit Illn 1998;13:311 [table].
118. Hobbs WR, Rall TW, Verdoorn TH. Hypnotics and sedatives: ethanol. In: Hardman JG, Limbird LE, Molinoff PB, et al, editors. Goodman and Gillman's the pharmacological basis of therapeutics. 9th edition. New York: Macmillan; 1996. p. 361–96.
119. Young GP, Rores C, Murohy C, et al. Intravenous phenobarbital for alcohol withdrawal and convulsions. Ann Emerg Med 1987;16:847–50.

120. Horwitz RI, Gottlieb LD, Kraus ML. The efficacy of atenolol in the outpatient management of the alcohol withdrawal syndrome: results of a randomized clinical trial. Arch Intern Med 1989;149:1089–93.
121. Blum K, Eubanks JD, Wallace JE, et al. Enhancement of alcohol withdrawal convulsions in mice by haloperidol. Clin Toxicol 1976;9:427.
122. Chance JF. Emergency department treatment of alcohol withdrawal seizures with phenytoin. Ann Emerg Med 1991;20:520–2.
123. Stuppaeck CH, Pycha R, Miller C, et al. Carbamazepine versus oxazepam in the treatment of alcohol withdrawal: a double-blind study. Alcohol Alcohol 1992;27: 153–8.

Index

Note: Page numbers of article titles are in **boldface** type.

Emerg Med Clin N Am 28 (2010) 707–717
doi:10.1016/S0733-8627(10)00065-9
0733-8627/10/$ – see front matter

emed.theclinics.com

C

D

F

G

H

N

O

P

Q

R

S

W

Printed and bound by CPI Group (UK) Ltd, Croydon, CR0 4YY
03/10/2024
01040457-0012